D1558637

R E V I E W   C O P Y

Please submit two tear sheets of review.

U.S. list price: $95.00

With the compliments of
FUTURA PUBLISHING COMPANY, INC.
135 Bedford Road, PO Box 418,
Armonk, NY 10504-0418
Web Site: www.futuraco.com

Current Concepts in Diagnosis and Management of Arrhythmias in Infants and Children

edited by

Barbara J. Deal, MD
Director of Electrophysiology Services
Division of Cardiology
Children's Memorial Hospital
Chicago, Illinois
and
Associate Professor of Pediatrics
Northwestern University Medical School
Chicago, Illinois

and

Grace S. Wolff, M.D.
Professor of Pediatrics
Director of Pediatric Cardiology
Department of Pediatrics
University of Miami School of Medicine
Miami, Florida

and

Henry Gelband, M.D.
Professor of Pediatrics
Vice President of Clinical Affairs
Department of Pediatrics
University of Miami School of Medicine
Miami, Florida

Futura Publishing
Company, Inc.
Armonk, NY

Library of Congress Cataloging–in–Publication Data

Current concepts in diagnosis and management of arrhythmias in infants
  and children/edited by Barbara J. Deal and Grace S. Wolff and Henry
  Gelband.
        p.   cm.
    Includes bibliographical references.
    ISBN 0-87993-687-8 (alk. paper)
    1. Arrhythmia in children. I. Deal, Barbara J. II. Wolff, Grace
S. III. Gelband, Henry.
    [DNLM: 1. Arrhythmia—in infancy & childhood. 2. Arrhythmia—
diagnosis. 3. Arrhythmia—therapy. WG 330 C9762 1998]
RJ426.A7C88   1998
818.92′128—dc21
DNLM/DLC
for Library of Congress

                                                                98-9638
                                                                    CIP

Copyright 1998
Futura Publishing Company, Inc.

Published by
Futura Publishing Company, Inc.
135 Bedford Road
Armonk, New York 10504-0418

LC #: 98-9638
ISBN #: 0-87993-687-8

Printed in the United States of America.

This book is printed on acid-free paper.

Dedicated to my teachers and colleagues,
José Gallastegui, MD and Daniel Scagliotti, MD.

-Barbara J. Deal, MD

Dedicated to my parents.

-Grace S. Wolff, MD

Dedicated to my colleagues and fellows.

-Henry Gelband, MD

Contributors

Carl L. Backer, MD   Associate Professor of Surgery, Northwestern University Medical School, Attending Surgeon, Division of Cardiovascular-Thoracic Surgery, Children's Memorial Hospital, Chicago, Illinois

Michael P. Carboni, MD   Fellow Pediatric Cardiology, Duke University Medical Center, Durham, North Carolina

Christopher L. Case, MD   South Carolina Children's Heart Center, Medical University of South Carolina, Charleston, South Carolina

Macdonald Dick II, MD   Professor of Pediatrics, University of Michigan, Ann Arbor, Michigan

Peter L. Ferrer, MD   Professor of Pediatrics (Cardiology), Diagnostic Radiology and Obstetrics, University of Miami School of Medicine, Miami, Florida

Richard A. Friedman, MD   Associate Professor of Pediatrics, Baylor College of Medicine, Chief, Arrhythmia and Pacing Services, Texas Children's Hospital, Houston, Texas

Arthur Garson, Jr., MD, MPH   Professor of Pediatrics (Cardiology), Dean for Academic Operations, Baylor College of Medicine, Houston, Texas

Paul C. Gillette, MD   South Carolina Children's Heart Center, Medical University of South Carolina, Charleston, South Carolina

John D. Kugler, MD   Professor of Pediatrics and Chief, Joint Division of Pediatric Cardiology, University of Nebraska/Creighton University, Omaha, Nebraska

Constantine Mavroudis, MD   Professor of Surgery, Northwestern University Medical School, Division Head, Cardiovascular-Thoracic Surgery, Children's Memorial Hospital, Chicago, Illinois

James C. Perry, MD   Children's Heart Institute, Children's Hospital San Diego, San Diego, California

Mark W. Russell, MD   Michigan Congenital Heart Center, S. Mott Children's Hospital, Ann Arbor, Michigan

Michael J. Silka, MD   Clinical Care Center for Congenital Heart Disease, Doernbecher Memorial Hospital for Children, Oregon Health Sciences University, School of Medicine, Portland, Oregon

Mary C. Sokolaski, MD   South Carolina Children's Heart Center, Medical University of South Carolina, Charleston, South Carolina

Dolores F. Tamer, MD   Professor, University of Miami School of Medicine, Miami, Florida

Edward P. Walsh   Department of Cardiology, Children's Hospital, Boston, Mass

Ming-Lon Young, MD, MPH   Professor, University of Miami, Miami, Florida

Preface

In 1975, two conventionally trained pediatric cardiologists, who a few years earlier in their careers became intrigued with the diagnosis and management of cardiac arrhythmias in the pediatric population, decided to undertake the task of compiling the knowledge of pediatric cardiac arrhythmias into a text. That resulted in the publication of *Cardiac Arrhythmias in the Neonate, Infant and Child* in 1977, with a revision in 1983. Since then, there have been and continue to be revolutionary advances at an astonishing rate in the understanding, diagnosis, and modalities of treatment for the pediatric patient with a cardiac arrhythmia. These extraordinary developments and expanded knowledge base are responsible for our effort.

The contributors to this edition are nationally recognized, dedicated scholars who are enthusiastic, innovative investigators and exhibit excellence in clinical care. They are responsible for many of the major advances presented in this text.

In contrast to our previous publications, this is a comprehensive clinical text intended for our colleagues and paraprofessionals whose daily cardiological activities are concerned with evaluation and management strategies. The clinical electrophysiological (EP) bases for specific arrhythmias are detailed in each indicated chapter. However, we purposely did not include basic detailed investigative chapters such as those describing the advances in the EP and ionic channel kinetics of the developing myocardium. New scientific clinical discoveries responsible for specific cardiac rhythm abnormalities are presented (genetics of long QT syndrome). Chapter topics such as syncope, long QT syndrome, emergency management, and ablation therapy are new or have been significantly expanded, whereas the chapter dealing with surgical therapy was revised to reflect the many changes in this mode of therapy. Current technological advances have been included in the chapter on device therapy.

Pediatric cardiologists with an interest (sometimes passion) for cardiac arrhythmias have accomplished much in 20 years. We no longer empirically manage our patients based on anecdotal experience or translation of adult cardiological strategies. Pediatric cardiac EP sessions at national and international meetings (AHA, ACC, NASPE) are well recognized, and we have evolved into a cohesive cooperative worldwide Pediatric Electrophysiology Society, which has grown in stature and function since its inception 18 years ago. We are proud, and rightly so.

Finally, as stated in the preface in our book of 1977, "We realize that this text does not represent the final word." We sincerely hope it does not.

Acknowledgments: We remain extremely grateful to our expert contributors, who have been wise, cooperative, and diligent in their tasks. We owe our gratitude for advice and assistance in the preparation of this text to the staff of Futura Publishing Company. Our thanks go to Ms. Melanie Gevitz, who assisted us continuously throughout the preparation of the text by making the contributors and us keep up with specific demanding schedules. Finally, one editor (H.G.) expresses a special ''thank you'' to Grace S. Wolff, MD, and Barbara J. Deal, MD, who, in their wisdom, foresaw the need for this text and whose effort, dedication, and hard work made its publication possible.

Henry Gelband, MD
Department of Pediatrics
University of Miami School of Medicine

Contents

Clinical Evaluation of the Child with an Arrhythmia

Ann Dunnigan, MD

Introduction

Many factors are involved in the clinical evaluation of the young patient with an arrhythmia. As many arrhythmias do not happen in any predictable way, the ability to document, interpret, and treat them depends on paying careful attention to the three important determinants of arrhythmias, namely, the arrhythmogenic substrate, the modulating factors, particularly changes in autonomic tone, and the occurrence of triggers that initiate the arrhythmia. Although each of these three factors is important individually, it is the relation of the three together that permits initiation of a reentrant tachycardia. For example, patients with ventricular preexcitation have the anatomic substrate for an arrhythmia, and exercise changes autonomic tone so that the reentrant circuit can sustain itself. However, if there is not a critically timed atrial or ventricular extrasystole (the so-called "trigger" or initiating event) during exercise, then the patient will not have an arrhythmia. Conversely, if a trigger such as an atrial extrasystole occurs, but autonomic tone is weak, the arrhythmia will not be sustained (Figure 1). It is the importance of these three factors that limits the value of diagnostic tests in these patients. Some tests, such as ambulatory monitoring, may allow visualization of the triggers, while others, such as exercise testing, primarily modulate autonomic tone. It is the discussion of the utility of

From Deal B, Wolff G, Gelband H, (eds.). *Current Concepts in Diagnosis and Management of Arrhythmias in Infants and Children.* Armonk, NY: Futura Publishing Co., Inc.; © 1998.

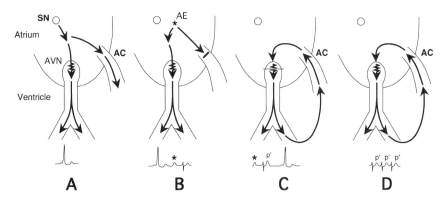

Figure 1. Drawing summarizing the relation among the anatomic substrate needed for an arrhythmia, the initiating event, and the modulating factors such as autonomic tone. In **A,** both the atrioventricular node (AVN) and accessory connection (AC) are utilized to activate the ventricle during normal sinus rhythm; tachycardia does not occur, although the anatomic substrate necessary for tachycardia occurrence (the AC) is present. In **B,** an atrial extrasystole (AE) serves as a trigger or initiating event to dissociate the two antegrade connections by blocking in the AC and conduction to the ventricle via the normal conduction system. The occurrence of antegrade block in the AC illustrated in **B** permits retrograde atrial activation to occur over the AC as seen in **C.** Perhaps due to absence of sympathetic tone (or to enhanced parasympathetic tone), in **C,** antegrade block of the AV node occurs following the single echo beat (p'), and orthodromic reciprocating tachycardia does not occur. In **D,** all three factors necessary for tachycardia occurrence and maintenance are present, and the orthodromic reciprocating tachycardia circuit is active. SN = sinus node.

each particular aspect of evaluation of the young patient with an arrhythmia that forms the basis of this chapter. Specifically, the importance of the history and physical examination, how electrocardiographic (ECG) testing may be helpful, and the role of transesophageal and intracardiac pacing and recording studies are discussed.

History and Physical Examination

The evaluation of young patients with possible arrhythmias is generally prompted by the frequency and severity of clinical symptoms. The type of symptoms present in young patients depends on the patient's age, the presence of associated structural or congenital cardiac disease, the activity being pursued when the arrhythmia occurs, and, of course, the heart rate during the arrhythmia. As in the evaluation of any potential medical problem, a careful history is important. Older children and adolescents are likely to notice paroxysmal rapid heart beating and will therefore be able to give a history of palpitations, defined as an awareness of one's heartbeat. Teenagers frequently notice atrial or ventricular extrasystoles, another cause of palpitations, and may become alarmed because they were not previously aware of their hearts at all. Younger children are usually not such good historians, and they may complain of headache or stomachache during an episode of paroxysmal tachycardia. Occasionally, a young patient will be able to relate to a parent that his or her heart is "beeping", but this may or may not mean that an arrhythmia is present. While a history of palpitations may be helpful and suggests the need for further evaluation, such a history may not always be available in young patients.

Additional symptoms that may be caused by arrhythmias include dizziness or presyncope, as well as syncope and cardiac arrest. When these symptoms occur, additional evaluation is always warranted, whether or not other symptoms such as palpitations are present. In addition to the history of the symptomatic events, a detailed cardiac family history is important, as many arrhythmias, including some associated with sudden cardiac death, may be familial.

Following the history, the physical examination should be performed to reveal the presence of structural heart disease, and heart rate and rhythm should be noted. Further evaluation will depend on the severity and frequency of symptoms, the age of the patient, and the presence of structural heart disease. In some patients, there are no symptoms during the arrhythmia, and the presence of an arrhythmia (too fast, too slow, or irregular heart rhythm) is noticed during physical examination. Often, even when there are only signs of arrhythmia without symptoms, further evaluation is warranted.

Electrocardiographic Evaluation

12-Lead Electrocardiogram

For a patient with a history of an arrhythmia, a complete 12-lead electrocardiogram (ECG) during which three simultaneous channels are recorded is the ideal place to start the evaluation. Frequently, clues as to the type of clinical problem the patient has are evident on the initial ECG (Figure 2). For example, the presence of ventricular preexcitation, QT interval prolongation, or ventricular hypertrophy with diffuse ST-T wave changes will indicate that further testing and treatment are essential. While an abnormal ECG is very sensitive, a normal 12-lead ECG is not nearly as helpful. Since cardiac rate, intervals, axis, and even hypertrophy assessment are age related, tables of normal ECG values for young patients must be consulted.[1,2]

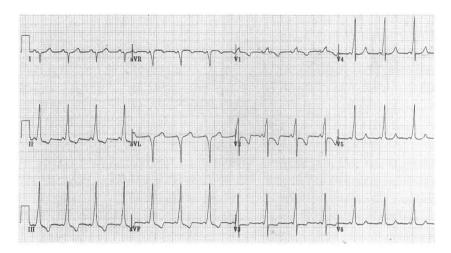

Figure 2. A 12-lead ECG obtained in a 9-year-old girl with a history of palpitations. There is a short PR interval, slurring to the onset of the QRS (the delta wave), and the QRS is wide. This patient has typical ECG features of WPW syndrome.

Ambulatory Electrocardiographic Monitoring

Following the baseline ECG, the most important part of the clinical evaluation of patients with arrhythmias is to obtain ECG documentation during symptoms or in asymptomatic patients during the presence of the heart rhythm problem itself. The recent development of reliable, portable ECG recording devices has facilitated this part of patient evaluation. In patients whose symptoms occur daily or nearly every day, 24-hour ambulatory ECG monitoring (Holter) may be helpful to obtain ECG documentation during symptoms. If symptoms do not occur during the monitoring period, clues as to the type of heart rhythm abnormality existing may be apparent nonetheless (Figure 3). Although too heavy for very young children to carry, these monitors offer very high fidelity recordings, are easy to use, and will document symptomatic as well as asymptomatic arrhythmias. In addition, information related to the average daily heart rate as well as the high and low heart rate can be obtained with these recorders. In normal, asymptomatic young patients, atrial and ventricular extrasystoles occur commonly, and even ventricular couplets may occur and be unrelated to the clinical problem.[3–5] In patients with permanent pacemakers implanted, ambulatory electrocardiography may be particularly helpful in screening for the possibility of intermittent pacemaker capture or sensing problems. However, unless the patient's symptoms are duplicated during the time the ambulatory monitoring is being performed, no additional information that assists in arrhythmia diagnosis is obtained.

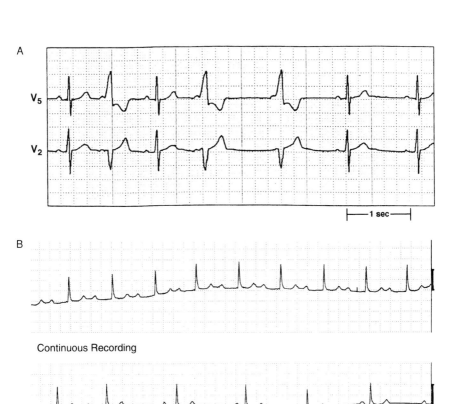

Figure 3. A: A sample of a continuous ambulatory monitor recording from a 12-year-old boy known to have ventricular preexcitation and palpitations. In this simultaneous two-channel recording, intermittent ventricular preexcitation is illustrated. V$_5$, V$_2$: modified ECG chest leads V$_5$ and V$_2$. **B**: A sample of a continuous ambulatory monitor recording from a 17-year-old girl with a history of palpitations, but normal sinus rhythm ECG. Although she did not have palpitations during the 24-hour ambulatory monitoring period, the occurrence of two populations of PR intervals illustrated here suggests the presence of dual AVN pathways and the possibility that this patient's tachycardia symptoms may be due to AVN reentry tachycardia. Note that, in the upper recording, the PR interval is 0.4 seconds at a time when the heart rate is 75 beats per minute (bpm); when the heart rate changes abruptly to 56 bpm, the PR interval shortens abruptly to 0.16 seconds.

Cardiac Event Recorders

Typical young patients with arrhythmias have paroxysmal symptoms; that is, symptoms tend to occur in clusters in an unpredictable manner, with days, weeks, or even months separating symptomatic events. The availability of patient-activated (or parent-activated) recorders capable of storing ECGs lasting from 1–5 minutes during symptomatic events and subsequently performing transtelephonic transmission has greatly improved the ability to document the etiology of symptoms.[6–8] Several types of event recorders were developed, and appropriate selection from those available will increase success in documenting symptoms. For example, in patients with recurrent syncope, a continuous-loop event monitor will show the cardiac rhythm for up to 1 minute prior to activation of the device. Patients (or their parents) can activate the device and, following recovery from the syncopal episode, transmit their ECG by telephone. For patients without loss of consciousness, but with sustained (at least a few minutes) palpitations secondary to paroxysmal tachycardia, a recorder similar to a wristwatch is available. For very brief or transient symptoms, this recorder is not effective since it requires some coordination and several seconds at least to position both arms to obtain a recording. However, in spite of this difficulty,

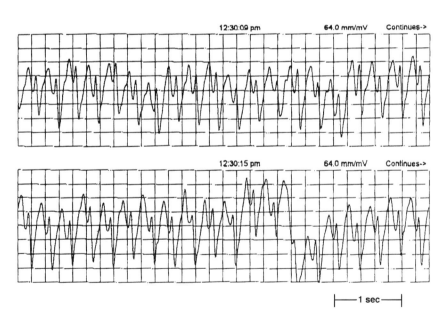

Figure 4. Sample recording from a cardiac event recorder received via telephone in a young patient experiencing symptoms of palpitations while watching television. Although there is some baseline artifact, the recording is of adequate quality to determine that the heart rate is approximately 195 bpm.

its use is well received by young patients and adolescents. For very young patients, a recorder the size of a playing card exists, with electrodes on the back. This device can be applied to the young patient's chest by parents, with the memory activated and an ECG recording stored in the device. Although the fidelity of many transient event recording devices is not of the quality of continuous recording devices, it is usually sufficient to determine whether an arrhythmia exists at the time of symptoms (Figure 4).

Signal-Averaged Electrocardiography

As with many advances in medicine, new techniques are frequently developed and studied first in adult patients with coronary artery disease. Subsequently, these techniques are applied to young patients to determine what normal values are for young and small patients and to see if there is clinical utility of the new technique in the diagnosis or management of pediatric patients.[9] Such has been the case with signal-averaged electrocardiography. It is recognized that the presence of ventricular late potentials (low-amplitude, high-frequency potentials at the end of the QRS complex) can predict malignment ventricular arrhythmias in patients with coronary artery disease and cardiomyopathy. Since young patients who had surgical repair of tetralogy of Fallot and other congenital defects that require right ventricular surgery are recognized to be at risk for clinically important ventricular arrhythmias, attempts were made to assess the utility of signal-averaged electrocardiography in predicting the occurrence of ventricular arrhythmias in this group of patients.[10–12] At this point, the indications and utility of signal-averaged electrocardiography in young patients is unclear, with some studies[10] suggesting that an abnormal signal-averaged ECG may correlate with the presence of inducible ventricular tachycardia (VT) in patients after tetralogy of Fallot surgery, while, in other studies,[12] an abnormal signal-averaged ECG did not correlate with the presence of clinically significant ventricular arrhythmias.

Provocative Testing

Exercise Testing

Since children and adolescents are normally very active during waking hours, it is extremely common to obtain a history of arrhythmia symptoms that occurred with exercise. An example would be the story of the 6-year-old child who is outside running and playing and subsequently returns home because his or her heart is racing. This type of history suggests that the arrhythmia is triggered only by exercise. Although this may occasionally be the case, it is much more common for the arrhythmia to onset at times other than during exercise. In addition, because children are active so frequently, other factors besides the activity or exercise itself must be responsible for the arrhythmia occurring. In practice, classical exercise testing does not usually induce common types of tachycardia, possibly because it does not duplicate the effect on autonomic tone of competitive sports. However, it may be that, although autonomic tone was modulated, a needed trigger, such as an atrial or ventricular extrasystole, did not occur during the 10- to 15-minute period of exercise that was being monitored. For that reason, exercise testing is frequently not helpful for obtaining ECG documentation during symptoms. However, exercise testing may be indicated in patients who have had syncope with exercise or in those patients who always experience arrhythmia symptoms with any exercise.[13,14] Patients in the latter group may most likely have VT, which has abnormal or triggered automaticity as its mechanism, and therefore may only be seen during exercise testing and not during any other type of ECG evaluation (Figure 5).

In addition, in patients with congenital complete heart block or patients who had surgical repair of congenital heart disease, exercise testing may uncover chronotropic incompetence, as well as the presence of ven-

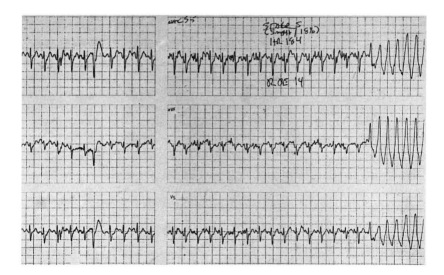

Figure 5. Simultaneous three-channel ECG recording during peak treadmill exercise utilizing a Bruce protocol in a 14-year-old boy with a history of presyncope and syncope with exercise. Note that, at stage 5 of exercise, on the left side of the figure, the sinus rate is 180 bpm. While exercise continues, a regular wide QRS tachycardia with probable ventriculo-atrial dissociation at a rate of 250 bpm abruptly starts and is sustained. The patient had reproduction of clinical symptoms of presyncope. CS_5, aVF, V_5: modified chest lead and standard ECG leads aVF and V_5.

tricular arrhythmias with exercise, which may suggest the need for closer follow-up or even therapeutic intervention.[15,16] In patients with structural heart disease, exercise testing may provide additional information that may not be available through other modes of ECG monitoring. Unfortunately, the occurrence of ventricular arrhythmias during exercise in some types of patients may be so frequent that the testing itself cannot help stratify patients at increased risk of clinically important arrhythmias.[17] The importance of arrhythmia suppression during exercise testing, such as ventricular extrasystole suppression, was not evaluated in a critical manner. However, in the absence of clinical symptoms, ventricular extrasystoles that suppress with exercise are purported to have a benign prognosis.

Upright Tilt Testing

Head-upright tilt table testing provides orthostatic stress by positioning the patient at a 70° to 90° angle for 15–60 minutes, sometimes including an isoproterenol infusion. The ability of upright tilt testing to reproduce clinical symptoms of presyncope and syncope in susceptible young patients prone to vasovagally mediated hypotension-bradycardia syndrome was demonstrated.[18–20] Unfortunately, the ideal protocol to minimize false-negatives and false-positives during upright tilt was not determined.[21] Studies are now available to suggest that upright tilt testing may not be sufficiently reproducible to be useful in assessment of therapy.[22] Realistically, in most young patients, vasovagal or neurally mediated syncope is a benign, self-limited condition that does not require definitive diagnosis or therapy. Circumstances and symptoms surrounding the syncopal event are important to note, as is the history from any eyewitness. In most cases, the prodrome and symptoms are so typical that no additional diagnostic testing is needed. Thus, although there was an initial flurry of activity and interest in upright tilt testing at the time it was developed to diagnose unexplained syncope, it is less frequently needed now to demonstrate the diagnosis of vasovagal syncope. In some patients, either where the etiology of syncope is not clear from the history or therapeutic interventions are being considered, upright tilt testing may be useful to provide a diagnosis in a patient with unexplained syncope. In addition, it is possible that a strategy for treatment might be apparent based on the results of the upright tilt test, specifically, whether the primary problem is hypotension secondary to vasodilation or whether the problem is primarily bradycardia. In most young patients, a response that consists of both hypotension and bradycardia occurs. Since no controlled therapeutic studies were performed, it remains difficult to judge the utility of serial upright tilt testing to judge efficacy of treatment. Nonetheless, upright tilt testing will be appropriate in select patients with recurrent syncope.

Transesophageal Atrial Pacing Studies

Transesophageal atrial pacing and recording techniques are particularly well suited to arrhythmia evaluation in the very young patient. The technique for optimal recording and stimulation was described.[23,24] These studies require minimal sedation, are relatively noninvasive, can provide a great deal of information regarding the patient's arrhythmia, and may be repeated with relative ease. For example, patients with Wolff-Parkinson-White (WPW) syndrome can undergo risk stratification with evaluation of antegrade accessory atrioventricular (AV) conduction using transesophageal atrial pacing techniques (Figure 6). In small patients, this information and other features of the tachycardia circuit may be helpful in selecting antiarrhythmic drug therapy. Moreover, provocative transesophageal atrial pacing studies can provide information about the natural history of the patient's arrhythmia substrate and answer the question, "Has the patient outgrown the tachycardia?"[25] Because both autonomic tone and the occurrence of triggers can be controlled during transesophageal pacing studies, arrhythmias that might not otherwise be captured with ECG monitoring can be diagnosed.[25,26] There are also reports of the application of transesophageal atrial pacing to evaluate older patients with palpitations.[27] When options for definitive treatment of tachycardia were limited to median sternotomy and epicardial mapping, knowing the tachycardia mechanism [ie, orthodromic reciprocating tachycardia with an accessory connection (AC) vs. tachycardia due to reentry in the AV node (AVN)] was helpful in deciding which patients should be subjected to further diagnostic testing prior to surgery. However, in the era of definitive tachycardia treatment with radiofrequency catheter ablation for essentially all common tachycardias, transesophageal atrial pacing is probably less helpful than it was previously for evaluation of palpitations after infancy. Indeed, because ventricular pacing cannot routinely be performed from the esophagus, this technique may result in false-negative studies, both for patients who have VT as the cause of their palpitations as well as for patients with concealed AC in whom tachycardia onset is dependent on retrograde conduction in the accessory connection.

In addition to being useful for obtaining a diagnosis about tachycardia mechanisms and natural history, transesophageal atrial pacing is a well-tolerated technique to use for tachycardia termination, especially in patients who have recurrent episodes of primary atrial reentrant tachycardias.[28,29] An example of this type of patient would be a patient who had atrial baffle surgery for D-transposition of the great arteries. These patients frequently have recurrent episodes of tachycardia that are poorly responsive to antiarrhythmic drug therapy, but they can frequently be treated with antitachycardia pacing. While information about whether permanent pacing could be useful in tachycardia termination is traditionally obtained by

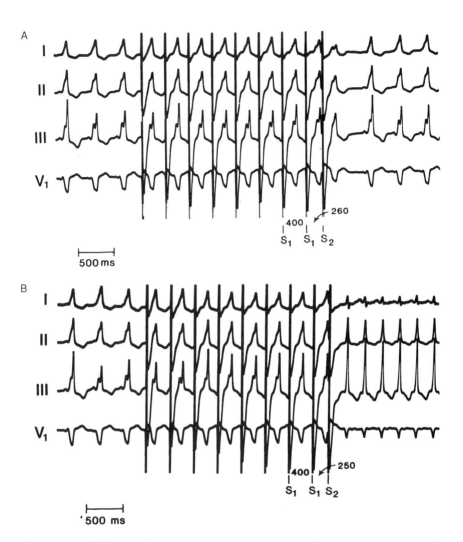

Figure 6. **A**: ECG recordings obtained during transesophageal atrial pacing and recording study in a 2-week-old infant with paroxysmal tachycardia and WPW syndrome. These recordings were obtained during an atrial refractory period determination at 400 milliseconds, with an S_1-S_2 interval of 260 milliseconds. Because the QRS following the S_2 is wide and similar in morphology to the sinus rhythm QRS, the S_2 conducts to the ventricle via the accessory connection. I, II, III, V_1: standard ECG leads I, II, III, V_1; S_1, S_2: stimulus artifacts. **B**: ECG recordings obtained during the same study as in **A.** Here, the S_1-S_2 interval was decreased from 260 milliseconds to 250 milliseconds, resulting in antegrade block in the accessory connection, conduction to the ventricle via the normal conduction system, and initiation of orthodromic reciprocating tachycardia. Thus, the antegrade effective refractory period of the accessory connection in this patient is 250 milliseconds.

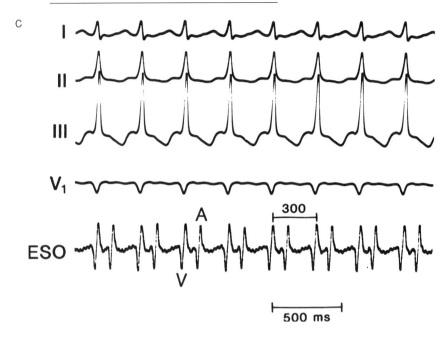

Figure 6. C: Simultaneous ECG recordings in addition to the ECG recorded from the esophageal catheter. The ventricular and atrial relation is clearly defined and supports the clinical impression of orthodromic reciprocating tachycardia as the tachycardia mechanism in this patient. The cycle length of the tachycardia is 300 milliseconds (equivalent to a heart rate of 200 bpm). A = atrial ECG from the esophagus; ESO = esophageal; V = ventricular ECG from the esophagus.

transvenous electrophysiology (EP) studies, in many patients who are veterans of congenital heart disease surgery and diagnostic procedures, venous access to the heart is no longer possible because of systemic venous obstruction. However, transesophageal atrial pacing can provide the needed information prior to pacemaker implantation and therefore is much more useful in helping plan treatment strategies than is the more traditionally used direct current cardioversion.

Intracardiac Electrophysiology Studies

Although ECG demonstration during arrhythmia symptoms is easily obtained in many patients, in others, provocative studies may be necessary. Again, noninvasive or minimally invasive testing may often be sufficient to obtain a diagnosis and treatment strategy, but, in some patients, invasive intracardiac EP studies are necessary. Generally, speaking, invasive diagnostic studies performed in patients with paroxysmal tachycardias are performed today most often in conjunction with a therapeutic procedure, ra-

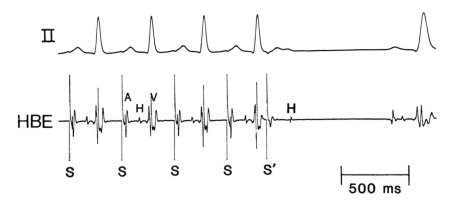

Figure 7. ECG recording and intracardiac electrogram from the low septal atrium in a 16-year-old boy who had episodes of recurrent syncope. He also has severe sickle cell hemoglobinopathy, status post-multiple transfusions and secondary cardiac hemochromatosis. This recording demonstrates the presence of infra-Hisian heart block during an atrial refractory period determination at 400 milliseconds. While not as helpful as ECG documentation obtained during symptoms of syncope, this finding at intracardiac EP study might support the presence of paroxysmal AV block below the His bundle recording site as the cause of syncope in this boy. Programmed ventricular stimulation did not demonstrate any arrhythmias. II = standard ECG lead II; H = His recording; HBE = recording obtained from the low septal atrium, the His bundle electrogram; S = stimulus artifact; A and V as defined in Figure 6.

diofrequency catheter ablation. This is true for patients with potentially life-threatening tachycardias as well as for patients with recurrent paroxysmal tachycardia who are not interested in chronic antiarrhythmic drug therapy.

In addition to diagnostic and therapeutic intracardiac EP procedures, patients with documented wide QRS tachycardias or patients who have symptoms of syncope or cardiac arrest are candidates for invasive EP studies. In these patients, sinus and AVN function, as well as His-Purkinje conduction can be assessed with programmed atrial stimulation and intracardiac recordings from the atrium and His bundle recording region (Figure 7). Guidelines were suggested for the appropriate use of intracardiac EP studies.[30] Programmed ventricular stimulation is helpful in young patients who have documented ventricular arrhythmias, but the optimal pacing protocol was not defined.[31] Moreover, the role of programmed ventricular stimulation in predicting future serious arrhythmias in susceptible but presently asymptomatic patients is unclear.[32,33] However, young patients with wide QRS tachycardias frequently have tachycardia mechanisms other than VT and deserve diagnostic EP study to determine their tachycardia mechanism, since this can have a profound influence on treatment and prognosis.[34]

Summary

Given the wide array of diagnostic techniques currently available, a careful clinical history will guide the judicious and cost-effective use of testing. For episodic symptoms in older children, event monitors typically provide more useful information than continuous ambulatory monitors or exercise testing. The neonate may be most expeditiously managed using transesophageal pacing techniques to guide efficacy of therapy. Patients with unexplained cardiac arrest will likely require intracardiac EP testing in addition to angiography, almost regardless of the results of noninvasive testing.

References

1. Liebman J, Plonsey R, Gillette PC, eds. Tables of normal standards. In: *Pediatric Electrocardiography*. Baltimore: Williams & Wilkins: 1982;82–133.
2. Davignon A, Rautaharju P, Boisselle E, et al. Normal ECG standards for infants and children. *Pediatr Cardiol* 1979/1980;1:123–131.
3. Southall DP, Johnston F, Shinebourne EA, et al. 24-hour electrocardiographic study of heart rate and rhythm patterns in population of healthy children. *Br Heart J* 1981;45:281–291.
4. Dickinson DF, Scott O. Ambulatory electrocardiographic monitoring in 100 healthy teenage boys. *Br Heart J* 1984;51:179–183.
5. Nagashima M, Matsushima M, Ogawa A, et al. Cardiac arrhythmias in healthy children revealed by 24-hour ambulatory ECG monitoring. *Pediatr Cardiol* 1987;8:103–108.
6. Goldstein MA, Hesslein P, Dunnigan A. Efficacy of transtelephonic electrocardiographic monitoring in pediatric patients. *Am J Dis Child* 1990;144:178–182.
7. Houyel L, Fournier A, Centazzo S, et al. Use of transtelephonic electrocardiographic monitoring in children with suspected arrhythmias. *Can J Cardiol* 1992;8:741–744.
8. Karpawich PP, Cavitt DL, Sugalski JS. Ambulatory arrhythmia screening in symptomatic children and young adults: comparative effectiveness of Holter and telephone event recordings. *Pediatr Cardiol* 1993;14:147–150.
9. Hayabuchi Y, Matsuoka S, Kubo M, et al. Age-related criteria for signal-averaged electrocardiographic late potentials in children. *Pediatr Cardiol* 1994;15:107–111.
10. Stelling JA, Danford DA, Kugler JD. Late potentials and inducible ventricular tachycardia in surgically repaired congenital heart disease. *Circulation* 1990;82:1690–1696.
11. Janousek J, Paul T, Bartáková H. Role of late potentials in identifying patients at risk for ventricular tachycardia after surgical correction of congenital heart disease. *Am J Cardiol* 1995;75:146–150.
12. Daliento L, Caneve F, Turrini P, et al. Clinical significance of high-frequency, low-amplitude electrocardiographic signals and QT dispersion in patients operated on for tetralogy of Fallot. *Am J Cardiol* 1995;76:408–411.
13. Rozanski JJ, Dimich I, Steinfeld L, et al. Maximal exercise stress testing in evaluation of arrhythmias in children: results and reproducibility. *Am J Cardiol* 1979;43:951–956.

14. Weigel TJ, Porter CJ, Mottram CD, et al. Detecting arrhythmia by exercise electrocardiography in pediatric patients: assessment of sensitivity and influence on clinical management. *Mayo Clin Proc* 1991;66:379–386.
15. Garson A Jr, Gillette PC, Gutgesell HP, et al. Stress-induced ventricular arrhythmia after repair of tetralogy of Fallot. *Am J Cardiol* 1980;46:1006–1012.
16. Karpawich PP, Gillette PC, Garson A Jr, et al. Congenital complete atrioventricular block: clinical and electrophysiologic predictors of need for pacemaker insertion. *Am J Cardiol* 1981;48:1098–1102.
17. Kavey RE, Blackman MS, Sondheimer HM. Incidence and severity of chronic ventricular dysrhythmias after repair of tetralogy of Fallot. *Am Heart J* 1982;103:342–350.
18. Pongiglione G, Fish FA, Strasburger JF, et al. Heart rate and blood pressure response to upright tilt in young patients with unexplained syncope. *J Am Coll Cardiol* 1990;16:165–170.
19. Thilenius OG, Quinones JA, Husayni TS, et al. Tilt test for diagnosis of unexplained syncope in pediatric patients. *Pediatrics* 1991;87:334–338.
20. Grubb BP, Temesy-Armos P, Moore J, et al. The use of head-upright tilt table testing in the evaluation and management of syncope in children and adolescents. *Pacing Clin Electrophysiol* 1992;15:742–748.
21. Benditt DG, Remole S, Bailin S, et al. Tilt table testing for evaluation of neurally-mediated (cardioneurogenic) syncope: rationale and proposed protocols. *Pacing Clin Electrophysiol* 1991;14:1528–1537.
22. Fish FA, Strasburger JF, Benson DW Jr. Reproducibility of a symptomatic response to upright tilt in young patients with unexplained syncope. *Am J Cardiol* 1992;70:605–609.
23. Benson DW Jr, Dunnigan A, Benditt DG, et al. Transesophageal study of infant supraventricular tachycardia: electrophysiologic characteristics. *Am J Cardiol* 1983;52:1002–1006.
24. Benson DW Jr, Sanford M, Dunnigan A, et al. Transesophageal atrial pacing threshold: role of interelectrode spacing, pulse width and catheter insertion depth. *Am J Cardiol* 1984;53:63–67.
25. Benson DW Jr, Dunnigan A, Benditt DG. Follow-up evaluation of infant paroxysmal atrial tachycardia: transesophageal study. *Circulation* 1987;75:542–549.
26. Biffi A, Ammirati F, Caselli G, et al. Usefulness of transesophageal pacing during exercise for evaluating palpitations in top-level athletes. *Am J Cardiol* 1993;72:922–926.
27. Pongiglione G, Saul JP, Dunnigan A, et al. Role of transesophageal pacing in evaluation of palpitations in children and adolescents. *Am J Cardiol* 1988;62:566–570.
28. Butto F, Dunnigan A, Overholt ED, et al. Transesophageal study of recurrent atrial tachycardia after atrial baffle procedures for complete transposition of the great arteries. *Am J Cardiol* 1986;57:1356–1362.
29. Dick M, Scott WA, Serwer GS, et al. Acute termination of supraventricular tachyarrhythmias in children by transesophageal atrial pacing. *Am J Cardiol* 1988;61:925–927.
30. Zipes DP, Akhtar M, Denes P, et al. Guidelines for clinical intracardiac electrophysiologic studies. A report of the American College of Cardiology/American Heart Association Task Force on Assessment of Diagnostic and Therapeutic Cardiovascular Procedures. *J Am Coll Cardiol* 1989;14:1827–1842.
31. Silka MJ, Kron J, Cutler JE, et al. Analysis of programmed stimulation methods in the evaluation of ventricular arrhythmias in patients 20 years old and younger. *Am J Cardiol* 1990;66:826–830.

32. Kugler JD, Pinsky WW, Cheatham JP, et al. Sustained ventricular tachycardia after repair of tetralogy of Fallot: new electrophysiologic findings. *Am J Cardiol* 1983;51:1137–1143.
33. Chandar JS, Wolff GS, Garson A Jr, et al. Ventricular arrhythmias in postoperative tetralogy of Fallot. *Am J Cardiol* 1990;65:655–661.
34. Benson DW Jr, Smith WM, Dunnigan A, et al. Mechanisms of regular, wide QRS tachycardias in infants and children. *Am J Cardiol* 1982;49:1778–1788.

Chapter 2

Fetal Arrhythmias

Peter L. Ferrer, MD

Introduction

Fetal cardiology is one of the newest and perhaps one of the most challenging fields in cardiology. An important aspect of this new field is the diagnosis and management of fetal cardiac arrhythmias.

This chapter provides the reader with information regarding fetal cardiac arrhythmias, including methods of detection, frequency, differential diagnosis, clinical implications, prenatal natural history, prognosis, and management. The information presented is based on a review of the literature as well as the author's own experience with more than 300 fetuses with fetal cardiac arrhythmias.

History

The use of fetal electrocardiography by Cremer[1] in 1906 marked a significant advancement in the study of fetal cardiac activity. During the following decade, fetal electrocardiograms (ECGs) were utilized in the evaluation of heart rate, diagnosis of twin pregnancies, and determination of fetal position.[2-4] Although recordings of ventricular depolarization were possible, ensuing difficulties in recording atrial depolarization (low-amplitude, high noise-to-signal ratio) precluded its utilization for the diagnosis of fetal cardiac arrhythmias. In 1953, Smyth[5] obtained fetal ECGs by use of a silver electrode wire introduced into the amniotic sac. Direct heart rate recordings were also possible in the intrapartum period when the membranes were ruptured, allowing leads to be placed on the fetal head or

From Deal B, Wolff G, Gelband H, (eds.). *Current Concepts in Diagnosis and Management of Arrhythmias in Infants and Children.* Armonk, NY: Futura Publishing Co., Inc.; © 1998.

buttocks. Several types of cardiac arrhythmias were diagnosed prenatally prior to the availability of fetal echocardiograms.[6–9] For detailed information on the technique of direct fetal ECG, the reader is referred to previous literature.[10–13] Major abnormalities in fetal heart rate and rhythm during pregnancy could be detected by auscultation and documented by phonocardiography. As early as 1973, Robinson and Shaw-Dunn[14] used M-mode echocardiograms (MMEs) to determine the fetal heart rate early in pregnancy. Beginning in the early 1980s, two-dimensional and M-mode echocardiography (MME) were utilized in the diagnosis of structural heart disease and fetal cardiac arrhythmias, as reported by multiple authors.[15–20] Since these early endeavors, numerous investigations contributed to our present knowledge of fetal cardiac arrhythmias. Specific contributions will be discussed as the different types of fetal cardiac arrhythmias are described.

The Fetal Conduction System and its Autonomic Control

Ventricular automaticity was observed in human fetuses as early as the end of the third week of gestation.[14,21] Shenker and associates[22] described evidence of cardiac activity by 4 weeks of gestation. The sinoatrial (SA) node originates from the sinus venosus and can be recognized by 7 weeks of gestation. The atrioventricular node (AVN) originates from primitive myocytes in the SA ring, atrioventricular (AV) ring, and septum primum, which can be recognized by the 10th week of gestation. As a result of the septation of the fetal atria and ventricles, the internodal pathways and AVN development take place. By the 10th to 12th week of gestation, the AVN, the junctional tissue, and its pathway to the ventricles are well developed. The conduction system of the ventricles probably develops from cells in the AV ring at approximately the same time as the interatrial and junctional conduction system.[23]

During this time, many changes take place in the fetal conduction system and its autonomic control. James[24] described a large number of P cells and a decrease in the number of transitional cells in the fetal and newborn SA node when compared with adults. In the early stages of fetal development, the SA node contains a small central artery that increases in size and prominence during childhood. The fetal SA node contains little collagen; this material increases progressively after birth. In addition, the location of the AVN migrates during fetal life, reaching its "adult" position postnatally.[24] According to James,[25] the AVN tissue and the His bundle undergo extensive postnatal "remodeling." The implication of all these changes in the functional electrical "instability" of the fetal and newborn heart remains controversial.

There is evidence that the regulation of the fetal and neonatal heart rate is predominantly cholinergic. It appears that cholinergic fibers are present by the sixth week of gestation.[26] Parasympathetic inhibition is present by 12–17 weeks of gestation.[27,28] Parasympathetic innervation is mediated by muscarinic cholinergic receptors that predominate at the SA and AVN and to a much lesser extent in the ventricular myocardium.[26] Others[28] demonstrated pacemaker inhibition by acetylcholine as early as the fourth week of gestation.

Sympathetic fibers were found in the fetal myocardium by 10 weeks of gestation[26]; sympathetic stimulatory effect was described by 22–23 weeks of gestation.[27,28] Several investigators[26,28,29] described increases in the fetal heart rate with norepinephrine as early as the fourth and fifth weeks of gestation.

Biochemical observation by Friedman and colleagues[30] is compatible with the concept that significant increases occur in the magnitude of sympathetic innervation postnatally. Studies of neonatal cardiac response to physiological events,[31] or responses associated with inhibitory reflexes,[32] suggest that the regulatory effect of the autonomic system is "immature." It could be postulated that this unbalanced autonomic innervation and the subsequent developmental changes affecting the conduction system are probably factors that play a role in the genesis and characteristics of some of the fetal cardiac arrhythmias.

Methodology of Detection of Fetal Cardiac Arrhythmias

The first stage in the evaluation of cardiac arrhythmias is documentation. Here the ECG is replaced by the echocardiogram as the method of detection in the fetus. Long-term detection of the fetal heart rate by Doppler ultrasound (cardiotachometer) provides only ventricular rate and, therefore, is limited compared with postnatal Holter monitoring.

M-Mode Echocardiography

The objective of arrhythmia analysis using MME is to evaluate the AV sequence by the simultaneous recording of two structures representing atrial and ventricular contractions, respectively (ie, the atrial wall and the ventricular wall on the apical four-chamber view or, alternatively, the atrial wall and an AV valve or a semilunar valve). An instrument capable of performing dual MME has the advantage of simultaneously recording two M-mode tracings (Figure 1). In general, ventricular contractility is easily recorded from multiple views. Recording of atrial contractions can be more easily obtained by a line of MME going through both atria, perpendicular to the foramen ovale, above the AV valves. This technique requires the

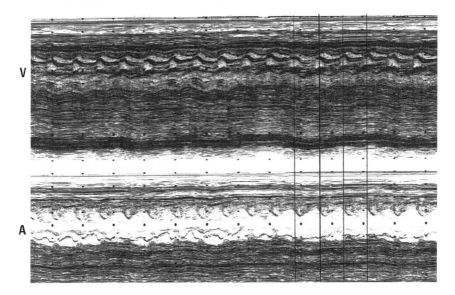

Figure 1. Simultaneous M-mode echocardiographic recordings (dual MME) of atria (A) and ventricles (V). Note the normal AV sequential contractions of atria and ventricles. Lines indicate early atrial contractions (A) coinciding with ventricular diastole (V). Time lines = 500 milliseconds/

apical four-chamber view perpendicular to the axis of the interatrial septum; recordings of the superior aspect of the atrial wall on the apical four-chamber view are less rewarding. The contractility of the atrial walls can be observed in a two-dimensional format, so to optimize the atrial recording, the cursor should be positioned at the point where the maximal atrial contractility occurs. An alternate approach is to record both atria on the sagittal view, with the right atrium (RA) located anteriorly and the left atrium (LA) located posteriorly.

Measurements of time intervals (cycle length, heart rate) can be easily obtained by measuring two consecutive atrial contractions (AA interval), similar to the measurement of the PP interval on an ECG. The ventricular rate (VV interval) can be measured from two consecutive ventricular contractions, similar to the RR interval of the ECG. An alternative estimate of ventricular rate can be obtained by measuring the interval between the two openings or two closings of an AV valve or semilunar valve. Measurement of multiple cycle lengths elucidate the variation of heart rate, the coupling period of extrasystoles, the presence of incomplete or complete compensatory pauses after ectopic beats, the existence of sinus pauses, and the frequency of atrial flutter (AF) or atrial tachycardia.

Simultaneous recordings of atrial contractility (atrial wall) and ventricular contractility (ventricular wall), or other systolic events such as opening and closing of the aortic and pulmonic valves, permit the observer to determine if blocked atrial extrasystoles (AEs), or any form of AV block, are present.

Doppler Echocardiography

Pulsed Doppler is useful in the diagnosis of fetal cardiac arrhythmias since it can be gated to a specific location, obtaining flow events that represent atrial and ventricular systole on the same tracing. For example, echocardiographic views such as the apical four-chamber view, the apical four-chamber view with aorta, or the apical two-chamber view offer the opportunity of simultaneous recordings of the left ventricular (LV) outflow (systole) and mitral valve inflow (atrial systole)[20] (Figure 2). Some researchers[33] suggested simultaneous Doppler recordings of the descending aorta (ventricular systole) and inferior vena cava (atrial systole), the ascending aorta and superior vena cava,[34] the pulmonary artery and a pulmonary vein[35] (the inferior vena cava or suprahepatic vein may be used instead of the pulmonary vein), or the umbilical artery and umbilical vein.[36] The reader interested in performing fetal echocardiograms should be prepared

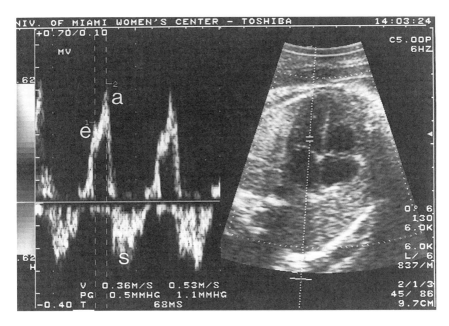

Figure 2. Spectral Doppler mapping of mitral valve inflow. Positive velocities (ventricular diastole) correspond to rapid ventricular filling (e) and atrial contraction (a); negative velocities correspond to flow in the LV outflow during ventricular systole (s). There is normal sequence of atrial and ventricular contractions. Time lines = 500 milliseconds.

to utilize all the techniques described. The author prefers to use M-mode echo recordings—based on their simplicity and the fact that they require lower levels of acoustic energy—and spectral Doppler recordings as a complementary procedure.

The utilization of ladder diagrams may facilitate the understanding of fetal arrhythmias by representing the AV sequence.[16,18,37] Once the diagnosis of arrhythmia is made, recordings of any arterial flow by spectral Doppler provide information regarding variability of ventricular rate due to ectopic beats, blocked supraventricular extrasystoles (SVEs), supraventricular tachyarrhythmias (SVTAs), AV block, or other forms of arrhythmia.

A fetal cardiac arrhythmia may be primary (absence of structural heart disease) or secondary (associated with congenital or acquired heart disease). Extensive descriptions of the methodology used to assess details of the anatomic features of the fetal heart (segmental approach) and the techniques used to obtain quantitative data, such as chamber size, wall thickness, and parameters of ventricular systolic and diastolic function, are available.[38,39]

Incidence

Shenker[40] and Elkayham and Gleicher[41] reported fetal rhythm disturbances in 1% to 2% of pregnancies. McCurdy and Reed[42] found that 10% of fetal cardiac arrhythmias may result in significant morbidity and mortality. Fetal arrhythmias may be responsible for 15% to 20% of cases referred for fetal echocardiography.[43,44] In our experience of 1078 patients (1700 fetal echocardiograms) referred for prenatal cardiac evaluation, 32% were referred for arrhythmias; in 75% of these cases the diagnosis was confirmed, while 25% had no arrhythmias at the time of observation. Among patients referred for reasons other than cardiac arrhythmias, 7% of these

_____ Table 1 _____

Diagnosis of Fetal Arrhythmias
University of Miami 1983–1996

	Patients	%
Extrasystoles	197	63
Brady/tachycardia	62	20
Supraventricular tachyarrhythmias*	37	12
Complete A-V block	13	5
Partial A-V block	2	
Total	311	100

* Includes 6 perinatology cases.

also presented arrhythmias. Hence, the frequency of cardiac arrhythmias in our entire (selected) referred population was 28%.[45]

Table 1 shows the types of arrhythmias in order of frequency. The most frequent arrhythmias are extrasystoles (63%), followed by sinus bradycardia/tachycardia (20%), SVTAs (12%), and second- or third-degree AV block (5%). Including 6 additional cases of perinatal SVTAs, we estimated that potentially lethal arrhythmias occurred in 50 of 311 patients (16%).[45,46]

Sinus Arrhythmia, Sinus Bradycardia, and Sinus Tachycardia

The fetal heart has a mean rate of 90 beats per minute (bpm) by approximately 4 weeks of gestation, increasing to a mean of 124 bpm by the 5th week,[22] and a maximum of 180 bpm by the 8th to 10th week of gestation. Thereafter, the mean heart rate decreases progressively toward birth.[14]

Sinus Arrhythmia

The heart rate in the fetus is constantly varying. Urbach and associates[47,48] introduced the term ''phasic'' or ''periodic variations.'' Sinus arrhythmia can be defined as phasic variations of the heart rate originating in the SA node. Echocardiographic recognition of sinus arrhythmia includes the gradual increase or decrease in the fetal heart rate with concordant atrial and ventricular contractions (ventricular beats are preceded by atrial beats).

Hammacher and colleagues[49] described an increase in heart rate variability preceding sinus tachycardia in fetuses with prolonged hypoxia. In general, sinus arrhythmia should be considered a normal variant.

Sinus Bradycardia

Sinus bradycardia was empirically defined as a heart rate less than 90 bpm in the newborn[50,51] and less than 90 bpm or more than 40 bpm below the baseline in the fetus for more than 1 minute.[52] Other investigators[18] defined bradycardia as a cardiac rhythm of less than 100 bpm. In the author's opinion, these empirical limits do not include fetuses referred with the diagnosis of fetal bradycardia with persistent heart rates ranging between 90 and 125 bpm. Thus, the author would like to extend the diagnosis of fetal bradycardia to include heart rates below 125 bpm, providing this heart rate is persistent. The term sinus bradyarrhythmia is used to define a variable heart rate in the presence of sinus bradycardia. In these cases, there is a normal AV sequence.

Bradycardia was detected in newborns and infants following physiological events such as defecating, hiccuping, and yawning, especially in the small premature infant; bradycardia as low as 32 bpm was reported during drowsiness or deep sleep.[31] Bradycardia was also observed following clamping of the umbilical cord, pressing of the anterior fontanel, stimulation of the ocular or carotid sinus,[32] as well as during nasopharyngeal stimulation,[53] perhaps a response to a cardioinhibitory reflex mediated by parasympathetic stimulation.[53] Fetal bradycardia can also be obtained by compression with the ultrasound transducer; spontaneous episodes of bradycardia are thought to be related to cord compression, probably mediated by parasympathetic stimulation.[54]

Echocardiographic characteristics of sinus bradycardia and sinus bradyarrhythmias include a normal AV sequence (Figure 3). The differential diagnosis includes second- or third-degree AV block or blocked AEs; in these cases, there are higher atrial rates in comparison with ventricular rates.

Short episodes of sinus bradycardia lasting less than 1–2 minutes are a frequent normal variant, particularly around 20 weeks of gestation, but can be observed throughout the pregnancy. Observation of this event by ultrasound can be quite "dramatic" as the heart stops and slowly starts again.[55]

The prognosis of fetal sinus bradycardia is related to its etiology. Persistent sinus bradycardia in association with nonimmune hydrops fetalis is an ominous sign that is probably related to fetal hypoxia.[55] Additional etiologies of sinus bradycardia include hypoxia or hypoperfusion,[56] prolonged QT syndrome,[57] and structural heart disease.[58,59] Lithium poisoning,[60] reserpine,[61] and potassium-iodide 131[62] were related to bradycardia in the newborn and probably in the fetus. Our experience, as well as the experience of others,[63] shows that in rare instances sinus bradycardia may occur in the absence of an obvious etiology and may result in a favorable outcome. Another form of bradycardia, with rates often ranging between 90 and 125 bpm, is the so called "coronary sinus rhythm,"[64–66] a form of shifting atrial pacemaker with echocardiographic characteristics similar to sinus bradycardia.[66]

Management. Transient sinus bradycardia is not of pathological significance and should not be treated. In cases of severe sinus bradycardia associated with nonimmune hydrops fetalis, particularly in the presence of other poor prognostic signs, premature delivery may be indicated, depending on the gestational age.[55]

Bradycardia related to coronary sinus rhythm is associated with polysplenia syndrome including interruption of the inferior vena cava, complex congenital heart disease, and heterotaxia.[66] This type of bradycardia should

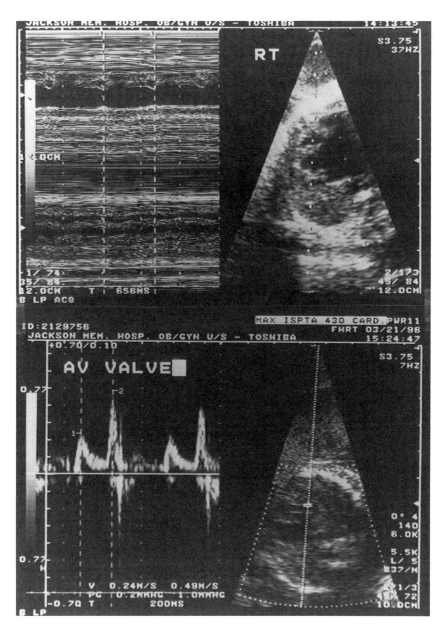

Figure 3. "Coronary sinus" rhythm in a fetus with complete AV septal defect and polysplenia syndrome, resulting in bradycardia of 81–92 bpm. The upper panel shows a dual MME of atria (**top**) and ventricles (**bottom**). Note the normal AV sequence with 1:1 conduction. The lower panel shows flow pattern at the common AV valve. Note the normal sequence of velocities during rapid ventricular filling (1) and atrial contraction (2). Time lines = 500 milliseconds.

be considered an intrinsic cardiac rhythm, and obstetricians should refrain from performing early delivery in these cases.[66]

Sinus Tachycardia

The rate of sinus tachycardia varies between 175 and 190 bpm between birth and 1 month of age and between 175 and 210 bpm in the fetus, depending on gestational age. Empirically, obstetricians defined tachycardia as fetal heart rate consistently above 160 bpm.[52] Transient heart rates above 160 bpm are frequently related to fetal movements and should be considered a normal variant. Persistent fetal tachycardia in utero was reported in association with certain conditions including cytomegalic inclusion disease[67] and maternal hyperthyroidism,[59] among others.

The fetal echocardiogram demonstrates concordance between atrial and ventricular contractions. While the fetal heart rate can easily reach 200 bpm, rates above 200 bpm are usually present with SVTAs. In the case of sinus tachycardia, the fetal heart rate has mild variations that can be detected by measuring PP or VV intervals, with gradual heart rate changes. In contrast, the heart rate in supraventricular tachycardia (SVT) is quite regular, with abrupt changes as the rhythm reverts to a sinus mechanism.[68] Changes in fetal ventricular rate may occur during SVT or AF in the presence of variable AV block or during the maternal administration of antiarrhythmic therapy.[46,68]

Management. The management of persistent sinus tachycardia involves treatment of the primary cause. Improvements in the fetal heart rate were demonstrated as maternal hyperthyroidism was controlled with propylthiouracil.[59]

Sinus Node Disorders

Sinus pauses can be observed in the fetus in association with sinus bradycardia. Sinus arrest can be observed in the so-called "coronary sinus rhythm," associated with polysplenia: poorly developed right side structures, including the SA node, create a predisposition toward a more primitive atrial rhythm with lower rates. Although atrial depolarization occurs in an abnormal direction, as demonstrated by the postnatal ECG,[65] the fetal echocardiogram shows AV concordance similar to cases of sinus bradycardia.[66]

Sick Sinus Syndrome

In this syndrome there is abnormal function of the SA node, manifested as bradycardia, which may manifest as a lower escape mechanism or tachycardia. The youngest baby described with this syndrome was seen for the first time at 21 days of age; it was hypothesized the condition was congenital in origin.[69] To our knowledge, no fetal cases were reported.

Shifting Pacemaker

This condition is characterized by shifting of the pacemaker site between the sinus node and a secondary pacemaker within the atria, probably related to an increase in parasympathetic tone and suppression of the SA node. The secondary pacemaker generally produces a lower heart rate.[68] The rhythm probably occurs in the fetus as a transitional rhythm during development of, or recovery from, severe transient bradycardia. The echocardiogram shows a normal sequence of atrial and ventricular contractions and, therefore, cannot be distinguished from sinus arrhythmia. This type of rhythm should be suspected when the fetal heart rate shifts between two frequencies, with the higher rate corresponding to the SA node. Postnatally, the rhythm can be recognized on ECG by the different P morphologies and P axes of the two pacemakers.

Ectopic Beats

Ectopic beats can be generated by abnormal pacemaker tissue located in the atria, junctional tissue, or ventricles. Ectopic beats may occur as escape beats when the SA node slows down, or they may be premature extrasystoles caused by increased automaticity.[68] The frequency of escape beats in the fetus was not established; this is due mainly to limitations in the echocardiographic diagnosis. Premature extrasystoles are easily detectable and can be present as an isolated rhythm or in association with other arrhythmias.

The frequency of extrasystoles in the population of healthy fetuses was not established. Similarly, the frequency and type of extrasystoles reported in newborns, as well as in infants, varies greatly. In general, the frequency of extrasystoles reported in healthy premature newborns was between 21% and 31% and in full-term neonates between 2% and 23%. One explanation for these wide-ranging percentages may be the different techniques and durations of observation used for documentation of the arrhythmias,[51,70] with higher values obtained with longer periods of observation. Similar limitations exist in the evaluation of fetal extrasystoles. As in the newborn, fetal SVEs are more frequent than ventricular extrasystoles (VEs).[39,45]

Supraventricular Extrasystoles

SVEs may be atrial or junctional. Premature AEs in the newborn are preceded by an early P wave of abnormal configuration on the ECG. SVEs occurring very early in the cardiac cycle may be blocked, or they may result in aberrant conduction with a pattern of right or left bundle branch block; both situations are frequently found in neonates.[71] Both atrial and junctional extrasystoles in the fetus have concordant AV contractions and incomplete compensatory pauses (Figure 4). Blocked SVEs are demonstrated by premature atrial contractions that are not followed by ventricular contractions in MMEs or Doppler recordings (Figures 5 and 6). Limitations in the present detection techniques preclude the diagnosis of SVEs conducted aberrantly.

Doppler samples at the junction of the mitral inflow and LV outflow tract (LVOT) will identify rapid ventricular filling (E wave during early ventricular diastole), atrial contractions (A wave during late ventricular diastole), and ventricular contractions (systole). SVEs conducted to the ventricles can be identified as an early diastolic flow across the mitral valve

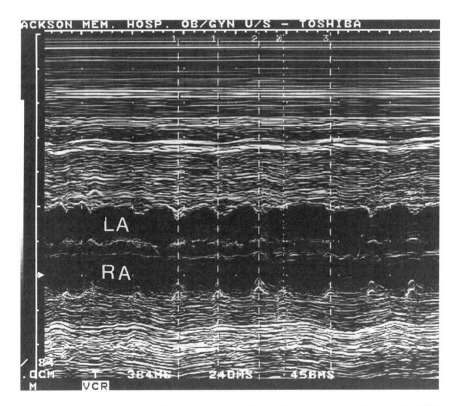

Figure 4. M-mode echocardiographic recording of both atria in a fetus with SVE (RA = right atrium; LA = left atrium). The first two cycles marked with dotted lines are sinus beats (cycle length = 384 milliseconds). Note the SVE (fourth dotted line) with a coupling interval of 240 milliseconds, followed by an incomplete compensatory pause of 456 milliseconds. Time lines = 500 milliseconds.

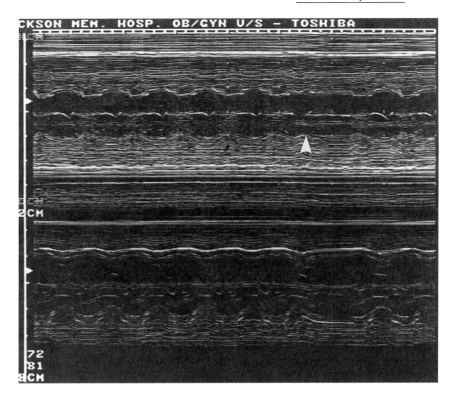

Figure 5. Dual M-mode echocardiographic recording of atria (**top**) and ventricles (**bottom**). Note the normal sequence of atrial and ventricular contractions consistent with a normal sinus rhythm of approximately 133–148 bpm. The seventh beat from left to right (arrow) is a SVE followed by an incomplete compensatory pause and not conducted to the ventricles (blocked SVE on bottom). Time lines = 500 milliseconds.

corresponding to atrial contractions (passive ventricular filling is obscured). This is followed by systolic ejection detected at the LVOT (Figure 7). The postextrasystolic beats demonstrate prolonged diastole. A similar pattern can be obtained in the tricuspid valve inflow; nonetheless, the right ventricular (RV) inflow and outflow are in different planes precluding the demonstration of RV systole. In our population of 200 fetuses with SVEs, a pattern of bigeminy, trigeminy, or quadrigeminy was noted in 33% of cases, and blocked extrasystoles were present in 28% of cases.

In the past, it was suggested that the fetal and neonatal heart were relatively lacking in the mechanism for postextrasystolic potentiation.[72] With time, this was proven not to be the case; fetal postextrasystolic potentiation of flow velocity demonstrates a normal Frank-Starling mechanism.[73,74]

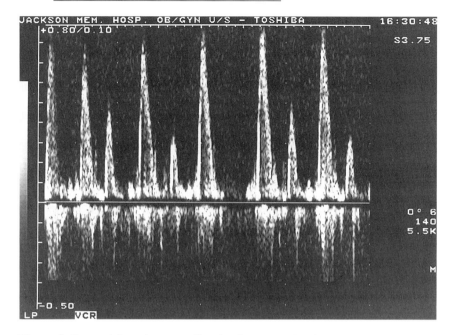

Figure 6. Spectral Doppler recording in the aorta of a fetus with frequent SVE (atrial bigeminy, atrial trigeminy). The first two beats from left to right are sinus, followed by an extrasystole with incomplete compensatory pause. The fourth and fifth beats correspond to a sinus beat and an extrasystole, respectively. Note that a blocked extrasystole follows the sixth sinus beat. The last four beats correspond to atrial bigeminy. This fetus had intervals of bradycardia when all extrasystoles were blocked. Time lines = 500 milliseconds.

The majority of cases of SVEs are not associated with structural heart disease. In isolated cases, SVEs may be the cause of referral for a fetal echocardiogram which then results in the diagnosis of an underlying heart disease. We have not seen a consistent link between SVEs and a specific congenital heart disease. It was postulated that atrial redundancy, or aneurysm, is associated with an increased frequency of SVEs.[75,76] We believe this aneurysm is a normal variant since, in the majority of cases, the condition is no longer present postnatally. It is possible that an aneurysm of the interatrial septum may be a contributing factor rather than a cause. Approximately half of our cases with aneurysms in the interatrial septum were associated with SVEs, but these cases corresponded to only a minimal number from our total group of patients with extrasystoles.

In our experience, SVEs may occur in fetuses with cardiac tumors. Three of our four patients with rhabdomyomas diagnosed prenatally had SVEs. One fetus developed SVT and hydrops, and a second fetus developed SVT postnatally; both had Wolff-Parkinson-White (WPW) syndrome. A

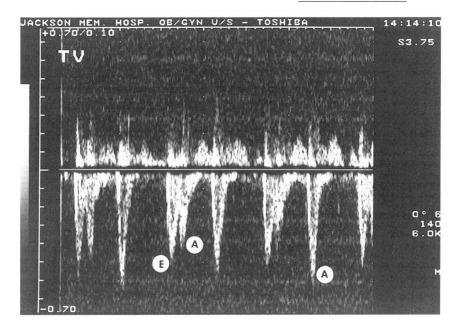

Figure 7. Spectral Doppler recording at the tricuspid valve inflow in a case of atrial bigeminy. Bimodal pattern of flow corresponds to sinus beats with the first wave representing rapid ventricular filling (E) and the second wave representing atrial contraction (A) (beats No. 1, 3, 5, 7 from left to right). The beats represented by a single wave correspond to AEs (A waves only), followed by an incomplete compensatory pause (beats No. 2, 4, 6 from left to right). Time lines = 500 milliseconds.

third fetus with SVEs prenatally developed incessant ventricular tachycardia (VT) at 3 months of age. All the patients survived.[77] Transplacental lithium poisoning is a rarely reported etiology.[78]

Traditionally, the obstetrics community considered SVEs a benign form of cardiac arrhythmia that resolves spontaneously. It was stated that SVEs were not proven to be the precursors of SVT.[55] Isolated premature SVEs were reported as prodromal echocardiographic observations in SVT in the neonate[79,80] as well as in the fetus.[81,82] In addition, SVEs are frequently associated with sinus rhythm following the conversion of SVT.[46,83] Kleinman and associates[84] suggested an association between SVEs and SVT in approximately 1% to 2% of cases. In our own experience[85] this association occurs in 6% of cases and may precede SVT as well as AF (Figures 8 and 9). More recently, Simpson and coworkers[86] reported an association of 5%.

Very early SVEs may result in blocked extrasystoles. The presence of blocked extrasystoles and SVT was reported by Silver and colleagues[79] and, more recently, emphasized by Simpson and associates.[86] These authors reported that SVT occurred in 2% of cases with multiple atrial ectopic beats

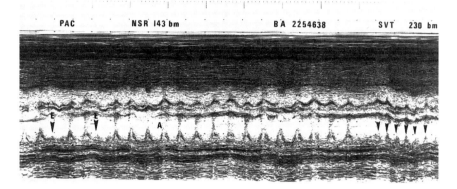

Figure 8. M-mode echocardiographic tracing of an atria (A) and the posterior great artery of a fetus. The cycle length of atrial contractions indicated sinus rhythm (143 bpm), interrupted by isolated SVE (E arrows). Note on the right the appearance of SVT (230 bpm) (arrows). Time lines = 500 milliseconds.

compared with 13% of cases with blocked atrial ectopic beats. Based on our experience of 200 cases of fetal SVEs, the relative risk of SVTAs (SVTAs include SVT and AF) is 3% for isolated SVEs, 12% for frequent SVEs (bi-

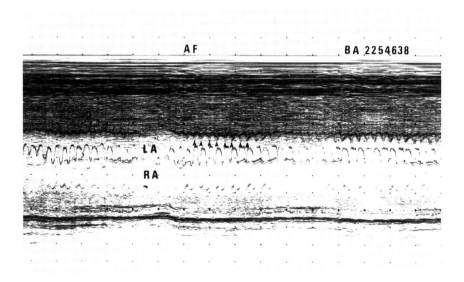

Figure 9. M-mode echocardiographic recording of the atria of the same fetus depicted in Figure 8; the tracing shows a fast atrial rate (arrows) consistent with AF with an atrial rate of 428 bpm. AF = atrial flutter; LA = left atrium; RA = right atrium. Time lines = 500 milliseconds.

geminy, trigeminy, and quadrigeminy), and 9% for blocked SVEs, resulting in an average risk of 6%. SVEs associated with SVTAs, on average, presented slightly earlier (25.1 weeks) than those not associated with SVTAs (29.7 weeks). However, this difference was not significant.

Management. SVEs do not require treatment. During counseling, mothers should be informed that SVEs are benign ectopic beats that occur in all ages and resolve spontaneously during pregnancy, or during the neonatal period, in the vast majority (94%) of cases.[85] Our protocol includes checking the fetal heart rate 2 or 3 times a week to detect the possibility of sustained tachycardia. A few minutes of simple auscultation by the obstetrician or obstetrical RN will suffice. This protocol can be discontinued if the SVEs subside or can become more strict if the SVEs are blocked or are very frequent.

If the surveillance is performed at longer intervals, sustained tachycardia may be undetected for several days and may result in hydrops fetalis. Bradycardia due to blocked SVEs may be severe if associated with atrial bigeminy or atrial trigeminy; early delivery should be avoided. As an added precaution during pregnancy, we agree with the recommendations that mothers should avoid stimulants such as caffeine, adrenergic derivatives (common in cough and decongestive preparations), tobacco, and, of course, any other form of substance abuse.[39]

Ventricular Extrasystoles

Our experience,[45] as well as the experience of others,[39] suggests that fetal VEs are rare, accounting for only 2% of extrasystoles. In the fetus, the diagnosis is based on a premature contraction in the ventricles followed by a complete compensatory pause associated with normal atrial sequence (normal AA interval) (Figure 10).

Doppler samples taken at the mitral or tricuspid inflow show a normal diastolic pattern (E and A waves) during normal beats. During VEs, there is an absence of flow through the AV valve; the postextrasystolic beat will show a prolonged diastole and a complete compensatory pause. The diagnosis is more difficult when there is an incomplete compensatory pause.[87]

VEs may be primary (not associated with heart disease) or secondary. The etiology of this rhythm disturbance may involve multiple factors including hypoxia, metabolic abnormalities, viral infections, long QT syndrome, or compromise of the myocardium. The risk of VT developing in fetuses with VEs is unknown.

Management. The management of ventricular ectopic beats should be conservative, with attention directed to excluding predisposing causes or structural heart disease.

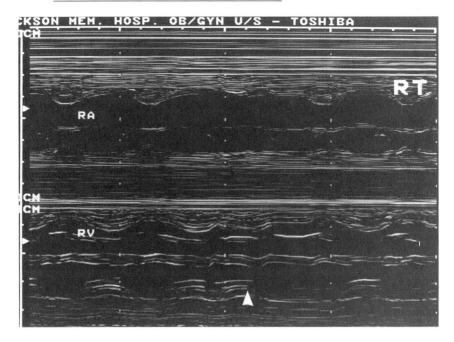

Figure 10. Dual mode echocardiographic recordings of atria (**top**) and ventricles (**bottom**). Note a VE (arrow) followed by a complete compensatory pause. Top panel demonstrates no VA conduction; thus, no discharge of the SA node occurs. RA = right atrium; RV = right ventricle. Time lines = 500 milliseconds.

Supraventricular Tachyarrhythmias

The term SVTAs includes several forms of fast atrial rhythm, including SVT, AF, and atrial fibrillation. Some investigators[88] make no distinction between SVT (SVT with 1:1 AV conduction) and AF (SVT with AV block). The author prefers to use the term AF, since the differential diagnosis may have therapeutical implications. The combined statistics of three centers published by van Engelen and coworkers[89] ($n =$ 49), plus our own experience ($n = 37$) showed 53 fetuses (62%) had SVT, 26 fetuses (30%) had AF, and 7 fetuses (8%) had both episodes of SVT and AF (the latter 7 fetuses were considered in the statistics of both SVT and AF; thus, the total number of cases was 93). These three forms of tachyarrhythmias are potentially lethal because they may produce congestive heart failure in utero (hydrops fetalis).[90–94] Therefore, the diagnosis and management is of paramount importance because maternal administration of antiarrhythmic therapy can be life saving for the fetus.

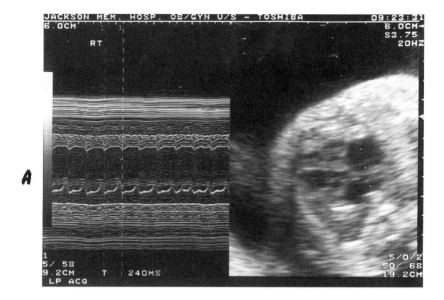

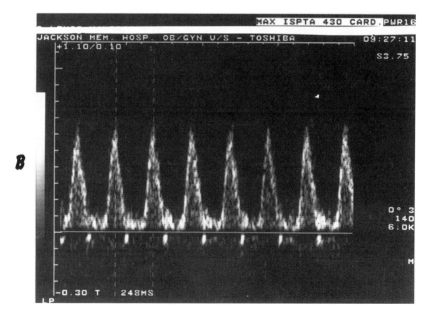

Figure 11. A: M-mode echocardiographic tracing of both atria; the dotted lines correspond to the AA interval with a cycle length of 240 milliseconds (atrial rate 250 bpm), consistent with a SVT. The panel on the right depicts the line of insonation on a two-dimensional format background. **B**: Spectral Doppler in the ascending aorta of the same fetus depicted in **A**. There is a SVT with a ventricular rate of approximately 250 bpm. Time lines = 500 milliseconds.

Supraventricular Tachycardia

The average ventricular rate during SVT is very fast, ranging between 220 and 320 bpm in the neonate[95,96] and with similar rates in the fetus.[16,18,97–103] In our experience of 20 cases of fetal SVT, the average ventricular rate was 250 bpm (Figure 11).

Mechanisms of SVT are extensively reviewed in Chapter 5 and Mehta et al.[104] Reentrant tachycardia involving an accessory connection is the most common mechanism of SVT in the young. Automatic forms of SVT, including ectopic atrial and junctional tachycardia, account for less than 20% of SVT in childhood. An isolated case of junctional tachycardia was reported.[105] The frequency of these forms of tachycardia in the fetus is unknown.

Reentrant Supraventricular Tachycardia

The most common forms of reentrant SVT include AV reentry utilizing an accessory connection and AVN reentry. The distinction between these two forms of tachycardia cannot presently be made in utero, therefore, estimates of their frequency are based on postnatal evaluation. Zales and colleagues[106] demonstrated postnatally the presence of accessory pathways leading to reciprocating tachycardia in 12 cases of fetal tachycardia. Naheed and coworkers,[88] utilizing postnatal transesophageal electrophysiologic (EP) procedures, reported 30 cases of SVT, managed pre- and postnatally, in which the mechanism of tachycardia was AV reciprocating tachycardia or intraatrial reentrant tachycardia. Based on these postnatal studies, AVN reentry tachycardia occurs rarely in the neonate and presumably in the fetus. SVT utilizing an accessory connection accounted for approximately 90% of SVT in infants with in utero tachycardia studied postnatally.[88]

Reentrant Supraventricular Tachycardia Related to Anomalous Atrioventricular Connections

According to Kleinman and Copel,[105] and our own data, the incidence of manifest WPW syndrome (preexcitation) on the surface ECG at birth of patients with fetal SVT is 8% to 15%. Naheed and coworkers[88] reported a 27% incidence of preexcitation including patients with AF. Preexcitation cannot be recognized in utero with the present technology but may be suspected. Three of our 20 cases (15%) of SVT and 2 of our 17 cases (12%) of AF demonstrated a preexcitation pattern postnatally. Three fetuses with SVT were also diagnosed with diseases involving the myocardium: two with multiple rhabdomyomas[77] and one with oncocytic cardiomyopathy.[59] WPW syndrome and SVT may occur in association with structural heart disease such as Ebstein's malformation of the tricuspid valve, corrected transposition of the great arteries, tetralogy of Fallot, ventricular septal defect, cardiomyopathies, and rhabdomyomas of the heart.[68]

Atrial Flutter and Atrial Fibrillation

Atrial Flutter

AF may be defined as a rapid, regular, atrial rhythm with atrial rates ranging between 360 and 480 bpm in the newborn[107,108] and between 430 and 530 bpm in the fetus.[83] Six of our 17 cases of AF showed transient atrial rates with 1:1 conduction. The rate and regularity of the ventricular complexes depend on the AV conduction. The most frequent form of AV conduction is 2:1 in which the ventricular rate is half that of the atrial rate. Nonetheless, variable AV conduction may result in variable or irregular ventricular rate. Thus, this form of arrhythmia should be given consideration in a fetus with irregular rhythm. Vagal maneuvers may increase the severity of AV block and improve visualization of the AF on the ECG postnatally.

Prenatally, the diagnosis of AF is made by direct recordings of the atrial wall, which show the fast atrial contractions. Measurements of the PP interval of the flutter waves represent the atrial rate. Simultaneous recordings of atrial and ventricular contractions by MME will demonstrate the associated second-degree AV block, which is most frequently 2:1 (Figure 12). Blumenthal and associates[109] demonstrated AF in the fetus by obtaining a fetal ECG on the fetal head at the time of delivery. Moller and colleagues[110] reported that 43% of cases of AF in children showed signs of arrhythmia before delivery. We have diagnosed, prenatally, 17 cases (5%) of AF among 311 fetuses with cardiac arrhythmias. AF was present in 46% of the 37 fetuses with SVTAs. In these cases, fetal flutter was diagnosed at a mean of 33 weeks of gestation (between 25 and 40 weeks), with the majority having sustained AF (16 of 17 patients). Atrial rates for these fetuses ranged between 414 and 530 bpm, with a mean of 460 bpm. Ventricular rates ranged between 210 and 288 bpm; the majority had 2:1 conduction, but a few cases had variable AV conduction and variable ventricular rate.[83]

The association of fetal AF with accessory connections and AV reentry tachycardia was reported by several authors.[88,111-113] Naheed and coworkers[88] reported eight cases of SVT and AV block (AF); seven were inducible during postnatal transesophageal EP evaluation. Five had AV reciprocating tachycardia, and two had intraatrial reentrant tachycardia. These authors speculated that rapid, retrograde atrial depolarization during reciprocating tachycardia initiates atrial reentrant tachycardia.

Postnatally, AF was reported in association with several structural heart diseases, including endocardial fibroelastosis, cardiomyopathy, as well as

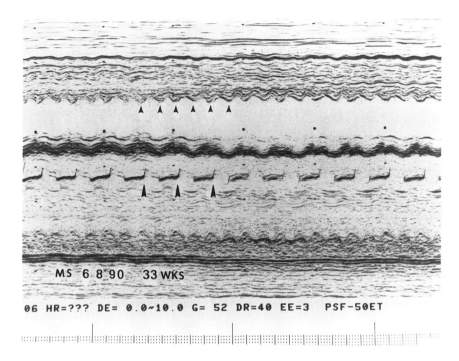

Figure 12. Fetal AF. M-mode echocardiographic recording of an atria (**top**) and a ventricle (**bottom**). Small arrows indicate atrial rate (480 bpm); large arrows indicate ventricular rate (240 bpm). Thus, there is AF with 2:1 conduction. Time lines = 500 milliseconds.

congenital heart disease. The same may occur prenatally. One of 15 cases reported by van Engelen[89] and colleagues had a hypoplastic LV and a dilated LA. Kleinman and Copel[105] reported 3 cases of congenital heart disease in 12 cases of AF. Included among these was one case of RV outflow tract obstruction and tricuspid insufficiency, one case of Ebstein's malformation of the tricuspid valve and tricuspid insufficiency, and one case of AV septal defect and AV valve insufficiency. In the latter case, the AF was associated with complete AV block. All three cases had marked RA enlargement. None of our 17 cases of AF were associated with structural heart disease, and only two demonstrated manifest WPW syndrome postnatally. Six of our 17 cases (35%) were associated with congestive heart failure in utero (hydrops fetalis).[83] This association has significant implications in terms of therapy as well as prognosis. Of the 36 fetal and perinatal cases described by Moller[110] and associates, 11 (31%) died and several had AF as well as atrial fibrillation. This was not our experience. None of our 17 cases had atrial fibrillation; 6 had, at times, transient SVT, and 17 of 17 patients (100%) survived.[83]

Atrial Fibrillation

Atrial fibrillation is an extremely rapid, chaotic, and irregular atrial rhythm with atrial rates within a 500- to 700-bpm range. The postnatal characteristics revealed by ECG include P waves of variable amplitude, morphology, and duration and an irregular ventricular cycle length (RR interval) with a variable ventricular rate.[114,115] The fast atrial fibrillatory waves may result in decrease of the ventricular response, particularly during drug therapy or vagal maneuvers, thereby adopting characteristics of AF.

Prenatally, detection of atrial activity may be difficult by M-mode echo or Doppler procedures. The atrial rate is higher in cases of atrial fibrillation than in cases of AF. The ventricular rate (VV interval) is constantly varying. Isolated cases of atrial fibrillation were reported.[116,117] Kleinman and Copel[105] described two cases (0.2% of all their fetal arrhythmias): gestational ages were 19 and 38 weeks, respectively, no hydrops was present, one was controlled in utero, and both survived. Postnatally, atrial fibrillation was associated with a number of heart diseases such as Ebstein's malformation of the tricuspid valve, endocardial fibroelastosis, cardiomyopathy, atrial tumors, and thyrotoxicosis.[68]

Supraventricular Tachyarrhythmias and Hydrops Fetalis

It was hypothesized that fetuses with SVTAs and congestive heart failure in utero have, primarily, diastolic dysfunction produced by the fast ventricular rate that limits the ventricular diastolic filling.[105] The fetal heart is susceptible to congestive heart failure; it has limited reserves because it works at a high level on the Starling curve. Further, intrinsic properties of the immature myocardium probably play a role in this propensity. These factors, such as a less-developed adrenergic autonomic system and fewer contractile elements per unit of myocardial tissue when compared with mature myocardium, contribute to this vulnerability.

Compromise of the ventricular diastolic function is supported by our own observations. Doppler spectral recordings at the ventricular inflow, after conversion of the SVTA to sinus rhythm, showed a reverse in the pattern of flow at the inflow of both ventricles (E > A waves). This profile normalizes (A > E waves) when the sinus rhythm persists.[83] During SVT, there is a decrease in velocity in the great arteries.[74] These findings suggest that the decrease in forward ventricular stroke volume is probably secondary to limitations in diastole rather than systole. During SVT, the RV diastolic pressure and RA pressure probably increase, as evidenced by the dilatation of the RV, the RA, and the systemic veins; there may be functional tricuspid insufficiency, and the flow pattern in the systemic veins may show an increase in retrograde flow velocities and a decrease in anterograde flow velocities.[118] As a consequence of the increased systemic venous pressure, hydrops fetalis develops (Figure 13).

Data from a collaborative study of three institutions published by Van Engelen and associates,[89] plus our own experience, showed that hydrops was present in 43% of fetuses with SVTAs (47% in fetuses with SVT and 36% in fetuses with AF). Valerius and Jacobsen[119] reported an increased incidence of hydrops fetalis when ventricular rates were above 230 bpm, but other investigators[120] found no correlation between the development of hydrops and increases in ventricular rate. In another study, Naheed and coworkers[88] found no correlation between ventricular rate, or the mechanism of fetal SVT (including AF), and hydrops; they found that gestational age was lower in hydropic fetuses ($m = 33$ weeks) compared with nonhydropic fetuses ($m = 38$ weeks) and that hydrops fetalis was related to the duration of the SVT, independent of gestational age. Further, these authors reported that hydrops occurred in their cases of sustained SVTAs, but not in their small series of nonsustained tachycardia.[88] However, this study was limited by its retrospective nature and by the fact that 13 of their 30 cases were first managed postnatally. Newburger and Keane[121] found that neither the duration of SVT nor the ventricular rate predicted the clinical outcome at birth. In our experience, hydrops occurred almost exclusively in cases of sustained SVTA; our main difficulty was in establishing the duration of tachycardia prior to the development of hydrops because the majority of cases had hydrops at the time of the first evaluation. Furthermore, the median gestational age of our hydropic fetuses and nonhydropic fetuses was the same (33 weeks).

The diagnosis of congestive heart failure in utero has management and prognostic implications. In the combined statistics of Van Engelen and colleagues[89] with our own experience, which will be described later in more detail, successful control of SVTAs occurred in 71% of the hydropic fetuses compared with 90% in the non-hydropic fetuses. Among the hydropic fetuses, successful control was higher in cases of SVT (78%) compared with cases of AF (60%) (Table 2). Kleinman and Copel[105] reported that decreasing the ventricular rate in cases of AF was not sufficient to decrease the severity of congestive heart failure. They attributed this failure to the volume overload of the right heart, with a relatively restrictive myocardium. In addition, persistence of the AF, resulting in atrial contraction with partially or completely closed AV valves, could result in persistence of RA and systemic venous hypertension, thereby retarding the resolution of fetal hydrops.[93]

We agree with the principle that the therapeutic end point of antiarrhythmic therapy is the restoration of sinus rhythm with 1:1 conduction. Nonetheless, we saw cases of persistent AF in which pharmacologic intervention decreased the ventricular rate and the severity of hydrops.[83] In these cases, delivery could be postponed to decrease morbidity related to

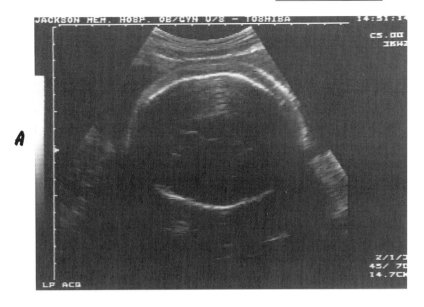

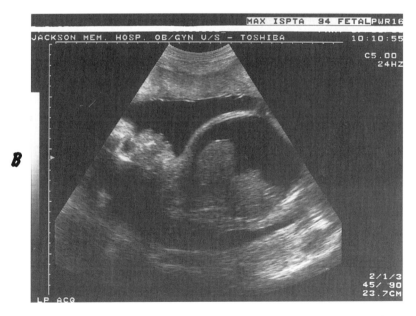

Figure 13. Hydrops fetalis of cardiac origin (congestive heart failure) in a fetus at 32 weeks of gestation. **A** shows scalp edema; **B** shows marked ascites. (Courtesy of the Division of Obstetric Ultrasound.).

_____ Table 2 _____

Antenatal Control of Supraventricular Tachyarrhythmias* with Maternal Administration of Antiarrhythmic Therapy**

	Supraventricular Tachycardia (n = 40)		Atrial Flutter (n = 19)	
	Hydrops # (%)	Nonhydrops # (%)	Hydrops # (%)	Nonhydrops # (%)
Antenatal control	14/18 (78%)	20/22 (91%)	6/10 (60%)	8/9 (89%)
Total antenatal control	34/40 (85%)		14/19 (74%)	

* Tachyarrhythmias include supraventricular tachycardia and atrial flutter.
** Combined statistics of four centers.

premature birth. Our statistics, combined with those of Van Engelen and coworkers,[89] showed the risk of death for hydropic fetuses with SVTAs was 13% (SVT 14%, AF 8%).

Management of Fetal Supraventricular Tachyarrhythmias

The diagnosis of SVTAs in the fetus signals an emergency situation requiring immediate action since these arrhythmias are potentially lethal.[92,117] In management, several factors should be taken into consideration: gestational age; duration of the tachyarrhythmia; type of SVTA; ventricular rate; presence and severity, or absence, of hydrops fetalis; existence of structural heart disease; and fetal well being.[55]

A brief fetal echocardiogram should be performed in order to diagnose the SVTA and to determine the presence and severity of pericardial effusion. This should be complemented with a limited obstetric scan to evaluate for other signs of hydrops fetalis (such as ascites, pleural effusion, scalp edema, or placental edema), to estimate the severity of the hydrops, and to obtain a fetal biophysical profile. The mother should be admitted, and antiarrhythmic therapy should be considered as soon as the diagnosis is made. There is a consensus for immediate therapy in cases of sustained SVTAs with or without hydrops and also for what may appear to be a nonsustained SVTA associated with hydrops fetalis of cardiac origin.[55] There is controversy surrounding the use of antiarrhythmics in patients with nonsustained SVTA not complicated with hydrops. Allan[55] favors therapy in cases in which the fetus has tachycardia more than 50% of the time. In determining the duration of the tachycardia, it is important to keep in mind that fetal monitoring has its limitations. Monitoring may be considered reliable as long as the angle of insonation of the Doppler detects the flow in the great arteries; however, fetal movement may alter recordings. We favor a prolonged or repetitive observation by echocardiography combined with fetal monitoring. In the author's view, recurrent SVT or AF, particularly in the presence of a high ventricular rate, should be considered for treatment even when present less than 50% of the time. This view is controversial since some investigators[88] found that nonsustained SVT is not associated with hydrops fetalis. However, observation must be very closely maintained since it is difficult to predict whether the tachycardia will become sustained. In our experience, as well as in the experience of others, maternal administration of antiarrhythmic therapy is safe when the appropriate guidelines are followed (M. L. Young, MD, written communication, September 1996); therefore, only qualified cases of sporadic, nonsustained SVTAs should be observed without administering treatment.

Treatment of the mother and fetus should proceed as a team approach between pediatric cardiologists and perinatologists. The therapy could be carried out on the labor floor or in the intensive care unit with experienced nurses and adequate instrumentation for maternal and fetal monitoring. Prior to pharmacologic treatment, a baseline maternal ECG should be obtained as well as baseline laboratory values to evaluate renal and liver function. We favor the use of an intravenous catheter to avoid the multiple punctures required for intravenous administration of antiarrhythmics or for obtaining drug levels. The initial fetal echocardiogram should be completed to assess ventricular systolic and diastolic function, to check for signs of systemic venous hypertension, and to detect the presence or absence of structural heart disease. The obstetric scan should also be completed to obtain information regarding gestational age and estimated fetal weight as well as to detect any congenital abnormalities.

Gestational age and estimated fetal weight are important considerations in treatment. Allan[55] advised delivering fetuses greater than 36 weeks of gestation—an option to consider especially if the fetus is hydropic. This indication can be extended to include cases of sustained SVTAs in which control of the arrhythmia was not obtained by 36 weeks of gestation or in cases of intermittent SVTA without hydrops in which the fetus is 36 weeks and deteriorating. Early delivery increases morbidity related to prematurity. Thus, before delivering fetuses with SVTA and hydrops, careful consideration of risks versus benefits for both mother and fetus is necessary within the context of experience of both therapist and institution. Delivery should not be performed before obtaining reasonable trials of antiarrhythmics with adequate maternal drug levels. Success may take days, and the utilization of more than one drug, or a combination of drugs, may be necessary. Steroids should be administered to accelerate lung maturation in anticipation of delivery.

In making the decisions that surround the maternal administration of an antiarrhythmic, the therapist must carefully weigh all factors involved. The primary goal of the therapist should be the mother's safety, as well as optimizing the chances of fetal survival.

Antiarrhythmic Drugs

Fetal therapy may be accomplished through maternal administration of drugs that reach the fetus through the placenta. Many pharmacologic aspects of such therapy need further study. Dosages appropriate for the nonpregnant woman may be inappropriately low during pregnancy due to expansion of blood volume or increased glomerular filtration rate. Alternatively, dosages may be inappropriately high because of decreased protein binding. Examples of factors to consider include dynamic gestational changes in maternal kinetics, placental drug passage, fetal body composition, and fetal drug metabolism and excretion.[122] A detailed review of all antiarrhythmic drugs that can be potentially utilized in the fetus is beyond the scope of this chapter. A list of dosage recommendations for the commonly used drugs, as well as other useful data, are presented in Table 3. Conversion to sinus rhythm, or tachycardia control, can be achieved through the use of cardiac glycosides (digoxin)[123–127]; class IA antiarrhythmic agents (procainamide[127,128] and quinidine[129,130]); class IC (flecainide[131–133]); class II, β-blockers (propranolol)[134,135]; class III (amiodarone,[136,137] sotalol[138–142]); or class IV, calcium channel blockers (verapamil).[121,143]

In cases of nonhydropic fetuses with sustained SVTAs, treatment can be initiated with the physician's drug of choice. In the combined experience of three centers, Van Engelen and colleagues[89] with our own, 59 patients (or 69%) received antiarrhythmic therapy. SVTAs were controlled in 28 of 31 (90%) nonhydropic fetuses: 71% with digoxin alone; 16% with flecainide alone; 3% with digoxin plus verapamil; the remaining 10% were controlled postnatally (Table 4).

The best drugs for use in hydropic fetuses with SVTA is still under investigation. Digoxin, when used alone, was less effective in hydropic than in nonhydropic fetuses. Some of the antiarrhythmic drugs used instead of digoxin include verapamil,[121,143] flecainide,[131,132] and amiodarone,[136,137] but their usage was limited, resulting in insufficient data to establish a superior choice. In addition, side effects, including fetal demise (flecainide), were reported.[133] In the combined experience of Van Engelen[89] with our own, tachycardia control in hydropic fetuses was achieved in only 19 of 28 patients or (68%): 14% with digoxin alone; 7% with flecainide alone; 40% with digoxin plus an added drug (verapamil, quinidine, procainamide, flecainide, propranolol, sotalol); 7% with flecainide plus added digoxin; the remaining 32% were either not controlled until birth or died (Table 4).

Table 3

Fetal Supraventricular Tachyarrhythmias: Antiarrhythmic Therapy

	Maternal Administration	Half-Life	Therapeutic Levels	Toxic Levels	Placental Transfer	Advantages	Disadvantages
Digoxin IV	Digitalization 1.5–2.0 mg/24 h 0.500 mg slow (10–15 min) 0.250 mg q 4–6 hrs (10–15 min)	24–48 hrs	2.0–2.5 Ng%	>3.5 Ng%	80–100%; Decreased with Hydrops	Fast placental transfer action 30 min. Positive inotropic drug	Slow conversion Small difference between the threshold of fetal action and maternal intoxication Fetal demise reported Proarrhythmic (mother) GI symptoms
IV	Maintenance 0.500–1.25 mg/24 hrs		2.0–2.5 Ng%				
P.O.	0.500–1.25 mg/24 hrs Divided q 6–8 hrs						
CLASS IA Procainamide IV	500–600 mg over 20 min.; check levels. Maintenance 2–6 mg/min				25%	Atrial Flutter	GI symptoms Hypotension Proarrhythmic blood dyscraisias

Table 3

Fetal Supraventricular Tachyarrhythmias: Antiarrhythmic Therapy

	Maternal Administration	Half-Life	Therapeutic Levels	Toxic Levels	Placental Transfer	Advantages	Disadvantages
P.O.	Initially 1250 mg, followed in 1 hr by 750 mg. Then 250–1000 mg q 3–6 hrs	2.5–5.0 hrs	4–10 mcg/ml	>10 mcg/ml			
Quinidine	200–400 mg P.O. q 4–6 hrs	4–10 hrs	3–7 mcg/ml	>9 mcg/ml	100%	Atrial Flutter	Neonatal thrombocytopenia GI symptoms (mother) Proarrhythmic (mother) Hepatic toxicity (mother)
CLASS IC Flecainide P.O.	100–300 mg/ 24 hrs Divided q 12 hrs	12–27 hrs Mean 20 hrs	0.2–1.0 mcg/ ml	>1.0 mcg/ ml	80%	Effective even if hydops is present, fast conversion	Fetal deaths reported Increased ventricular rate in atrial flutter Proarrhythmic (mother) Visual and CNS symptoms

	Dose	Half-life	Therapeutic level	Placental transfer	Indications	Side effects
CLASS II beta-blockers						
Propanolol IV	1 mg/min, max 3 mg	2–4.5 hrs				
PO	40–320 mg/24 hrs Divided q 6–8 hrs		25–150 Ng/ml adult >100 Ng/ml child	20–100%	SVT Atrial Flutter Ventricular arrhythmias	Bradycardia Hypoglycemia Reported low birth weight
CLASS III						
Amiodarone P.O.	800–1000 mg/24 hrs Divided with meals Dec. to 600–800 mg/24 hrs for 4 weeks Maint. 400 mg (200–800 mg)/24 hrs Divided with meals	Weeks	0.7–2.8 mcg/ml	4:1 maternal/fetal	Effective when other drugs have failed	Depression maternal and fetal thyroid Proarrhythmic GI symptoms Acute pulmonary toxicity, CNS symptoms
Sotalol P.O.	160–320 mg/24 hrs Divided q 12 hrs	12 hrs	N/A	Information scarce; assumed to have good placental transfer	Information scarce on efficacy	Maternal proarrhythmic effects
CLASS IV calcium channel blockers						
Verapamil p.o.	240–320 mg/24 hrs Divided q 6–8 hrs	3–13 hrs	0.1–0.4 mcg/ml	3:1 maternal/fetal	Effective isolated or associated with Digoxin fast conversion	Negative inotropic Uterine contractions Labor dysfunction Fetal demise reported

_____ Table 4 _____

Efficacy of Maternal Administration of Antiarrhythmics in the Control of Fetal Supraventricular Tachyarrhythmias*

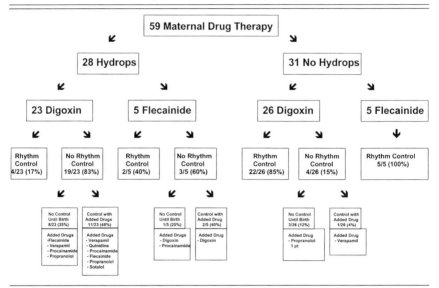

* Combined Statistics of Four Centers—Adapted with permission from Reference 89.
* Tachyarrhythmias include supraventricular tachycardia and atrial flutter.

Our approach was to start with digoxin intravenously at high doses, aiming for maternal digoxin levels of 2.0 to 2.5 ng percent or greater if tolerated without digoxin intoxication. If conversion is not achieved within 48–72 hours of adequate maternal levels, a second antiarrhythmic, such as verapamil, sotalol, or flecainide, is added. The amount of digoxin should be decreased if verapamil, quinidine, amiodarone, or flecainide are added.

In cases of hydropic fetuses with AF, antenatal conversion to sinus rhythm was less effective than in hydropic fetuses with SVT (60% vs. 78%; Table 2). In AF, digoxin and/or verapamil can be used to increase AV block and decrease ventricular rate; in many cases, this approach will result in conversion to sinus rhythm. If conversion is not obtained, a type IA antiarrhythmic drug (procainamide, quinidine), a β-blocker, or a class III agent (sotalol) can be added.

From an informal survey (Table 5) of 105 members of the North American Society of Pacing and Electrophysiology (NASPE) from 15 centers around the United States, information was obtained regarding frequency of use of antiarrhythmics, as well as maternal and fetal side effects, in 190 cases of fetal SVTAs. The survey did not separate SVT from AF, nor did it include drug efficacy. The percentage of time each drug was utilized in the entire popula-

Table 5

Frequency of Utilization of Antiarrhythmic Drugs in Fetal Supraventricular Tachyarrhythmias*
Survey of 15 Centers, 190 Cases

Medication	#	% of Pts	#	%	Maternal Complications	#	%	Fetal Complications
Digoxin	149	78%	7	5%	4 GI, 2 uterine irritability, 1 Wenckebach	1	0.6%	1 died 96 hrs after Digoxin, 35 wks, myocarditis
Flecainide	16	8%	2	13%	1 GI, 1 CRBBB	1	6%	1 slow SVT, 3 wks, no SVT after discontinuation
Verapamil	13	7%	1	8%	1 visual symptoms and uterine irritability	0	0	
Procainamide	11	6%	0	0		0	0	
Quinidine	11	6%	2	18%	1 GI, 1 thrombocytopenia	0	0	
Amiodarone	9	6%	1	11%	1 thrombocytopenia, photosensitivity rush	2	22%	2 borderline hypothyroidism
Propranolol	4	2%	0	0		0	0	
Sotalol	3	2%	0	0		0	0	
Adenosine	2	1%	0	0		0	0	
Total	218	**	13	6.8%		4	2.1%	

GI = gastrointestinal symptoms, nausea and/or vomiting (digoxin, quinidine), acidity (flecainide); CRBBB = complete right bundle branch block; Pts = patients.

* Tachyarrhythmias include supraventricular tachycardia and atrial flutter.

** Several antiarrhythmic drugs used in sequence or in combination.

tion was digoxin (78%), flecainide (8%), verapamil (7%), procainamide (6%), quinidine (6%), amiodarone (6%), propranolol (2%), and sotalol (2%). (Note: Some patients received more than one drug, accounting for the sum of percentages greater than 100%.) Maternal side effects occurred in 13 instances (6.8%), with higher percentages in order of frequency for quinidine, flecainide, amiodarone, verapamil, and digoxin. Fetal complications were rare (2.1%) (M. L. Young, written communication, 1996).

Alternative Therapies in Fetal Supraventricular Tacharrythmias

Martin and associates[144] reported two cases of successful conversion of SVT by transabdominal cord massage, probably mediated through parasympathetic stimulation. Fernandez and colleagues[145] reported a similar case. Other alternative therapies include antiarrhythmic administration through the amniotic fluid or direct fetal therapy by either intramuscular injection to the fetus or cordocentesis.[146–149] These techniques, though not exempt from complications such as lacerations or hemorrhage, may be useful in boosting drug levels or terminating the tachycardia. However, they are less suitable for avoiding recurrences by repeated administration. Amiodarone was used in direct intravenous therapy and has the advantage of a long half-life.[150] Direct fetal intravenous administration of adenosine could be considered for termination of sustained SVT; however, its very short half-life precludes its use as a prophylactic drug, which is accomplished with other antiarrhythmics. Adenosine is ineffective in terminating automatic SVT or AF.[105,151]

Allan[55] discussed the possibility of cardioversion by direct current to the fetus through the maternal abdomen. In this situation, the mother would require general anesthesia, and there is a risk of premature labor or placental abruption.

Fetal Ventricular Tachycardia

Ventricular tachyarrhythmias include VT, ventricular flutter, and ventricular fibrillation. VT is a rare arrhythmia in the fetus.[16,18,40,45,89] Ventricular flutter and fibrillation may be associated with fetal demise.

The fetal echocardiogram will usually show a ventricular rate below 200 bpm, not preceded by atrial contractions in a regular manner, and the ventricular rate will be higher than the atrial rate. This AV dissociation is also present in junctional tachycardia, although junctional tachycardia appears to be very rare in the fetus.[105] The differential diagnosis of ventricular from SVTs may be impossible if retrograde ventriculo-atrial (VA) conduction occurs, since the AV sequence in this case (depending on the time interval required to depolarize the atria retrogradely) may be normal.

In the past, rare cases of fetal VT were reported even before echocardiography was available as a diagnostic tool. Kleinman and Copel[105] found four cases (0.4%) among fetuses referred for fetal cardiac arrhythmias. Three of the four cases were not associated with hydrops and were not treated in utero. Postnatally, episodes of VT were infrequent. These infants were asymptomatic and were not treated. The fourth fetus developed prolonged VT during labor, with an enlarged RA and RV thought to be related to arrhythmogenic RV dysplasia. Therapy after delivery was performed with intravenous lidocaine, followed by oral mexiletine.

Stevens and coworkers[152] reported three cases of fetal VT diagnosed retrospectively from among 14 neonatal cases of VT. One infant died postnatally of myocarditis. The remaining infants had a benign course. As evidenced in these cases, the diagnosis of VT does not imply inevitable death.

Of our 311 patients with fetal cardiac arrhythmias, none demonstrated VT in utero. One fetus with VEs showed a low rate VT as a newborn; thus, it is possible this fetus presented VT in utero which was not recognized. A second fetus, diagnosed with perinatal hydrops fetalis and SVT, converted to normal sinus rhythm shortly after birth. Nonetheless, this infant developed VT and ventricular fibrillation and died; the autopsy showed oncocytic cardiomyopathy.[59] A third fetus, diagnosed at 32 weeks of gestation with multiple rhabdomyomas and SVEs in utero, developed incessant VT at 3 months of age which was nonresponsive to antiarrhythmic therapy. This infant underwent a lifesaving ablation at the site of origin of the VT in the RV.[153]

Management

In the rare event of prenatal diagnosis of sustained VT, pharmacologic intervention may be warranted, particularly when high ventricular rates are present. Consideration should be given to the maternal administration of procainamide, sotalol, propranolol, or amiodarone at the same dosage recommended for SVT (Table 3). In cases of VT with evidence of congestive heart failure, Kleinman and Copel[105] suggested the use of direct umbilical vein infusion of lidocaine, followed by maternal therapy with mexiletine, quinidine, procainamide, flecainide, or propranolol. There are insufficient data to favor any specific antiarrhythmic therapy for VT in the fetus.

Lidocaine

There is limited information regarding the direct use of this class IB antiarrhythmic drug in the fetus. The half-life for this drug is probably longer in the fetus compared with the premature infant (3.2 hours) or children (1.8 hours). The protein binding capabilities of this drug range between 20% and 60%. Guidelines for infants and children could be utilized but should be undertaken with caution. The recommended bolus dose for children is 1 mg/kg. A similar or lower dose could be used in the fetus considering the estimated fetal weight with a maintenance of 10–50 μg/kg per minute.

Maternal doses of procainamide, quinidine, flecainide, propranolol and sotalol are the same as shown in Table 3 for SVT. Mexiletine, a type IB drug, could be used in initial doses of 100–200 mg every 8 hours, aiming for an effective plasma concentration of 0.5–2.0 μg/mL. Maintenance oral doses are 100–300 mg every 6 to 12 hours to a maximum 1200 mg every 24 hours.

Conduction Disturbances

Second-Degree Atrioventricular Block and Complete Atrioventricular Block

The diagnosis of conduction disturbances in the fetus is limited to second-degree and third-degree AV block. The diagnosis of first-degree AV block, or intraventricular conduction block, requires a fetal ECG. The incidence of partial AV block is approximately 0.6% of cases of fetal cardiac arrhythmias. Some of these cases with second-degree AV block (Mobitz type II) may progress to complete AV block, and some may resolve postnatally. The incidence of complete AV block was estimated at 1 case per 20,000 live-born infants.[154] We can assume that this incidence is higher in the fetus since a number of them die in utero.

The echocardiographic features of the diagnosis of second-degree AV block include detection of atrial contractions not followed by ventricular contractions (blocked). This arrhythmia may correspond to a second-degree AV block Mobitz type I (Wenckebach periodicity) or Mobitz type II (2:1, or other form of partial AV block). As in the case of blocked AEs, second-degree AV block may result in bradyarrhythmia; however, in contrast to blocked AEs, atrial contractions not conducted to the ventricles are not premature, and they are not followed by incomplete compensatory pauses.[68]

The echocardiographic diagnosis of complete AV block includes AV discordance with atrial rates higher than ventricular rates (Figure 14).

A review of the two largest series in the literature,[155,156] plus our own experience with complete AV block, provided information on 105 fetuses from 5 institutions: 57 patients (or 54%) had complete AV block associated with structural heart disease. This is in contrast to postnatal data from international studies in which structural heart disease was present in only 25% of cases with complete AV block.[154] This discrepancy may be related to the high fetal and early neonatal mortality of these patients (88%).

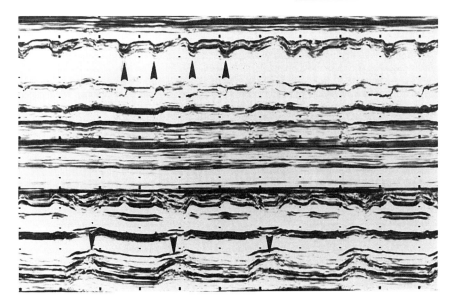

Figure 14. Dual MME of atria (**top**) and ventricles (**bottom**) in a fetus at 32 weeks of gestation. Note the discordance between atrial contractions (arrows, 143 bpm) and ventricular contractions (arrows, 67 bpm) consistent with complete AV block. Time lines = 500 milliseconds.

Seventy-four percent of these cases were associated with LA isomerism (polysplenia syndrome) and complex forms of AV septal defect, 12% were related to AV discordance, and 14% were related to other defects, including AV septal defects, tetralogy of Fallot, and pulmonic stenosis. The remaining 48 fetuses had normal cardiac anatomy; the majority of these were associated with maternal connective tissue disease, including lupus erythematosus, rheumatoid arthritis, Raynaud's syndrome, and Sjorgren's syndrome.

Considering all 105 cases, the survival rate in fetuses with complete AV block and structural heart disease was 7 of 57 fetuses (12%) compared with 40 of 48 fetuses (83%) with isolated complete AV block (Table 6). An important risk factor for death in these cases was the presence or absence of associated congestive heart failure in utero. In the combined statistics, hydrops fetalis developed in 36 of 57 fetuses (63%) with complete AV block and structural heart disease, with no survivals in the hydropic cases. Conversely, hydrops developed in only 8 of 48 fetuses (17%) with isolated complete AV block, with a 13% survival rate in the hydropic cases (Table 6). Additional factors contributing to a poor prognosis include the presence of low ventricular rates (equal to or less than 55 bpm) and low atrial rates (equal to or less than 120 bpm). The atrial rate is not an independent factor since it is asssociated with LA isomerism (polysplenia syndrome) and

_____ Table 6 _____

Outcome of Fetuses with Complete A-V Block*

	Total Group		Hydropic Group	
	No. Pts.	Survival %	No. Pts.	Survival %
Isolated CAVB	48	83	8	13
CAVB associated with structural heart disease	57	12	36	0
Total	105 Pts	45%	44 Pts	2%

* Combined Statistics of 5 Centers, CAVB = Complete Atrioventricular Block, Pts = patients (fetuses).

complex congenital heart disease. A contributing factor in the production of hydrops in fetuses is the presence of cardiomyopathy, secondary to maternal diabetes.[66]

Management

Fetuses with partial or complete AV block not associated with structural heart disease, and in the presence of maternal anti-Ro and anti-La antibodies, can be treated with steroids (dexamethasone or betamethasone). However, resolution of the hydrops without improvement in the AV block was reported.[157] Digoxin and furosemide were used with limited success.[158,159]

Maternal administration of β-adrenergic receptor agonists, such as terbutaline or ritodrine, may be associated with an increase in the fetal heart rate but was not shown to improve hydrops fetalis with or without the presence of structural heart disease.[105] Isolated cases of successful therapy with maternal salbutanol and direct fetal administration of isoproterenol were reported.[160,161] These drugs should be administered only after maternal heart disease is excluded and a baseline maternal ECG is obtained.

Terbutaline sulfate (Brethine) is a sympathomimetic drug that increases both the maternal and the fetal heart rate and produces maternal bronchodilatation. It has a half-life of approximately 3–4 hours or greater and can potentiate other sympathomimetic drugs. The possibility of adverse reactions, particularly during labor, should be kept in mind; reactions could include hypoglycemia, hypocalcemia, arrhythmias, myocardial ischemia, and elevations of liver enzymes. This drug can also produce neonatal hypoglycemia. The recommended dosage is 0.25 mg subcutaneously. This can be repeated in 30 minutes but should be discontinued if no response is obtained. Orally, the recommended dosage is 2.5–5.0 mg three times daily during waking hours.

Ritodrine hydrochloride (Yutopar) is a β-adrenergic agonist that may increase the fetal heart rate and inhibit the contractility of the uterine smooth muscle. This drug was used in the management of preterm labor. It is contraindicated before 20 weeks of pregnancy and has several other contraindications including maternal diabetes and hyperthyroidism. Care should be taken in using this drug intravenously. The suggested oral dosage is 10–20 mg every 4–6 hours; the dosage depends on the effect on the fetal heart rate as well as the appearance of any unwanted side effects. The recommendation for maternal intravenous administration of salbutamol is reported as 4–64 μg per minute.[160]

At present, different methodologies for experimental fetal pacing were described.[162,163] Carpenter and associates[164] paced a fetus with complete AV block and hydrops by direct ventricular puncture. Although pacing was achieved, the fetus subsequently died. Fetuses with complete AV block and without structural heart disease should be followed prospectively for the possibility of congestive heart failure, although this is an infrequent complication. If the fetus is mature and has complete AV block associated with hydrops, delivery is indicated. Steady improvement in morbidity and mortality rates in preterm infants suggests that delivery may be a consideration in selective cases prior to 36 weeks of gestation.

In cases of complete AV block, monitoring with Doppler shows bradycardia. However, since this technique represents only ventricular rates, it will not change with asphyxia and, therefore, is unreliable as an indicator of fetal well-being.[55]

At birth, infants with complete AV block, structural heart disease, and hydrops should be treated aggressively. Treatment should include drainage of ascites and pleural effusions, oxygen administration, ventilatory support, and correction of acidosis. Bedside external pacing can be done transiently (skin burns were noted with external pacing for as short as 30 minutes) and may be replaced by temporary epicardial wires or permanent pacemaker implantation. In the premature infant, a staged approach to pacing using temporary epicardial wires until the infant has grown enough to accommodate a permanent generator was described.[165] Postnatally, infants with complete AV block without heart disease, evidence of heart failure or ventricular arrhythmia, and with average ventricular rates greater than 55 bpm can be treated conservatively without immediate implantation of a pacemaker. Studies of the natural study of complete heart block demonstrated a progressive decrease in survival in childhood[154] and adulthood.[166] Hence, these studies show the importance of prospective reevaluations to determine the ultimate need of pacing.

Conclusion

Progress in the application of ultrasound has revolutionized the process of diagnosis in many fields of medicine. Ultrasound permits a reliable, noninvasive, and safe methodology for the diagnosis of fetal cardiac arrhythmias never before possible. Further, through the use of ultrasound, we are able to distinguish benign from potentially lethal arrhythmias, and, at the same time, we are provided with a methodology for optimal surveillance.

This chapter summarizes the present knowledge and experience in fetal cardiac arrhythmias including frequency, etiology, the relation with structural heart disease when present, echocardiographic characteristics, and clinical presentation. An effort was made to present combined statistics from several centers whenever possible as well as providing a consensus of the modalities of therapy presently available.

Much remains to be learned in this challenging and ever-expanding field. Carefully designed, multidisciplinary, collaborative studies from different centers of research will be necessary to improve our understanding of, for example, the pharmacokinetics of fetal drug treatment through the mother and to obtain additional information on the efficacy of antiarrhythmic drugs and alternative modes of therapy.

Acknowledgments: The author thanks the ultrasonographers and the clinical staff for their skillful assistance, as well as Ms. Aurora Couzo and Mrs. Cecilia Schmid for secretarial assistance in the preparation of this chapter. I also acknowledge the expert editorial assistance of Ms. Debra Bowling.

References

1. Cremer MV. Ueber die direkte ableitung der akionsstrome des menschlichen herzens vom oesophagus und uber das electrokardiogramm des fotus. *Muench Med Wochensch* 1906;53:811–813.
2. Ibarra-Polo AA, Guiloff E, Gomez-Rogers C. Fetal heart rate throughout pregnancy. *Am J Obstet Gynecol* 1972;113:814–818.
3. Larks SD. The fetal electrocardiogram in multiple pregnancy. *Am J Obstet Gynecol* 1959;77:1109–1115.
4. Larks SD, Faust R, Longo L, et al. Experiences in the diagnosis of fetal life with fetal electrocardiogram. *Am J Obstet Gynecol* 1960;80:1143–1150.
5. Smyth CN. Experimental electrocardiography of the foetus. *Lancet* 1953; 1:1124–1126.
6. Plant RK, Stevens RA. Complete AV block in the fetus. *Am Heart J* 1945;30:615.
7. Stadler HE. Prenatal auricular flutter. *J Pediatr* 1948;33:624.
8. Sancetta SM, Reading TH, Hanbvich WS. Supraventricular tachycardia in the fetus: report of a case. *N Engl J Med* 1952;247:943.
9. Freistadt H. Fetal bigeminal rhythm. Report of a case. *Am J Obstet Gynecol* 1962;84:13.
10. Bell GH. The human foetal electrocadiogram. *Br J Obstet Gynaecol* 1938;45:802–809.

11. Hon EH, Hess OW. The clinical value of fetal electrocardiography. *Am J Obstet Gynecol* 1960;79:1012–1023.
12. Figueroa-Longo JG, Poseiro JJ, Alvarez LO, et al. Fetal electrocardiogram at term labor obtained with subcutaneous fetal electrodes. *Am J Obstet Gynecol* 1966;96:556–564.
13. Komaromy B, Gaal J, Lampe I. Fetal arrhythmia during pregnancy and labour. *Br J Obstet Gynaecol* 1977;84:492–496.
14. Robinson HP, Shaw-Dunn J. Fetal heart rates as determined by sonar in early pregnancy. *J Obstet Gynaecol Br Commonw* 1973;80:805–809.
15. Kleinman CS, Hobbins JC, Jaffe CC, et al. Echocardiographic studies of the human fetus: prenatal diagnosis of congenital heart disease and cardiac dysrhythmias. *Pediatrics* 1980;65:1059–1066.
16. Kleinman CS, Donnerstein RL, Jaffe CC, et al. Fetal echocardiography: a tool for the evaluation of in utero cardiac arrhythmias and monitoring of in utero therapy. Analysis of 71 patients. *Am J Cardiol* 1983;51:237–243.
17. Kleinman CS, Valdes-Cruz LM, Weinstein EM, et al. Two dimensional Doppler echocardiographic analysis of fetal cardiac arrhythmias. *Pediatr Res* 1984;18:124A.
18. Allan LD, Anderson RH, Sullivan ID, et al. Evaluation of fetal arrhythmias by echocardiography. *Br Heart J* 1983;50:240–245.
19. Wladimiroff JW, Struyk P, Stewart PA, et al. Fetal cardiovascular dynamics during cardiac dysrhythmia. Case report. *Br J Obstet Gynaecol* 1983;90:573.
20. Strasburger JF, Huhta JC, Carpenter RJ, et al. Doppler echocardiography in the diagnosis and management of persistent fetal arrhythmias. *J Am Coll Cardiol* 1986;7:1385–1391.
21. Sissman NJ. Developmental landmarks in cardiogenic morphogenesis: comparative chronology. *Am J Cardiol* 1970;25:141–148.
22. Shenker L, Astle C, Reed KL, et al. Embryonic heart rates before the seventh week of pregnancy. *J Reprod Med* 1986;31:333–335.
23. Anderson RH, Becker AE, Arnold CG, et al. The development of the cardiac specialized tissue. In: Wellens HJJ, Lie KI, Janse MJ, eds. *The Conduction System of the Heart*. Philadelphia: Lea & Febiger; 1976:3–28.
24. James TN. Cardiac conduction system: fetal and postnatal development. *Am J Cardiol* 1970;25:213–216.
25. James TN. Sudden death in babies: new observations in the heart. *Am J Cardiol* 1968;22:479–506.
26. Long WA, Henry GW. Autonomic and central neuroregulation of fetal cardiovascular function. In: Polin RA, Fox WW, eds. *Fetal and Neonatal Physiology*. Philadelphia: WB Saunders Co; 1992:629–645.
27. Wolfson RN, Sorokin Y, Rosen MG. Autonomic control of fetal cardiac activity. In: Elkayam U, Gleicher N, eds. *Cardiac Problems in Pregnancy*. New York: Alan R Liss; 1982:365–379.
28. Papp JG. Autonomic responses and neurohumoral control in the human early antenatal heart. *Basic Res Cardiol* 1988;83:2–9.
29. Papp JG. Age-related changes in cardiac responsiveness to positive ionotropic agents. In: Patron W et al, eds. *Symposium on Cardiac Ionotropic Agents. IUPHAR 9th International Congress of Pharmacology*. London: Macmillan; 1984:21–27.
30. Friedman WF, Poole PE, Jacobwitz D, et al. Sympathetic innervation of the developing rabbit heart: biochemical and histochemical comparisons of fetal, neonatal, and adult myocardium. *Circ Res* 1968;23:25.
31. Lipton EL, Steinschneider A, Richmond JB. Autonomic function in the neonate. VIII. Cardio-pulmonary observations. *Pediatrics* 1964;33:212.

32. Phyllips SJ, Agate FJ Jr, Silverman WA, et al. Autonomic cardiac reactivity in premature infants. *Biol Neonate* 1964;6:225.
33. Chan FY, Woo SK, Ghosh A, et al. Prenatal diagnosis of congenital fetal arrhythmias by simultaneous pulsed Doppler velocimetry of the fetal abdominal aorta and inferior vena cava. *Obstet Gynecol* 1990;76:200–204.
34. Reed KL, Appleton CP, Anderson CF, et al. Doppler studies of vena cava flows in human fetuses. Insights into normal and abnormal cardiac physiology. *Circulation* 1990;81:498–505.
35. De Vore GR, Horenstein J. Simultaneous Doppler recording of the pulmonary artery and vein: a new technique for the evaluation of a fetal arrhythmia. *J Ultrasound Med* 1993;12:669–671.
36. Indik JM, Chen J, Reed KL. Association of umbilical venous with inferior vena cava blood flow velocities. *Obstet Gynecol* 1991;77:551–557.
37. De Vore GR, Siassi B, Platt LD. Fetal echocardiography. III. The diagnosis of cardiac arrhythmias using real-time-directed M-mode ultrasound. *Am J Obstet Gynecol* 1983;146:792.
38. Allan LD. *Color Atlas of Fetal Cardiology*. St. Louis: Mosby; 1994.
39. Silverman NH. *Pediatric Echocardiography*. Baltimore: Williams & Wilkins; 1993:534–552.
40. Shenker L. Fetal cardiac arrhythmias. *Obstet Gynecol Surv* 1979;34:561–572.
41. Elkayham U, Gleicher N. *Cardiac Problems in Pregnancy. Diagnosis and Management of Maternal and Fetal Disease*. New York: Alan R Liss; 1982:535–564.
42. McCurdy CM, Reed KL. Fetal Arrhythmias. In: Copel JA, Reed KL, eds. *Doppler Ultrasound in Obstetrics and Gynecology*. New York: Raven Press; 1995:253–270.
43. Copel JA, Kleinman CS. The impact of fetal echocardiography on perinatal outcome. *Ultrasound Med Biol* 1986;12:327–335.
44. Fyfe DA, Meyer KB, Case CL. Sonographic assessment of fetal cardiac arrhythmias. *Semin Ultrasound CT MR* 1993;14:286–297.
45. Ferrer PL, Quetel T, Bezjian A, et al. Outcome of fetal and perinatal cardiac arrhythmias, an eight year experience. *J Ultrasound Med* 1991;10(suppl):13S.
46. Ferrer PL, Gelband H. Perinatal experience with potentially lethal cardiac dysrhythmias. *Pediatr Res* 1992;31:234A.
47. Urbach JR, Phyvicht B, Zweizig HZ, et al. Instantaneous heart rate patterns in newborn infants. *Am J Obstet Gynecol* 1965;93:965.
48. Urbach JR, Zweizig HZ, Loveland MW, et al. Monitoring of fetal and neonatal arrhythmias. In: Dreifus LS, Likoff W, Moyer JH, eds. *Mechanisms and Therapy of Cardiac Arrhythmias*. New York: Grune & Stratton; 1966:642.
49. Hammacher K, Huter KA, Bokelmann J, et al. Foetal heart rate frequency and perinatal conditions of foetus and newborn. *Gynaecologia* 1968;166:349–360.
50. Valimaki I. Tape recordings of the electrocardiogram in newborn infants. *Acta Paediatr Scand* 1969;199(suppl):7.
51. Church SC, Morgan BC, Oliver TK, et al. Cardiac arrhythmias in premature infants: an indication of autonomic immaturity? *J Pediatr* 1967;71:542.
52. De Vore GR, Horenstein J. Evolution of ventricular function in the term and post-term fetus: the use of real-time, M-mode, color and pulsed Doppler echocardiography. In: Orduini D, Rizzo G, Romanini C, eds. *Fetal Cardiac Function*. New York: The Parthenon Publishing Group; 1995:51–71.
53. Cordero L Jr, Hon EH. Neonatal bradycardia following nasopharyngeal stimulation. *J Pediatr* 1971;78:441.
54. Young BK, Katz M, Klein SA, et al. Fetal blood and tissue pH with moderate bradycardia. *Am J Obstet Gynecol* 1979;135:45–52.
55. Allan LD. Fetal arrhythmias. In: Long WA, ed. *Fetal and Neonatal Cardiology*. Philadelphia: WB Saunders Co; 1990:180–184.

56. Gilstrap LC III, Hauth JC, Hankins GDV, et al. Second stage fetal heart rate abnormalities and type of neonatal acidemia. *Obstet Gynecol* 1987;70: 191–195.
57. Green DW, Ackerman NB, Lund G, et al. Prolonged QT syndrome presenting as fetal bradycardia. *J Matern Fetal Med* 1992;1:202–205.
58. Cameron A, Nicholson S, Nimrod C, et al. Evaluation of fetal cardiac dysrhythmias with two-dimensional, M-mode, and pulsed Doppler ultrasonography. *Am J Obstet Gynecol* 1988;158:286–290.
59. Ferrer PL, Quetel TA, Mas M, et al. Diagnosis and outcome of fetal myocardial diseases. *J Am Coll Cardiol* 1996;27:158A.
60. Tunessen WN Jr, Hertz CG. Toxic effects of lithium in newborn infants: a commentary. *J Pediatr* 1972;81:804.
61. Budnick IS, Leikin S, Hoeck LE. Effects in the newborn infant of reserpine administered antepartum. *Am J Dis Child* 1955;90:286.
62. Carswell F, Kerr MM, Hutchison JH. Congenital goitre and hypothyroidism produced by maternal ingestion of iodides. *Lancet* 1970;1:1241.
63. Minagawa Y, Akaiwa A, Hidaka T, et al. Severe fetal supraventricular bradyarrhythmia without fetal hypoxia. *Obstet Gynecol* 1987;70:454–456.
64. Momma K, Linde LM. Abnormal P wave axis in congenital heart disease associated with asplenia and polysplenia. *J Electrocardiol* 1969;2:395–402.
65. Freedom RM, Ellison RC. Coronary sinus rhythm in the polysplenia syndrome. *Chest* 1973;63:952–958.
66. Ferrer PL, Quetel TA, Salman F. Prenatal experience in patients with cardiosplenic syndrome. *J Ultrasound Med* 1994;13(suppl):22S.
67. Levy DL. Persistent fetal tachycardia in utero prior to labor in an infant with congenital cytomegalic inclusion disease: case report. *Am J Obstet Gynecol* 1972;112:859–860.
68. Ferrer PL. Arrhythmias in the neonate. In: Roberts NK, Gelband H, eds. *Cardiac Arrhythmias in the Neonate, Infant and Child.* New York: Appleton-Century-Crofts; 1977:265–316.
69. Onat A, Dominic N, Onat T. Sick sinus syndrome in an infant: severe disturbance of impulse formation and conduction involving the SA node and the AV junctional tissue. *Eur J Cardiol* 1974;2:79–83.
70. Valimaki I. Heart-rate variation in full-term newborn infants. *Biol Neonate* 1971;18:129–139.
71. Ferrer PL, Gelband H, Garcia OL, et al. Occurrence of arrhythmias in the newborn period. *Clin Res* 1977;25:64A.
72. Arcilla RA, Lind J, Zetterqvist P, et al. Hemodynamic features of extrasystoles in newborn and older infants. *Am J Cardiol* 1966;18:191–199.
73. Tonge HM, Wladimiroff JW, Noordam MJ, et al. Fetal cardiac arrhythmias and their effect on volume blood flow in descending aorta of human fetus. *J Clin Ultrasound* 1986;14:607–612.
74. Reed KL, Sahn DJ, Marx GR, et al. Cardiac Doppler flows during fetal arrhythmias: physiologic consequences. *Obstet Gynecol* 1987;70:1–6.
75. Stewart PA, Wladimiroff JW. Fetal atrial arrhythmias associated with the redundancy/aneurysm of the foramen ovale. *J Clin Ultrasound* 1988;16: 643–650.
76. Toro L, Weintraub RE, Shiota T, et al. Relation between persistent atrial arrhythmias and redundant septum primun flap (atrial septal aneurysm) in fetuses. *Am J Cardiol* 1994;73:711–713.
77. Kholi V, Ferrer PL, Rodriguez M. Clinical experience with cardiac tumors diagnosed in utero. Proceedings of the XV InterAmerican Congress of Cardiology; 1995; Santiago, Chile. Reviewed in *Chile NA Cardiol* 1995;14:97.

78. Stevens D, Burman D, Midwinter A. Letter: Transplacental lithium poisoning. *Lancet* 1974;7:595.
79. Silver W, Joos HA, Lamazor E, et al. Prodromal arrhythmias preceding the onset of paroxysmal supraventricular tachycardia in the newborn. *Pediatrics* 1973;52:871.
80. Ferrer PL, Sung RJ, Garcia OL, et al. Repetitive supraventricular tachycardia in a newborn with concealed Wolff-Parkinson-White syndrome. *Clin Res* 1977;25:4A.
81. Bernstine RL, Winker JE, Callagan DA. Fetal bigeminy and tachycardia. *Am J Obstet Gynecol* 1968;101:856–857.
82. Klapholz H, Schifrin BS, Rivo E. Paroxysmal supraventricular tachycardia in the fetus. *Obstet Gynecol* 1974;43:718.
83. Ferrer PL, Wolff GS, Young ML. Clinical experience and management of fetal atrial flutter. *Cardiol Young* 1997;7:118.
84. Kleinman CS, Copel JA, Weinstein EM, et al. In utero diagnosis and treatment of fetal supraventricular tachycardia. *Semin Perinatol* 1985;9:113–129.
85. Ferrer PL, Gelband H. Are fetal supraventricular extrasystoles always benign? Proceedings of the Southwestern Pediatric Cardiology Society; 1992; Orlando, Fla. Reviewed in *Cardiol Young* 1994;4:20.
86. Simpson JM, William R, Yates M, et al. Irregular heart rate in the fetus—not always benign. *Cardiol Young* 1996;6:28–31.
87. Ehlers KH. Supraventricular and ventricular dysrhythmias in infants and children. *Cardiovasc Clin* 1972;4:59.
88. Naheed ZJ, Strasburger JF, Deal BJ, et al. Fetal tachycardia: mechanisms and predictors of hydrops fetalis. *J Am Coll Cardiol* 1996;27:1736–1740.
89. Van Engelen AD, Weitjens O, Brenner JI, et al. Management outcome and follow-up of fetal tachycardia. *J Am Coll Cardiol* 1994;24:1371–1375.
90. Silber DL, Durnin RE. Intrauterine atrial tachycardia associated with massive edema in a newborn. *Am J Dis Child* 1969;117:722.
91. Van Der Horst RL. Congenital atrial flutter and cardiac failure presenting as hydrops foetalis at birth. *S Afr Med J* 1970;44:1037.
92. Bratteby L. Intrauterine death due to supraventricular tachycardia. *Acta Obstet Gynecol Scand* 1973;52:381.
93. Kleinman CS, Donnerstein RL, De Vore GR, et al. Fetal echocardiography for evaluation "in utero" congestive heart failure: a technique to study nonimmune fetal hydrops. *N Engl J Med* 1982;306:568.
94. Ferrer PL, Quetel T, Bezjian A. Congestive heart failure in utero, etiology and prognostic implications. *J Ultrasound Med* 1992;11(suppl):22S.
95. Nadas AS, Daeschner CW, Roth A, et al. Paroxysmal tachycardia in infants and children. Study of 41 cases. *Pediatrics* 1952;9:167.
96. Lubbers WJ, Losekoot TG, Anderson RH, et al. Paroxysmal supraventricular tachycardia in infancy and childhood. *Eur J Cardiol* 1974;2:91.
97. Wilburne M, Mack EG. Paroxysmal tachycardia in the newborn with onset in utero. *JAMA* 1954;154:1337.
98. Hilrich NM, Evrad JR. Supraventricular tachycardia in the newborn with onset in utero. *Am J Obstet Gynecol* 1955;70:1139.
99. Kesson CW. Foetal paroxysmal auricular tachycardia. *Br Heart J* 1958;20:552.
100. Levkoff AH. Perinatal outcome of paroxysmal tachycardia of the newborn with onset in utero. *Am J Obstet Gynecol* 1969;104:73.
101. Tuxen P, Kaplan EL, Ueland K: Intrauterine paroxysmal atrial tachycardia. *Am J Obstet Gynecol* 1971;109:958.
102. Hedvall G. Congenital paroxysmal tachycardia—a report of three cases. *Acta Paediatr Scand* 1973;62:550.

103. Carretti NG, Galli PA, Pellegrino P. Fetal paroxysmal supraventricular tachycardia. Report of a case documented by transvaginal electrocardiogram during fetal distress in labor. *Acta Obstet Gynecol Scand* 1974;53:275.

104. Mehta AV, Castro A, Wolff GS. Supraventricular tachycardia. In: Roberts NK, Gelband H, eds. *Cardiac Arrhythmias in the Neonate, Infant, and Child.* Norwalk, Conn: Appleton-Century-Crofts; 1983:105–146.

105. Kleinman CS, Copel JA. Fetal cardiac arrhythmias: diagnosis and therapy. Proceedings of the 9th International Fetal Cardiology Symposium; 1996:326–341; Orlando, Fla.

106. Zales VR, Dunnigan A, Benson DW. Clinical and electrophysiologic features of fetal and neonatal paroxysmal atrial tachycardia resulting in congestive heart failure. *Am J Cardiol* 1988;62:225–228.

107. Herin P, Thoren C. Congenital arrhythmias with supraventricular tachycardia in the perinatal period. *Acta Obstet Gynecol Scand* 1973;52:381.

108. Rodriguez-Coronel A, Sueblingvong V, Hastreiter HR. Clinical forms of atrial flutter in infancy. *J Pediatr* 1968;73:69.

109. Blumenthal S, Jacobs JC, Steer CM, et al. Congenital atrial flutter: report of a case documented by intrauterine electrocardiogram. *Pediatrics* 1968;41:659.

110. Moller JH, Davachi F, Anderson RC. Atrial flutter in infancy. *J Pediatr* 1969;75:643.

111. Till J, Wren C. Atrial flutter in the fetus and young infant: an association with accessory conduction. *Br Heart J* 1992;67:80–83.

112. Johnson WH Jr, Dunnigan A, Fehr P, et al. Association of atrial flutter with orthodromic reciprocating tachycardia. *Am J Cardiol* 1987;59:374–375.

113. Bellhaussen B, Pauzner D, Bleidun L, et al. Intrauterine and postnatal atrial fibrillation in WPW syndrome. *Circulation* 1982;66:1124–1128.

114. Edeiken J, Rugel SJ. Auricular fibrillation in infancy with fluttering paroxysm. *J Pediatr* 1946;28:471.

115. Zaldivar N, Gelband H, Tamer D, et al. Atrial fibrillation in infancy. *J Pediatr* 1973;83:821.

116. Reygaerts J. Un nouveau probleme de cardiologie foetale: la fibrillation auriculaire in utero. *Gynecol Obstet* 1959;58:208.

117. Smyth CN. Notes on foetal paediatrics. *Bull Soc R Belge Gynecol Obstet* 1960;30:207.

118. Gembruch U, Krapp M, Baumann P. Changes of venous blood flow velocity wave forms in fetuses with supraventricular tachycardia. *Ultrasound Obstet Gynecol* 1995;5:394–399.

119. Valerius NH, Jacobsen RJ. Intrauterine supraventricular tachycardia. *Acta Obstet Gynecol Scand* 1978;57:407–410.

120. Maxwell DJ, Crawford DC, Allan LD, et al. Obstetric importance, diagnosis and management of fetal tachycardia. *BMJ* 1988;297:107–110.

121. Newburger JW, Keane JF. Intrauterine supraventricular tachycardia. *J Pediatr* 1979;95:780–786.

122. Ward RM. Drug therapy of the fetus. *J Clin Pharmacol* 1993;33:780–789.

123. Lingman G, Ohrlander S, Ohlin P. Intrauterine digoxin treatment of fetal paroxysmal tachycardia. *Br J Obstet Gynaecol* 1980;87:340.

124. Kerenyi TD, Gleicher N, Meller J, et al. Transplacental cardioversion of intrauterine supraventricular tachycardia with digitalis. *Lancet* 1980;11:393.

125. Kleinman CS, Copel JA, Weinstein EM, et al. Treatment of fetal supraventricular tachyarrhythmias. *J Clin Ultrasound* 1985;13:265–273.

126. Mimura S, Suzuki C, Yamazaki T. Transplacental passage of digoxin in a case of nonimmune hydrops fetalis. *Clin Cardiol* 1987;10:63–65.

127. Given BD, Phillippe M, Sander SP, et al. Procainamide cardioversion of fetal supraventricular tachyarrhythmia. *Am J Cardiol* 1984;53:1460.
128. Triedman JK, Walsh EP, Saul JP. Response of fetal tachycardia to transplacental procainamide therapy. *Cardiol Young* 1996;6:235–238.
129. Spinnato JA, Shaver DC, Flinn GS, et al. Fetal supraventricular tachycardia: in utero therapy with digoxin and quinidine. *Obstet Gynecol* 1984;64:730–735.
130. Killeen AA, Bowers LD. Fetal supraventricular tachycardia treated with high-dose quinidine: toxicity associated with marked elevation of the metabolite, 3(s)-3-hydroxy quinidine. *Obstet Gynecol* 1987;70:445–449.
131. Perry JC, Ayres NA, Carpenter RJ Jr. Fetal supraventricular tachycardia treated with flecainide acetate. *J Pediatr* 1991;118:303–305.
132. Allan LD, Chita SK, Sharland GK, et al. Flecainide in the treatment of fetal tachycardias. *Br Heart J* 1991;65:46–48.
133. Allan LD: Fetal tachycardia. Editorial comment. *Cardiol Young* 1996;6:197.
134. Gladstone GR, Hordof A, Gersony WM. Propranolol administration during pregnancy: effects on the fetus. *J Pediatr* 1975;86:962.
135. Teuscher A, Bossi E, Imhof P, et al. Effect of propranolol on fetal tachycardia in diabetic pregnancy. *Am J Cardiol* 1978;42:304.
136. Lusson JR, Beytout M, Jacquetin B, et al. Traitment d'une tackycardie supra-ventriculaire foetale: association digoxine-amiodarone. *Coeur Med Interne* 1985;15:315.
137. Arnoux P, Seyral P, Llurens M, et al. Amiodarone and digoxin for refractory fetal tachycardia. *Am J Cardiol* 1986;59:166–167.
138. Colin A, Chabaud JJ, Poinsot J, et al. Les tachycardies supraventriculaires foe-tales et leur traitement: a propos de 23 cas. *Arch Fr Pediatr* 1989;46:335–340.
139. Meden H, Neeb U: Transplazentare kardioversion bei fetaler supraventriku-larer tachykardie mit sotalol. *Z Geburtshilfe Perinatol* 1990;194:182–184.
140. Meijboom EJ, van Engelen AD, van de Beek EW, et al. Fetal arrhythmias. *Curr Opin Cardiol* 1994;9:97–102.
141. Bowman E, Paes BA, Way RC. Oral sotalol in neonatal supraventricular tachy-cardia. *Acta Paediatr Scand* 1988;77:171.
142. Maragnes P, Tipple M, Fournier A. Effectiveness of oral sotalol for treatment of pediatric arrhythmias. *Am J Cardiol* 1992;69:751–754.
143. Wolff F, Breuker KH, Schlenker KH, et al. Prenatal diagnosis and therapy of fetal heart rate anomalies: with a contribution on the placental transfer of verapamil. *J Perinat Med* 1980;8:203.
144. Martin CB, Nijhuis JG, Weijer AA. Correction of fetal supraventricular tachy-cardia by compression of the umbilical cord: report of a case. *Am J Obstet Gynecol* 1984;150:324–326.
145. Fernandez C, De Rosa GE, Guevara E, et al. Reversion by vagal reflex of a fetal paroxysmal atrial tachycardia detected by echocardiography. *Am J Obstet Gynecol* 1988;159:860–861.
146. Daffos F, Capella-Pavlovsky M, Forestier F. Fetal blood sampling during preg-nancy with needle guided by ultrasound. A study of 606 consecutive cases. *Am J Obstet Gynecol* 1985;153:655–659.
147. Weiner CP, Thompson MIB. Direct treatment of fetal supraventricular tachycardia after failed transplacental therapy. *Am J Obstet Gynecol* 1988;158:570–573.
148. Hallak M, Neerhof MG, Perry R, et al. Fetal supraventricular tachycardia and hydrops fetalis: combined intensive, direct and transplacental therapy. *Obstet Gynecol* 1991;78:523–525.
149. Hansmann M, Gembruch U, Bald R, et al. Fetal tachyarrhythmias: transpla-cental and direct treatment of the fetus: a report of 60 cases. *Ultrasound Obstet Gynecol* 1991;1:162–170.

150. Gembruch U, Manz M, Bald R. Repeated intravascular treatment with amiodarone in a fetus with refractory supraventricular tachycardia and hydrops. *Am Heart J* 1989;118:1335–1338.
151. Kohl T, Tercanli S, Kececioglu D, et al. Direct fetal administration of adenosine for the termination of incessant supraventricular tachycardia. *Obstet Gynecol* 1995;85:873–874.
152. Stevens DC, Schriener RL, Hurwitz PA, et al. Fetal and neonatal ventricular arrhythmia. *Pediatrics* 1979;63:771–777.
153. Kohli V, Mangru N, Pearse LA, et al. Radiofrequency ablation of ventricular tachycardia in an infant with cardiac tumors. *Am Heart J* 1996;132:198–200.
154. Michäelsson M, Engle MA. Congenital complete heart block: an international study of the natural history. *Cardiovasc Clin* 1972;4:85–101.
155. Machado MVL, Tynan MJ, Curry PVL. Fetal complete heart block. *Br Heart J* 1988;60:512–515.
156. Schmidt KG, Ulmer HE, Silverman NH. Perinatal outcome of fetal complete atrioventricular block: a multicenter experience. *J Am Coll Cardiol* 1991; 17:1360–1366.
157. Buyon JP, Winchester R. Congenital complete heart block. A human model of passively acquired autoimmune injury. *Arthritis Rheum* 1990;33:609–614.
158. Harris JP, Alexson CG, Manning JA, et al. Medical therapy for the hydropic fetus with congenital complete atrioventricular block. *Am J Perinatol* 1993; 10:217–219.
159. Anandakumar C, Biswas A, Chew SS, et al. Direct fetal therapy for hydrops secondary to congenital atrioventricular block. *Obstet Gynecol* 1996;87:835–837.
160. Groves AM, Allan LD, Rosenthal E. Therapeutical trial of sympathomimetics in three cases of complete heart block in the fetus. *Circulation* 1995;92:3394–3396.
161. Lopez LM, Cha SC, Leone C, et al. Use of sympathomimetic agents in fetal atrioventricular block. *Arg Bras Cardiol* 1994;63:297–298.
162. Assad RS, Jatene MB, Moreira LF, et al. Fetal heart block: a new experimental model to assess fetal pacing. *Pacing Clin Electrophysiol* 1994;17:1256–1263.
163. Kikushi Y, Shiraishi H, Igarashi H, et al. Cardiac pacing in fetal lambs: intrauterine transvenous cardiac pacing for fetal complete heart block. *Pacing Clin Electrophysiol* 1995;18:417–423.
164. Carpenter RJ Jr, Strasburger JF, Garson A Jr, et al. Fetal ventricular pacing for hydrops secondary to complete atrioventricular block. *J Am Coll Cardiol* 1986;8:1434–1436.
165. Weidling SN, Saul JP, Triedman JK, et al. Staged pacing therapy for congenital complete heart block in premature infants. *Am J Cardiol* 1994;74:412–413.
166. Michäelsson M, Jonzon A, Riesenfeld T. Isolated congenital complete atrioventricular block in adult life. A prospective study. *Circulation* 1995;92:442–449.

Chapter 3

Benign Arrhythmias: Neonate Throughout Childhood

John D. Kugler, MD

Introduction

The definition of benign, when discussing and classifying arrhythmias, can be approached in several ways. One can be from an approach that implies that nothing serious currently exists, no treatment is indicated, no follow-up is necessary, and the prognosis is so good that the condition will virtually never be associated with, or develop into, any future health problem. At the other end of the spectrum, a definition might include that nothing serious exists and no treatment is indicated currently; however, with variable degrees of certainty or uncertainty, serious future consequences may require extensive further evaluation and/or treatment; that is, the condition may be benign now, but the potential exists for variable degrees of change to a nonbenign situation, and some form of follow-up therefore is required. In this chapter, the emphasis will be closer to the former definition because many of the conditions that may relate to the latter definition are discussed in the respective chapters pertaining to the specific arrhythmia. Because of the spectrum inherent in this approach to the definition, overlap exists and it will be described when relevant. As with virtually all arrhythmias in infants, children, and adolescents, age-related considerations will be emphasized. An "Indications for Treatment" section for each arrhythmia will not be included in this chapter by virtue of the definition of benign.

Sinus Arrhythmia

Incidence

According to several reported studies of 24-hour ambulatory electro-cardiogram (ECG) monitoring in various age groups involving young sub-

From Deal B, Wolff G, Gelband H, (eds.). *Current Concepts in Diagnosis and Management of Arrhythmias in Infants and Children.* Armonk, NY: Futura Publishing Co., Inc.; © 1998.

jects, virtually all normal children and young adults have evidence of sinus arrhythmia.[1-7] In Brodsky and coworkers'[6] study of 50 healthy medical students, 50% had marked sinus arrhythmia (defined as spontaneous changes in adjacent cycle lengths of 100% or more).[6,8]

Electrocardiogram Criteria

Irregular rhythm with gradual variation in PP intervals.

Sinus P wave precedes each QRS.

Rates vary with phase of respiration: increase with inspiration, and decrease with expiration.

Clinical Correlation

Sinus arrhythmia, in earlier writings, was referred to as respiratory sinus arrhythmia to distinguish it from ventriculophasic sinus arrhythmia during atrioventricular (AV) block[9] (Figure 1). The periods of faster rates are noted toward the end of inspiration, whereas the periods of slower rates occur toward the end of expiration,[9] related to changes in vagal tone. If the P-wave axis changes, wandering atrial rhythm may be present (see spe-

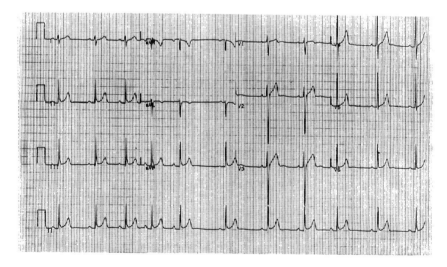

Figure 1. Twelve-lead ECG from an asymptomatic 13-year-old boy who was found to have an "irregular heart beat" when his nursing student older sister was listening to his chest. The ECG shows sinus arrhythmia manifested by sinus rhythm with gradual increase and decrease of the P-P intervals with the P-wave morphology unchanged from beat to beat. All four horizontal recordings are simultaneous with the bottom recording, all lead II, whereas the top three recordings are from the six limb leads and six chest leads.

PAUSE   HR = 89   5:34.7P1

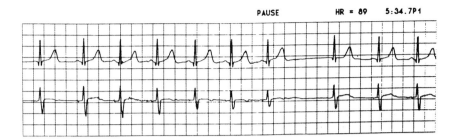

Figure 2. Rythm recording from a routine 24-hour ambulatory ECG monitor (**top**: lead II; **bottom**: lead V₁) in an 11-year-old who had previously undergone radio frequency catheter ablation. During sinus arrhythmia and 1.2-second pause, an asymptomatic junctional escape beat was recorded.

cific section below). Marked sinus arrhythmia was defined as changes of adjacent cycle lengths of 100% or more.[8] During increased vagotonia, sinus pauses of various degrees interrupted by escape beats and/or rhythms may be seen (Figure 2). The escape beats may be of sinus, atrial, junctional, or ventricular origin.[7–10]

Evaluation

Sinus arrhythmia alone is not associated with symptoms. Therefore, patients need no further evaluation when it is suspected on routine examination during auscultation or when it is noted on monitoring carried out for some other reason. At times, sinus arrhythmia may precipitate or be associated with other arrhythmias that require further evaluation. For example, paroxysmal supraventricular tachycardia can be precipitated by junctional escape beats during sinus arrhythmia. Sinus node (SN) dysfunction manifested by marked sinus or other bradycardia may be associated with marked sinus arrhythmia. Evaluation is then directed toward the specific problem rather than directly on the sinus arrhythmia.

Wandering Atrial Rhythm and Atrial Ectopic Rhythms

Incidence

The incidence of these rhythms was determined in several 24-hour ambulatory ECG studies of healthy children and adolescents as well as in Brodsky and associates' study of 50 medical students. Wandering atrial pacemaker rhythm was found in 25% of healthy newborn infants[1]; 34% of healthy 10- to 13-year-old boys[3]; 26% of 14- to 16-year-old boys[4]; and 54%

of medical students.[6] Atrial ectopic rhythm was not mentioned specifically in any of the studies in children, but the reporting of this rhythm may have been related to the definition, and therefore ectopic atrial rhythm conceivably was grouped with those who had more than one P-wave morphology change. Brodsky et al reported that 1 medical student (2%) had one asymptomatic episode of 12 consecutive beats of atrial ectopic rhythm.[6]

Electrocardiogram Criteria

1. Usually irregular rhythm with ongoing changes in P-wave morphology.
2. Associated changes in PP interval during more than two beats.
3. Usually noted during periods of low heart rates.

Clinical Correlation

Wandering atrial rhythm, commonly called wandering atrial pacemaker (Figure 3) is distinguished from the nonbenign chaotic atrial tachycardias by its occurrence during periods of lower heart rates.[11] In the study by Scott and colleagues,[3] the times of day were analyzed. The rhythm was found most often during sleep only (15% of all subjects) and less during other times (5% awake only; 13% both sleep and wake; 2% exercise).

Atrial ectopic rhythm is distinguished from wandering atrial pacemaker rhythm by its unchanging P-wave axis/morphology (Figures 4 and 5). The point at which atrial ectopic rhythm as a benign arrhythmia becomes a potentially nonbenign atrial ectopic tachycardia relates to the inherent characteristic rate of the rhythm corresponding also with the patient age. Although definitions were not established to distinguish these rhythms, there is virtually no disagreement when an atrial ectopic rhythm during sinus slowing and/or at the lower limits of heart rate for age are recorded (Figures 4 and 5). When somewhat faster rates of atrial ectopic rhythm are found, the duration of the rhythm also enters into factoring

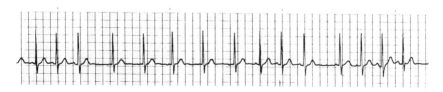

Figure 3. Recording of lead II rhythm in a 14-year-old girl with leukemia who was noted to have an irregular rhythm and "changing P waves" noted on an ECG monitor in the ICU. Wandering atrial rhythm is demonstrated by the variable P-wave morphologies and the irregular P-P intervals. The patient had no cardiovascular symptoms.

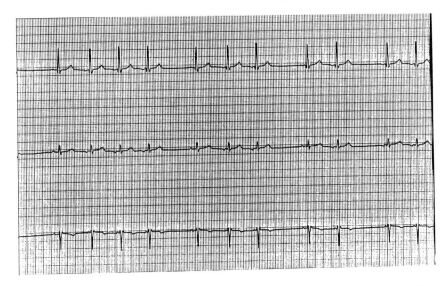

Figure 4. Simultaneous recording of leads I, II, and III in a 15-year-old girl who had undergone tricuspid valve replacement for Ebstein's anomaly at age 10 years. During a routine follow-up clinic visit, this asymptomatic girl had frequent slow ectopic atrial rhythm recorded during a preclinic ECG. After the first sinus beat, a short pause is interrupted by the first of three atrial beats with the same P-wave morphology but different from that of the sinus P wave. The second salvo of beats is similar in that only two beats of the atrial rhythm occur and the last two sets of beats alternate between the sinus and atrial origin.

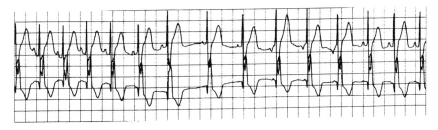

Figure 5. Rhythm recording in an asymptomatic 1-year-old boy who underwent routine 24-hour ambulatory ECG monitoring 9 months after undergoing tetralogy of Fallot repair. This rhythm (*top,* lead II; *bottom,* V₁) was recorded during a nap and shows sinus rhythm slowing, followed by three atrial escape beats, as depicted by the different P-wave morphology compared to that of the sinus beats before and after the atrial rhythm.

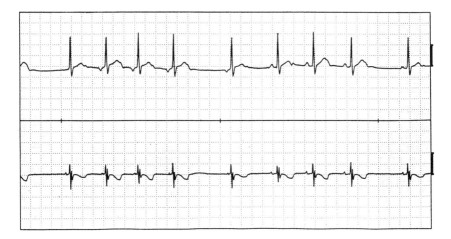

Figure 6. Rhythm recording (**top**: lead II; **bottom**: lead V_1) in a 4-year-old boy with intermittent atrial ectopic-focus tachycardia to demonstrate that it is sometimes difficult to distinguish between atrial escape beats and slow atrial ectopic tachycardia. The recording from a 24-hour ambulatory ECG monitor shows four beats of a different P-wave morphology with the P-P intervals of the first three beats shorter than those of any of the sinus P-P intervals. These beats are not escape beats and therefore represent a nonsustained short run of slow atrial ectopic tachycardia.

whether or not the arrhythmia is benign or more closely resembles atrial ectopic tachycardia (Figure 6). The upper limit of heart rates for age are not helpful in distinguishing some atrial ectopic tachycardias because many of these tachycardias are within the sinus tachycardia heart rate range for age.[12]

Evaluation

Wandering atrial rhythm is commonly detected on 12-lead ECG, rhythm strip recordings, or 24-hour ambulatory ECG monitoring carried out for various other indications. Further evaluation is not necessary unless the rate is faster than that expected for escape or vagotonic conditions, and therefore chaotic atrial tachycardia is a potential diagnosis.[11] Further testing with 24-hour ambulatory ECG monitoring and echocardiography to search for underlying atrial disease may then be helpful.

Atrial ectopic rhythm also does not need further investigation unless the rate suggests the possibility of tachycardia. When the rate suggests possible tachycardia rather than an escape rate, the potential is greater for the development of continuous or "incessant" tachycardia. Incessant tachycardia, even when the rates are well within sinus tachycardia rates for age, over months to years can lead to the development of ventricular enlargement and/or dysfunction.[13] Knowledge of patient activity is important when assessing whether the atrial ectopic rhythm may represent atrial ectopic tachycardia. For example, an atrial ectopic rhythm in a sleeping 6-month-old infant of 120 beats per minute (bpm) would suggest an ectopic atrial tachycardia, whereas a rate of 70 bpm would suggest an escape benign atrial ectopic rhythm. Another example in an older child: a heart rate of 120 bpm on resting ECG in a 12-year-old is higher than expected, and it might be predicted that this is an ectopic atrial tachycardia with the potential that the rhythm may also be faster than normal during activity. A 24-hour ambulatory ECG monitor recording is helpful in the evaluation because correlation of heart rate and activity can then be made. When the differential is in doubt and follow-up is recommended, an echocardiogram is indicated to obtain baseline measurement of ventricular size and function.

Premature Atrial Contractions

Incidence

Reported 24-hour ambulatory ECG surveillance studies in various pediatric age groups of normal subjects, as well as in the medical student series, showed that the incidence of premature atrial contractions (PACs) varies: 51% for newborns[5]; 14% to 64% for infants[1,5]; 62% for children 4–6 years old[5]; 21% for 7–11 years[3]; 59% for 9–12 years[5]; 13% for 10–13 years[2]; 77% for 13–15 years[4,5]; and 56% for medical students.[6]

Electrocardiogram Criteria

Premature P waves differing in axis and morphology from normal sinus P waves.

PR interval may be prolonged.

AV conduction may be normal, aberrant (bundle branch block), or blocked.

Clinical Correlation

The detection of the premature P wave can be difficult because it is often hidden within the T wave of the preceding ventricular conducted beat. Therefore, careful comparison of T waves in multiple ECG leads is required to detect subtle differences that uncover the buried P wave. Failure to do so often leads to the common misdiagnosis of "premature junctional beat."

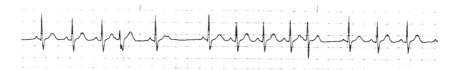

Figure 7. Recording of lead II rhythm in an asymptomatic 7-year-old girl who had an irregular rhythm detected on routine physical examination by her pediatrician. Frequent premature atrial contractions (PACs) were found. Variable conduction is illustrated in the recording. The first PAC (fourth beat in the recording) was aberrantly conducted, while the next beat shows a nonconducted, or blocked, PAC (P wave within the T wave but without a following QRS). The fourth-from-the-last beat shows a normally conducted PAC.

Conduction of the PAC to the ventricle is variable, ranging from a normally-conducted beat (normal QRS complex) when the PAC falls late after the specialized conduction system refractory periods, to a nonconducted PAC (sometimes referred to as "blocked") when the PAC arises so early that it falls within the refractory period of the AV node (AVN) and/or the His-Purkinje system, and therefore conduction to the ventricle is blocked (Figure 7). If nonconducted PACs arise in a bigeminal pattern, it is easy to mistake this rhythm for sinus bradycardia. When a PAC falls within the relative refractory period of the bundle branch-Purkinje system, still late enough so that depolarization of the ventricular myocardium occurs, the QRS is aberrant (Figure 7). Aberrantly conducted PACs are most common when the preceding RR interval is long because the length of this interval is directly proportional to the bundle branch refractory period; that is, the longer the RR, the longer the bundle branches take to recover.

Aberrant PACs commonly are mistaken for premature ventricular complexes (PVCs). Keys to avoiding this mistake are to carefully examine T waves for buried P waves and to remember that PACs and PVCs do not commonly occur in the same patient at the same time; therefore, when normally conducted or nonconducted P waves are noted along with aberrantly conducted beats, the latter are more likely to be PACs than PVCs. Another cause of aberrantly conducted PACs is in association with an otherwise inapparent ("concealed") Wolff-Parkinson-White (WPW) type of preexcitation. A PAC arising near the atrial insertion may conduct over the accessory pathway, thereby exposing its presence.[14] This type of aberrant PAC is distinguished by its shorter PR interval contrasted with the prolongation associated with the usual type of aberrantly conducted PAC.

Evaluation

Most patients with PACs are asymptomatic, and the PACs are detected during routine monitoring in the hospital, during outpatient evaluation for some other unrelated symptom or problem that requires standard or ambulatory ECG testing, or during a routine examination when an irregular rhythm is detected on auscultation (followed by ECG recording documenting the PAC). Occasionally, patients will present with a complaint of palpitations or some description thereof (eg, chest pain representing palpitations). If the symptoms are relatively infrequent, correlation of symptoms with rhythm is best accomplished by use of an event recorder.

Patients with underlying diseases or conditions may present with PACs, and/or the PACs may indicate atrial involvement. Examples include myocarditis and tumors associated with: tuberous sclerosis; stimulant drugs such as sympathomimetics, digitalis, caffeine, cocaine (including the fetus/newborn from maternal use); tricyclic antidepressants (imipramine/desipramine); mechanical devices (central intravenous/intracardiac catheters); hypokalemia, hypercalcemia, hypoxia, and hypoglycemia.[15–17] Atrial myocardial trauma from incisions for open heart surgery or from central line catheters also commonly cause PACs.[15] Evaluation of the patient with PACs is therefore directed toward detection of possible underlying disease or condition. For example, echocardiography is indicated for patients who may have presenting signs or risk factors for myocarditis. Echocardiography also may detect atrial rhabdomyomas in patients with tuberous sclerosis.

Unless the PACs are associated with some other related condition that requires evaluation and/or treatment, testing and therapy are not needed solely for the PACs. Patients with palpitations due to PACs are virtually always successfully managed with reassurance and without specific treatment other than avoidance of stimulants or conditions that correlate with provoking individual symptoms.

Junctional Rhythm

Incidence

Because junctional beats or rhythm are found during times of sinus arrhythmia, especially marked sinus arrhythmia, they are found commonly in the pediatric population (see Sinus Arrhythmia). Junctional rhythm appears more often in age groups of children who have more vagotonia; for example, it was found in 13% of 131 10- to 13-year-old boys during sleep in the study of Scott et al.[3] In 104 7- to 11-year-old children, Southall and associates[2] found junctional rhythm in 45% and the longest duration was 25 minutes during sleep. In infants, junctional beats or rhythm are also relatively common, as noted in 19% of the study population reported by Southall and colleagues.[1] They were notable during sinus bradycardia and following sinus pauses. Endurance athletes have a 20% incidence of junctional rhythm.[7] Scott and associates[3] reported that single junctional escape beats were noted after single-cycle episodes of sinoatrial block that occurred in 8% of normal 10- to 13-year-old boys.

Electrocardiogram Criteria

Usually a regular rhythm with narrow QRS (or QRS resembling patient's normal QRS).

Rates typically 40–100 bpm (vary with age).

P waves may be dissociated or follow each QRS (retrograde conduction).

Clinical Correlation

For this rhythm, the standard definition of the junction will be used: either the AVN or the His bundle. Therefore, the origin of junctional rhythm is assumed to be from either of these two areas. During junctional rhythm, the QRS complexes are identical to those from the individual's sinus or atrial conducted beats. Therefore, although the QRS complexes of most patients are normal, if right bundle branch block is present during sinus rhythm, the same right bundle branch would be expected during junctional rhythm. If any change in the QRS occurs, the rhythm would originate distal to the junction and would not be classified as junctional unless the QRS change could be attributed to tachycardia-related aberrancy. In this case, the junctional rhythm would not be classified as simple, completely benign junctional rhythm. The point at which the rate of the junctional rhythm becomes suspicious for a tachycardia is age related, and the same criteria apply as described above for atrial ectopic rhythm and atrial ectopic tachycardia.

Evaluation

Junctional rhythm is usually detected coincidentally during times of vagotonia while patients undergo routine monitoring in the hospital or on 24-hour ambulatory ECG testing carried out for other reasons (Figures 8 and 9). As was discussed above for other benign supraventricular rhythms, the common normal benign junctional rhythms are those resulting as escape rhythms from slowing of higher pacemakers during these vagotonic conditions.[10,18] The rate, relative to age and activity, is an important factor when deciding whether the junctional rhythm is normal and benign or if the rate is faster than expected for an escape rhythm (and therefore junctional tachycardia should be considered).[19] When it is unequivocal that the junctional rhythm is an escape rhythm appropriate for age, no further evaluation is needed. This includes when very low rates for age are found during sleep in an asymptomatic patient with an otherwise normal heart; that is, even when rates are in the 20- to 30-bpm range during sleep. However,

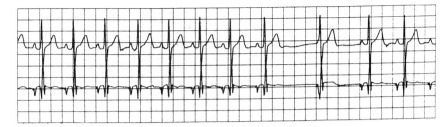

Figure 8. Recording in an asymptomatic 8-year-old boy who had undergone tetralogy of Fallot repair at 1 year of age. During a routine 24-hour ambulatory ECG, this rhythm (**top**: lead II; **bottom**: lead V₁) was recorded showing a single junctional escape beat following a sinus pause during sinus arrhythmia. The junctional beat falls on an unrelated P wave.

when the rate is slow, further evaluation is based on the presence of other associated heart disease and/or symptoms. In the case of slow heart rates, the evaluation is directed toward SN function (see Chapter 4). When the rate is equivocally or definitely too fast for an escape rhythm, further evaluation is indicated. This would include 24-hour ECG ambulatory monitoring and echocardiogram to evaluate possible tachycardia-induced ventricular dilation and/or dysfunction.

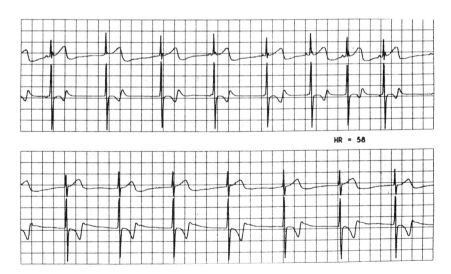

Figure 9. Rhythm recording during sleep in an asymptomatic 3-year-old boy who underwent surgical repair of total anomalous pulmonary venous connection to a left superior vena cava at 3 months of age. This rhythm (**top**: lead II; **bottom**: lead V₁) was recorded by routine 24-hour ambulatory ECG monitor and shows junctional escape rhythm at approximately 60 bpm with intermittent sinus beats at approximately 90 bpm.

Ventricular Rhythm

Incidence

Two types of ventricular rhythm will be discussed: ventricular escape beats or rhythm and accelerated ventricular rhythm. The incidence is unknown in childhood for each rhythm but it appears to be low. Neither of these rhythms was reported in all of the published 24-hour ambulatory ECG studies carried out in normal infants, children and adolescents.[1–5] However, accelerated ventricular rhythm was found in 3% to 7% of adolescent and adult athletes undergoing surveillance 24-hour ambulatory ECGs,[6,7] and some investigators attributed these ventricular rhythms to vagotonia.[20] The heart rate in athletes ranged predominantly between 40 and 100 bpm, but occasionally higher rates were found.[6,21–23] For example, 5 beats of 136 bpm ventricular rhythm were recorded during sleep in a medical student.[6] Premature ventricular beats were not uncommon in subjects in these studies and, although not specifically mentioned, it is possible that some of these single beats were not "premature" but rather escape beats during vagotonia. Therefore, if attention is taken to analyze degree of prematurity (or, saying it the opposite way, lateness), it is possible that escape beats may be more common than current data imply. Idioventricular rhythm in children is rare and is found in nonbenign conditions of AV block (see Chapter 4 for discussion of AV block).

Electrocardiogram Criteria-Ventricular Escape Beats

Wide QRS beats occurring in setting of sinus and junctional bradycardia.

Rates typically 20–60 bpm.

No preceding P wave.

Clinical Correlation

For benign ventricular escape beats or rhythm, the same criteria apply as for junctional escape rhythms, but, since the junction is also vagotonic, the ventricle may provide the escape beat or beats (Figure 10). The diagnostic dilemma, however, is to determine whether junctional disease is present to explain the absence of junctional escape.

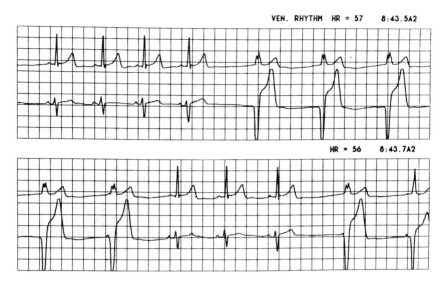

Figure 10. Continuous rhythm (**top**: lead II; **bottom**: lead V_1) recording during sleep in an asymptomatic 15-year-old boy with exercise-induced asthma who had an ECG (not shown) done before participating in a drug protocol study. The ECG had shown beats with "bundle branch block." Subsequent 24-hour ambulatory ECG monitor revealed several episodes similar to this recording, which shows 5 beats of a ventricular escape rhythm at 57 bpm following a sinus pause. After resumption of three beats of sinus rhythm, two additional ventricular escape beats follow another sinus pause (**bottom**). The evaluation, which included history and physical examination, standard 12-lead ECG, and echocardiogram, revealed no abnormalities. No treatment or follow-up was recommended.

Electrocardiogram Criteria-Accelerated Ventricular Rhythm

Three or more successive wide QRS beats at a rate close to baseline rhythm.

Initiation with an escape or fusion beat.

Mild acceleration or deceleration prior to termination with return to sinus rhythm.

AV dissociation usually present at onset; retrograde VA conduction may develop.

Clinical Correlation

For accelerated ventricular rhythm, conventional descriptions and definitions focused on the rate of the ventricular rhythm as it compares to the rate of the sinus rhythm.[24-28] Van Hare and Stanger[27] found that the rate

Time: 06:11:34   Date: 24-APR-96

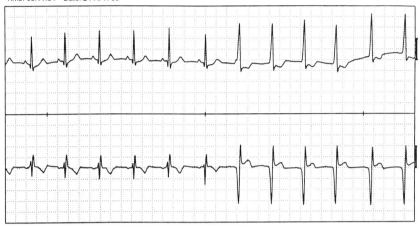

Figure 11. Rhythm recording during sleep in a 13-year-old girl with relapsed rhabdomyosarcoma (primary from oral pharynx) metastatic to the base of the cardiac interventricular septum. Echocardiogram showed a 1.5 cm by 2.5 cm echo-dense mass. A 24-hour ambulatory ECG monitor recording was carried out following the recording of asymptomatic wide-QRS rhythm during routine inpatient monitoring. The recording (**top**: lead II; **bottom**: lead V_1) shows several beats of sinus rhythm at approximately 88–90 bpm followed by an accelerated ventricular rhythm at 93–95 bpm.

of the ventricular rhythm was <12% of the sinus rhythm and all rates were less than 200 bpm for the 12 infants in their series. Zipes'[29] and Fisch's definition was slightly different in adult patients; they found that the accelerated ventricular rhythm was within 10 bpm faster than the sinus rate.[29]

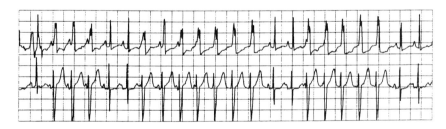

Figure 12. Rhythm recording in an asymptomatic neonate who was noted on routine examination to have an irregular rhythm. The recording (**top**: lead II; **bottom**: lead V_1) from a 24-hour ambulatory ECG monitor shows a few sinus beats at approximately 166–188 bpm with frequent runs of accelerated ventricular rhythm at similar, only slightly faster, rates compared to the concomitant sinus beats. Evaluation, including history and physical examination and echocardiogram, was normal. Treatment was not instituted, and the accelerated ventricular rhythm resolved spontaneously during follow-up at 3 months of age.

Time: 15:00:00   Date: 24-APR-96

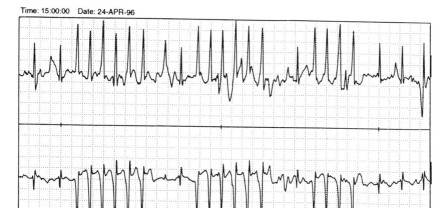

Figure 13. Rhythm recording from the same patient described in Figure 11. This rhythm was recorded at a different time but from the same 24-hour ambulatory ECG monitor as characterized in Figure 11. In this recording, the sinus beats (first two and last three) are faster (125–135 bpm), suggesting increased adrenergic and/ or parasympathetic withdrawal state. The corresponding runs of asymptomatic ventricular rhythm are much faster at 230–250 bpm, and the diagnosis appears to be no longer accelerated ventricular rhythm but rather nonsustained VT. With successful repeat chemotherapy and without administration of any antiarrhythmic drugs, the interventricular septal tumor and the ventricular arrhythmia simultaneously gradually regressed during the next few weeks. The follow-up 24-hour ambulatory ECG monitor recording at 2 months showed no ventricular arrhythmia, and the echocardiogram showed a 50% smaller, less-dense mass.

Typically, the rate of the accelerated ventricular rhythm varies with patient activity as does the sinus rate (Figures 11 and 12). Also, age-related accelerated ventricular rhythm rates follow those of age-related sinus rhythm rates. A diagnostic dilemma occasionally arises when the ventricular rhythm rate is considerably faster than that of the sinus rate and therefore the diagnosis of ventricular tachycardia (VT) is possible (Figure 13). As illustrated in Figures 11 and 13, accelerated ventricular rhythm and nonsustained VT may coexist. In such cases the clinician is therefore left with a borderline situation. Other clinical findings such as symptoms and echocardiographic and exercise data are used to make the distinction between the diagnoses. Accelerated ventricular rhythm is not associated with any symptoms or abnormal cardiac tests; therefore, if any are found the diagnosis of VT is likely.

Evaluation

Because the chance is probably high for coexistence of junctional disease (see Chapter 4) when ventricular escape beats are detected incidentally during vagotonia, the evaluation of patients with ventricular escape beats is focused on excluding underlying AVN and/or His-Purkinje conduction system disease. This is carried out by 24-hour ambulatory ECG monitoring and by evaluating AV conduction during exercise. Although a "benign" diagnosis of junctional disease may be found, truly benign vagotonia-induced ventricular escape beats may be found alone (without underlying AVN and/or His-Purkinje system disease) and therefore no further evaluation or treatment is needed.

The detection/presentation of accelerated ventricular rhythm also is usually incidental during routine examination or during monitoring for some unrelated indication.[24–27,30–32] The focus of evaluation for the patient with accelerated ventricular rhythm is related to distinguishing the arrhythmia from VT. Careful history for dizziness/syncope associated with palpitations is essential as is the physical examination and echocardiogram for signs of underlying disease. Because the heart rates of accelerated ventricular rhythm are only slightly faster than those of sinus rates, symptoms of dizziness would be unlikely to be related even if they were reported during the accelerated ventricular rhythm. Use of a memory-loop event ECG recorder is useful to assist in documenting rhythm at the time of symptoms. Other important testing includes 24-hour ambulatory ECG to determine the rate of the ventricular rhythm relative to that of the preceding and following sinus rhythm. As is illustrated in Figures 11 and 14, intramyocardial tumors can be associated with accelerated ventricular rhythm. Other types of ventricular arrhythmias such as premature beats or tachycardia (Figure 13) can be found in patients with tumors.[33,34]

During follow-up, accelerated ventricular rhythm spontaneously disappears in many children, but the resolution may be age related.[23–26,30–32] Spontaneous disappearance appears especially true for infants as illustrated by the study of Van Hare and Stanger[27] since no infant had evidence of the arrhythmia at last follow-up (median 48 months) and the median age at last detected episode was 9 days (range 1–150). Van Hare and Stanger therefore recommended that antiarrhythmic drug therapy should not be started. Gaum[24] and colleagues, in the first report of this benign arrhythmia in children, reported on four children 6–14 years of age. Three of the four patients still had evidence of the arrhythmia on short-term (8 months to 2 years) follow-up, so the spontaneous disappearance rate may be different for older children compared to infants, but large series of pediatric patients of any age group were not reported, and therefore the spontaneous rate of resolution is unknown. Regardless of the persistence in some older children, treatment is not recommended for this benign arrhythmia.

However, when the accelerated ventricular rhythm is frequent and/or associated with frequent ventricular ectopy (see following section), echocardiographic assessment of left ventricular size and function are important. Some patients may develop arrhythmia-induced left ventricular dila-

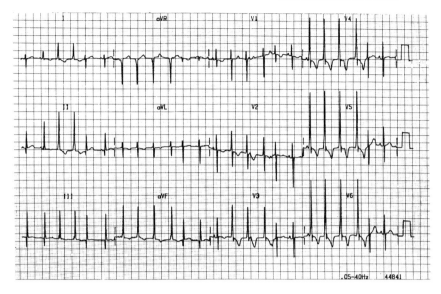

Figure 14. Standard 12-lead continuous ECG recording in a 1-day-old asymptomatic infant who had an irregular rhythm detected during routine examination. Accelerated ventricular rhythm is demonstrated: runs of venticular beats at 140–145 bpm are interspersed with beats of sinus rhythm at 135–150 bpm. Many fusion beats are produced because of the similar rates of the two rhythms. The echocardiogram showed a 4-mm, echo-dense nonobstructive mass in the anterior wall of the right ventricular outflow tract. The patient was not treated. The accelerated ventricular rhythm and the echo-dense mass consistent with a rhabdomyoma persisted until both were no longer detected at 2 years of age.

tion and/or dysfunction.[13,35,36] It is for this reason that patients with this otherwise benign arrhythmia should undergo periodic (1–2 years) follow-up to monitor for this possible adverse development.

Premature Ventricular Contractions

Incidence

Premature ventricular contractions/complexes (PVCs) were found during ambulatory ECG monitoring in healthy newborns, infants, children, adolescents, and medical students. Nagashima and coworkers,[5] in their study of 360 children from newborns to 15-year-old adolescents, found PVCs in each of 5 age groups: 18% of newborns; 6% of infants 1–11 months old; 8% of children 4–6 years of age; 14% of 9- to 12-year-olds; and 27% of 13- to 15-year-olds. Although statistics were not reported, they concluded that PVCs were more common in both newborns and in older adolescents. Southall and associates[1] reported only "extra-systoles," so it is unclear whether PVCs and PACs were distinguished or separated. In the study by Southall and colleagues[2] of 104 healthy, 7- to 11-year-old children, premature beat analysis was carried out by analyzing randomly selected 6-hour recordings. They found only one patient who had PVCs. Scott and coworkers,[3] in their study of 131 healthy 10- to 13-year-old boys, found that 26% had PVCs, but none had more than 4 beats per every 24 hours except for 2 boys who had 27 and 35 beats. Dickinson and Scott[4] found a 41% incidence of PVCs in 100 healthy 14- to 16-year-old boys; 75% had uniform beats and 25% had multiform beats. Brodsky[6] and colleagues found that 50% of medical students had PVCs and only one had more than 50 (86) for the 24-hour ECG recording. Palatani and associates[37] reported that 70% of well-conditioned, young athletes had PVCs and some had multiform beats, couplets and runs.

Electrocardiogram Criteria

Premature QRS complex without preceding conducted P wave.

QRS morphology differs from a sinus conducted beat.

QRS duration usually prolonged.

Clinical Correlation

Several ECG leads may be required to distinguish differences in the QRS compared to the sinus QRS. Unless the PVC occurs very late after the P wave of the next sinus beat, or in unusual situations such as second- or third-degree AV block, PVCs are unaccompanied by preceding P waves. The latest possible ventricular beat to fit the diagnostic criteria of a PVC is

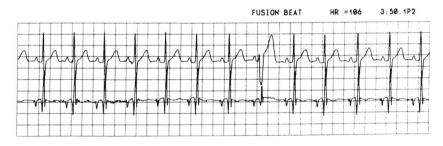

Figure 15. Continuous rhythm recording (**top**: lead II; **bottom**: lead V₁) by 24-hour ambulatory ECG monitor from an asymptomatic 9-year-old boy who had an irregular rhythm incidentally detected during monitoring while undergoing general anesthesia and surgery for a chronic ear problem. Note isolated PVC occurring at the time of sinus P wave.

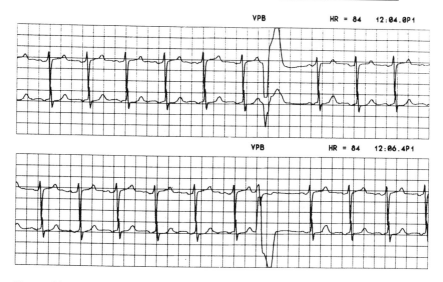

VPB   HR = 84   12:04.0P1

VPB   HR = 84   12:06.4P1

Figure 16. Rhythm recording in a 16-year-old boy who underwent aortic valve replacement for progressive aortic regurgitation from previous valvotomy for congenital aortic valve stenosis. This recording (**top**: lead II; **bottom**: lead V$_1$) was carried out 2 days postoperatively because PVCs were noted during routine monitoring. Multiform single PVCs were recorded as illustrated. The asymptomatic patient was not treated and the beats persist 6 months after surgery.

one that arises virtually coincident (ie, fusion beat) with the sinus-conducted QRS (Figure 15). When a late ventricular beat arises in the absence of a sinus beat because of a sinus pause, the beat would not be classified as premature but rather as an escape beat (see previous section).

Uniform PVCs are those that have the same morphology; multiform beats are of more than one morphology (Figure 16). No studies were reported comparing the specific morphologies of benign and nonbenign PVCs. Single uniform beats define simple ectopy as the standard of benign PVCs.[38] However, complex ectopy (such as bigeminy, couplets, or triplets, with or without multiform beats) also can be benign after evaluation is completed.[39–42]

Evaluation

Probably the most frequent mode of presentation for PVCs is incidental, during routine physical examination or during monitoring for unrelated reasons (eg, outpatient surgery such as myringotomy with tube insertion). Further investigation of history for symptoms, especially those of dizziness/syncope, is essential. Although symptoms of dizziness/syncope in older children and adolescents are most often due to a vasovagal mechanism, it is important to document the rhythm at the time of symptoms to exclude an arrhythmia by using a memory-loop event ECG recorder.

The type of arrhythmia is virtually impossible to determine by physical examination alone. Recording of the rhythm by standard ECG and/or by 24-hour ambulatory ECG is used to document whether the premature beats are of supraventricular or ventricular origin. Moreover, standard ECG recordings are used to determine the specific type of bundle branch block and QRS axis and to determine if other important problems exist such as a long QT interval and/or ventricular hypertrophy.

Benign PVCs are characteristically found in patients without underlying structural heart disease.[38–42] Although benign PVCs also are found in patients with underlying structural heart disease, it is imperative to search for the possibility of associated heart disease because, if present, further investigation, management, and follow-up are dependent on the specific underlying disease.

The investigation of underlying heart disease is best carried out by echocardiography. Echocardiographic examination is directed toward a search for congenital heart disease (including mitral valve prolapse), right ventricular size and function (especially for arrhythmogenic right ventricular dysplasia), left ventricular size and function, tumors, or coronary artery disease (eg, Kawasaki disease). Arrhythmia-induced left ventricular dilation and/or dysfunction from years of tens of thousands of PVCs per day is another reason for evaluating left ventricular size and function.[13,35,36] The issue of ectopy related to left ventricular false tendons is unsettled.[28,43] Although reports suggested an association, neither blinded nor prospective studies were reported.[44–46] The clinical significance of finding a false tendon with or without PVCs is unknown, but it is believed to be inconsequential.

The response of PVCs during exercise was used by many practitioners as a major marker for deciding on whether PVCs are benign.[47,48] Some investigators found exercise-induced VT as the only manifested abnormality in children with PVCs who then were found to have serious underlying heart disease (eg, arrhythmogenic right ventricular dysplasia, myocarditis, or cardiomyopathy).[48] No data were reported in children with underlying heart disease to show the converse (ie, suppression of PVCs with exercise means that the PVCs are benign). Nevertheless, when PVCs are suppressed with exercise, the implication is that the PVCs are benign; the theory that benign PVCs are suppressed with exercise is primarily held for subjects who do not have underlying structural heart disease. However, despite the correlation of an adverse prognosis of some patients with PVCs who demonstrated other evidence of underlying heart disease, the suppression of PVCs in these patients also is often taken as a favorable sign. Again, prospective studies were not reported to support this view.

The long-term follow-up is good for children with benign PVCs who have no underlying structural heart disease.[38–42] Moreover, among children without any evidence of structural heart disease who have infrequent, benign PVCs, the need for periodic evaluation was not established.[28,38–42] For example, it is possible that some children with tens of thousands of PVCs per 24 hours may develop an arrhythmia-induced left ventricular dilation and/or dysfunction, presumably if the very frequent ectopy continues over several years or decades.[13,35,36] Therefore, while asymptomatic children with frequent PVCs may have a completely benign situation when initially detected, it is unknown whether or not a problem may develop. Accordingly, it may be prudent to follow these children at 1- to 2-year intervals to assess left ventricular size and function if the PVCs continue at the same high frequency. During follow-up, there is no indication to restrict activities.

Acknowledgments: I am indebted to Gary Felix, BS, for his data analysis, Kris Houston, RN, BSN, for her assistance in data research, to Stacey Froemming, Sheila Urbach, and Mora Link for their patience and diligence in the recording of ECG rhythms in oftentimes restless children, and Louise Larsen for assistance in preparing the manuscript.

References

1. Southall DP, Richards J, Mitchell P, et al. Study of cardiac rhythm in healthy newborn infants. *Br Heart J* 1980;43:14–20.
2. Southall DP, Johnston F, Shinebourne EA, et al. 24-hour electrocardiographic study of heart rate and rhythm patterns in population of healthy children. *Br Heart J* 1981;45:281–291.
3. Scott O, Williams GJ, Fiddler GI. Results of 24 hour ambulatory monitoring electrocardiogram in 131 healthy boys aged 10 to 13 years. *Br Heart J* 1980; 44:304–308.
4. Dickinson DF, Scott O. Ambulatory electrocardiographic monitoring in 100 healthy teenage boys. *Br Heart J* 1984;51:179–183.
5. Nagashima M, Matsushima M, Ogawa A, et al. Cardiac arrhythmias in healthy children revealed by 24-hour ambulatory ECG monitoring. *Pediatr Cardiol* 1987;8:103–108.
6. Brodsky M, Wu D, Denes P, et al. Arrhythmias documented by 24 hour continuous electrocardiographic monitoring in 50 male medical students without apparent heart disease. *Am J Cardiol* 1977;39:390–395.
7. Viitasalo MT, Kala R, Eisalo A. Ambulatory electrocardiographic recording in endurance athletes. *Br Heart J* 1982;47:213–220.
8. Garson A Jr, Gillette PC, McNamara DG. *A Guide to Cardiac Dysrhythmias in Children.* New York: Grune & Stratton; 1980;117.
9. Schamroth L. Sinus arrhythmia. In: *The Disorders of Cardiac Rhythm.* Kent, England: Whitstable Litho Ltd; 1971;25–26.
10. Randall WC, Wehrmacher WH, Jones SB. Hierarchy of supraventricular pacemakers. *J Thorac Cardiovasc Surg* 1981;82;797–800.
11. Dodo H, Gow RM, Hamilton RM, et al. Chaotic atrial rhythm in children. *Am Heart J* 1995;129:990–995.
12. Naheed ZJ, Strasburger JF, Benson DW Jr, et al. Natural history and management strategies of automatic atrial tachycardia in children. *Am J Cardiol* 1995;75:405–407.
13. Kugler JD, Baisch SD, Cheatham JP, et al. Improvement of left ventricular dysfunction after control of persistent tachycardia. *J Pediatr* 1984;105:543–548.

14. Kugler JD. Evaluation of pediatric patients with preexcitation syndromes. In Benditt DG, Benson DW Jr, eds. *Cardiac Preexcitation Syndromes.* Boston: Martinus Nijhoff; 1986;361–411.

15. Garson A Jr. *The Electrocardiogram in Infants and Children: A Systematic Approach.* Philadelphia: Lea & Febiger; 1983;210–211.

16. Muhler EG, Turniski-Harder V, Engelhardt W, et al. Cardiac involvement in tuberous sclerosis. *Br Heart J* 1994;72:584–590.

17. Frassica JJ, Orav EJ, Walsh EP, et al. Arrhythmias in children prenatally exposed to cocaine. *Arch Pediatr Adolesc Med* 1994;148:1163–1169.

18. Urthaler F, Katholi CR, Macy J Jr, et al. Mathematical relationship between automaticity of the sinus node and the AV junction. *Am Heart J* 1973;86:189–195.

19. Kugler JD. Sinus node dysfunction. In: Gillette PC, Garson Jr A, eds. *Pediatric Arrhythmias: Electrophysiology and Pacing.* Philadelphia: WB Saunders Co; 1990;252.

20. Gallagher JJ, Damato AN, Lau SH. Electrophysiologic studies during accelerated idioventricular rhythms. *Circulation* 1971;44:671–677.

21. Chapman JH. Profound sinus bradycardia in the athletic heart syndrome. *J Sports Med Phys Fitness* 1982;22:45–48.

22. Hanne-Paparo N, Kellermann JJ. Long-term Holter ECG monitoring of athletes. *Med Sci Sports Exerc* 1981;13:294–298.

23. Zehender M, Meinertz T, Keul J, et al. ECG variants and cardiac arrhythmias in athletes: clinical relevance and prognostic importance. *Am Heart J* 1990; 119:1378–1391.

24. Gaum WE, Biancaniello T, Kaplan S. Accelerated ventricular rhythm in childhood. *Am J Cardiol* 1979;43:162–164.

25. Bisset GS III, Janos GG, Gaum WE. Accelerated ventricular rhythm in the newborn infant. *J Pediatr* 1984;104:247–249.

26. Scagliotti D, Kumar SP, Williamson GD. Ventricular rhythm with intermediate rate in the neonate without heart disease. *Clin Perinatol* 1988;15:609–618.

27. Van Hare GF, Stanger P. Ventricular tachycardia and accelerated ventricular rhythm presenting in the first month of life. *Am J Cardiol* 1991;67:42–45.

28. Yabek SM. Ventricular arrhythmias in children with an apparently normal heart. *J Pediatr* 1991;119:1–11.

29. Zipes DP, Fisch C. Accelerated ventricular rhythm. *Arch Intern Med* 1972; 129:650–652.

30. Eibschitz I, Abinader EG, Klein A, et al. Intrauterine diagnosis and control of fetal arrhythmia during labor. *Am J Obstet Gynecol* 1975;122:597–600.

31. Geggel RL, McInerny J, Estes NA III. Transient neonatal ventricular tachycardia associated with maternal cocaine use. *Am J Cardiol* 1989;63:383–384.

32. Lightfoot PR, Bhatt DR. Idiopathic recurrent parasystolic ventricular tachycardia in a child. *Pacing Clin Electrophysiol* 1983;6:587–591.

33. Nir A, Tajik AJ, Freeman WK, et al. Tuberous sclerosis and cardiac rhabdomyoma. *Am J Cardiol* 1995;76:419–421.

34. Holley DG, Martin GR, Brenner JI, et al. Diagnosis and management of fetal cardiac tumors: a multicenter experience and review of published reports. *J Am Coll Cardiol* 1995;26:516–520.

35. Carroll JD, Widmer R, Hess OM, et al. Left ventricular isovolumic pressure decay and diastolic mechanics after postextrasystolic potentiation and during exercise. *Am J Cardiol* 1983;51:583–590.

36. Stoddard MF, Pearson AC, Kern MJ, et al. The effect of premature ventricular contraction on left ventricular relaxation, chamber stiffness, and filling in humans. *Am Heart J* 1989;118:725–733.

37. Palatini P, Maraglino G, Sperti G, et al. Prevalence and possible mechanisms of ventricular arrhythmias in athletes. *Am Heart J* 1985;110:560–567.
38. Jacobsen JR, Garson A Jr, Gillette PC, et al. Premature ventricular contractions in normal children. *J Pediatr* 1978;92:36–38.
39. Montague TJ, McPherson DD, MacKenzie BR, et al. Frequent ventricular ectopic activity without underlying cardiac disease: analysis of 45 subjects. *Am J Cardiol* 1983;52:980–984.
40. Friedli B. Ventricular arrhythmias in children and adolescents. *Pediatrician* 1986;13:189–198.
41. Attina DA, Mori F, Falorni PL, et al. Long-term follow-up in children without heart disease with ventricular premature beats. *Eur Heart J* 1987;8:21–23.
42. Paul T, Marchal C, Garson A Jr. Ventricular couplets in the young: prognosis related to underlying substrate. *Am Heart J* 1990;119:577–582.
43. Perry LW, Ruckman RN, Shapiro SR, et al. Left ventricular false tendons in children: prevalence as detected by 2-dimensional echocardiography and clinical significance. *Am J Cardiol* 1983;52:1264–1266.
44. Suwa M, Hirota Y, Nagao H, et al. Incidence of the coexistence of left ventricular false tendons and premature ventricular contractions in apparently healthy subjects. *Circulation* 1984;70:793–798.
45. Malouf J, Gharzuddine W, Kutayli F. A reappraisal of the prevalence and clinical importance of left ventricular false tendons in children and adults. *Br Heart J* 1986;55:587–591.
46. Suwa M, Hirota Y, Kaku K, et al. Prevalence of the coexistence of left ventricular false tendons and premature ventricular complexes in apparently healthy subjects: a prospective study in the general population. *J Am Coll Cardiol* 1988;12:910–914.
47. Rozanski JJ, Dimich I, Steinfeld L, et al. Maximal exercise stress testing in evaluation of arrhythmias in children: results and reproducibility. *Am J Cardiol* 1979;43:951–956.
48. Bricker JT, Traweek MS, Smith RT, et al. Exercise-related ventricular tachycardia in children. *Am Heart J* 1986;112:186–188.

Sinus and Atrioventricular Conduction Disorders

Richard A. Friedman, MD

Disorders of Sinoatrial Node Function

Sinus Bradycardia

Definition

The definition of sinus bradycardia is a rhythm whose origin is the sinoatrial (SA) node and where the rate is less than normal for age. There are multiple methods of obtaining a resting heart rate including physical examination, ambulatory monitoring (Holter and transtelephonic event recorders), and standard 12- or 15-lead surface electrocardiograms (ECGs). Infants and children present a significant problem in the analysis of the resting heart rate as there is usually some anxiety or fear associated with the performance of these tests. This adds significant sympathetic input and may further complicate the ability to diagnose this problem. Holter monitoring, which adds significant expense, may be more helpful as the infant or child will accommodate to the presence of the recorder, allowing a more natural situation during measurement of the heart rate. We favor the measurement of the heart rate in the awake, resting state and use the following guidelines suggested by Kugler[1]:

From Deal B, Wolff G, Gelband H, (eds.). *Current Concepts in Diagnosis and Management of Arrhythmias in Infants and Children.* Armonk, NY: Futura Publishing Co., Inc.; © 1998.

Criteria for Sinus Bradycardia

Holter

1. Neonates/infants: <80 beats per minute (bpm) sleeping.
2. Children 2–6 years: <60 bpm.
3. Children 7–11 years: <45 bpm.
4. Adolescents >12 years: <40 bpm.
5. Endurance athletes: <30 bpm.

Surface Electrocardiogram

1. Neonates/infants: <100 bpm, awake, resting.
2. Children to 3 years: <100 bpm.
3. Children 3–9 years: <60 bpm.
4. Children 9–16 years: <50 bpm.

Etiology

The incidence of sinus bradycardia in the healthy pediatric population is not known. This is because the overwhelming majority of these patients are asymptomatic with their bradycardia (Figure 1). These patients rarely require any intervention. A frequent reason for evaluation of bradycardia in a newborn is the presence of premature atrial contractions (PACs). PACs are relatively common in newborns and are rarely of clinical significance.[2] However, when the PACs are nonconducted because their coupling interval to the last sinus beat is short, the appearance of the next sinus beat is "prolonged." These nonconducted PACs cannot be discerned on physical examination and, when examining the infant in the newborn nursery, a pulse below normal is noted. Even when the child is on a monitor, it takes a keen eye to note the blocked P waves in or at the end of the T wave from the preceding beat. This is especially true in blocked atrial bigeminy where every other atrial impulse is a PAC that is nonconducted (Figure 2). Careful examination of the T wave for deformities in the downstroke or in the

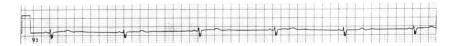

Figure 1. Sinus bradycardia. Record of an awake, asymptomatic 15-year-old boy who was referred after a school physical for the track team revealed a very slow heart rate. There was no history of exercise intolerance and a treadmill exercise test demonstrated a normal chronotropic response to exercise. The patient was released with recommendations to allow full participation in all school activities.

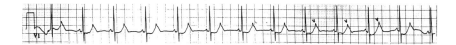

Figure 2. Bradycardia. This record is from an infant in the newborn nursery referred for episodes of sudden bradycardia. The ventricular rate is 75 bpm, which could be interpreted as sinus bradycardia for age. Careful inspection of the T waves demonstrates a "peaked" appearance. This is actually a case of blocked atrial bigeminy. Blocked premature atrial contractions are responsible for a significant number of consultations in newborns with sinus bradycardia.

appearance of the peak compared with T waves from a part of the rhythm strip where there are successive normal sinus beats will confirm the proper diagnosis. It is important to examine the T waves in as many leads as possible as the PACs may not be evident in all leads.

Sinus bradycardia in the absence of structural abnormalities and exclusive of the side effects of drugs can be seen in long QT syndrome (LQTS)[3] (Figure 3). This may present in the newborn period or any time thereafter. True sinus bradycardia in this condition must be differentiated from complete atrioventricular (AV) block with isochronic dissociation and 2:1 AV block. In the first

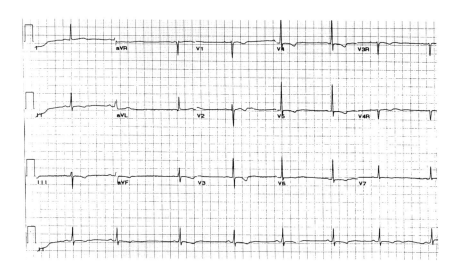

Figure 3. Sinus bradycardia and LQTS. This ECG was obtained at the time of the initial consultation on an 18-year-old female hospitalized for recurrent syncope that began 2 months prior. Sinus arrhythmia is present but the heart rate drops to as low as 38 bpm. The corrected QT interval is 630 milliseconds. Ambulatory monitoring did not reveal VT but did show persistent sinus bradycardia. Following initiation of β-blocker therapy, the patient required implantation of a permanent pacemaker. She had no further episodes of syncope.

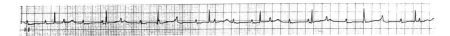

Figure 4. Congenital complete AV block. The record is from a 9-hours-old infant referred for bradycardia. A stable narrow QRS (junctional) escape rhythm is seen in the presence of AV dissociation. P waves that should conduct (ie, outside the T wave) do not, thus establishing the diagnosis of complete AV block. Examination of the QT interval shows that, when corrected using Bazett's formula, it is prolonged to 485 milliseconds. Frequently ventricular ectopy was seen and the infant was treated with β-blockers. An epicardial permanent pacing system was implanted.

situation both the sinus node (SN) and the AV junction have similar automaticity (spontaneous discharge rates). At times, the P wave may occur before the QRS and appear to be associated. Careful examination of a long rhythm strip will demonstrate that the PR intervals change and that the rhythms become dissociated at times. In the second situation, similar to blocked atrial bigeminy, there are P waves that fall into the T wave and are nonconducted. However, the P waves do not come prematurely. Rather, the P wave is nonconducted by virtue of the T wave being delayed as a result of prolonged repolarization. The P wave is nonconducted because the His-Purkinje system is still refractory to electrical stimulation (Figure 4). Rosenbaum and Acunzo[4] correctly pointed out that this is really pseudo-2:1 AV block as there is no evidence of any intrinsic abnormality of AV conduction. Rather, this is an example of simple interference.

When sinus bradycardia is present on surface ECG recordings, subsidiary pacemakers (ie, atrial, junctional, or ventricular) become apparent. Automaticity is usually greatest in the atrium, followed by the junction [AV node (AVN)-His bundle region] and finally the ventricle (Figure 5).

Some recent reports described other rare conditions that can cause sinus bradycardia. Mehta et al[5] described an adolescent with palpitations and exercise intolerance secondary to sinus bradycardia. The bradycardia was abolished with autonomic blockade and exercise testing. The patient's

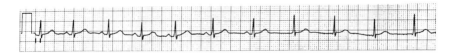

Figure 5. Sinus bradycardia with junctional escape rhythm. This ECG is from a 16-year-old female who underwent radiofrequency catheter ablation of a left-sided accessory connection. She was asymptomatic with this rhythm. Note the slight difference in the QRS complex beginning with the second junctional escape beat compared to the sinus conducted beats. A small "pseudo q wave" can be seen in lead II. This is actually rapid retrograde activation of the atrium from the junctional rhythm and represents an inverted P wave. A similar phenomenon may be noted in patients with typical AVNRT.

father and cousin had similar symptoms. The etiology was felt to be secondary to hypervagotonia, and all three patients received pacemaker therapy. SN dysfunction was also described in tuberous sclerosis.[6]

The majority of pediatric patients with sinus bradycardia will have this disorder as a result of surgery to correct or palliate congenital heart disease. The most prominent of these are patients who had atrial baffles (Mustard or Senning procedure) for transposition of the great arteries. Unfortunately, the presence of sinus bradycardia in this setting is frequently associated with atrial tachycardia and more commonly termed "tachy-brady syndrome." A multicenter study of patients who underwent the Mustard procedure showed a progressive deterioration in the presence of sinus rhythm in the decade following repair. Ten years postoperatively 60% of patients were predominantly in a "passive rhythm," ie, junctional or idioventricular escape, compared with 70% being in sinus rhythm in the year following their surgery.[7] The Senning procedure became popular partly due to the hopes that SN dysfunction was less likely to occur by virtue of the baffling procedure not involving the area of the SN and thus avoiding direct injury during surgery. Byrum et al[8] demonstrated that abnormal SN function was less common in patients who had the Senning operation than in those who had the Mustard operation. Unfortunately, later studies did not support this finding. Deanfield and colleagues[9] showed that both Mustard and Senning patients demonstrated a similar gradual decrease in sinus rhythm to between 56% and 66%. Late death was not correlated with this finding. The popularity of a more anatomic correction using the arterial switch technique resulted in a significant improvement in the preservation of normal sinus rhythm acutely and long term. Nearly all patients remained in sinus rhythm in one study up to 8.5 years after arterial switch.[10]

More recently, patients with single ventricle underwent the Fontan procedure. As in the Mustard or Senning procedures, extensive atrial surgery is performed. Significant SN dysfunction is seen in many of these patients. Use of the total cavopulmonary connection was demonstrated to result in a higher incidence of SN dysfunction, manifest as sinus bradycardia, compared with patients undergoing the "classic" Fontan operation.[11] Another recent study showed that a staged approach to Fontan using a cavopulmonary shunt results in a significantly higher risk for the development of SN dysfunction compared to a single-staged approach or after either of the two single interventions.[12] This is most likely due to inadvertent direct damage to the SN region during the additional surgery. All surgery in the atrium is not necessarily associated with high rates of SN dysfunction. Meijboom and colleagues[13] studied 135 children who underwent atrial septal defect repair (both secundum and sinus venosus types). At mean follow-up of 14.5 years, 89% were in sinus rhythm and 88% had normal exercise capacity. A somewhat surprising result of surgery for tetralogy of Fallot, which one would expect to emphasize late postoperative ventricular arrhythmias, highlighted a significant number of patients with atrial arrhythmias. Fifty-three patients who were operated on at a mean age of 9.1 years were studied. SN dysfunction was present in 36% of these adults, four of whom required a permanent pacemaker for therapy.[14]

Evaluation

Noninvasive studies of SN function are the mainstay in the evaluation of the child referred for bradycardia. Many centers routinely perform Holter studies on postoperative congenital heart surgical patients in order to screen for occult arrhythmias. Most of the asymptomatic patients referred to the arrhythmia service come from this group. It is important to obtain a careful history that includes subtle symptoms of exercise intolerance compared with that of the patient's peers. Children described as "exhausted" after school by the parents should heighten the suspicion that there is a likelihood of SN dysfunction. Obvious symptoms are dizziness, presyncope, or syncope, although our experience is that the majority of patients do not present in this manner. Rather, they may come to attention when presenting for evaluation of a tachyarrhythmia, such as atrial reentry tachycardia. Once the tachycardia is terminated, monitoring reveals the presence of a previously "asymptomatic" sinus bradycardia.

Besides the surface ECG and Holter monitor criteria mentioned earlier, our primary tool for the evaluation of sinus bradycardia is treadmill exercise testing. This method was found to be a more sensitive indicator of SN disease in these patients than was invasive electrophysiology (EP) testing.[15] The modified Bruce protocol used in this study is widely accepted as a reasonable standard. The protocol varies speed and work load (incline) progressively every 3 minutes until the patient complains of exhaustion. We generally perform this in children older than 5–6 years, as the test is somewhat intimidating and younger children are rarely cooperative enough to obtain a valid study. The advantage of this protocol is that it brings the patient to maximum heart rate and anaerobic threshold in a fairly short time. Continuous recordings of the ECG and oxygen consumption are made so that the rhythm can be evaluated. Although some patients fail to respond to the initial stress of the exercise with a reasonable increase in heart rate, many of the patients develop a delayed response with a slow increase in the sinus or junctional rate and then a more rapid response with conversion to sinus as sympathetic stimulation ensues. These patients either fail to reach a reasonable maximum heart rate (>180 bpm) or, if they do, rapidly revert to sinus bradycardia as soon as the sympathetic stimulus of exercise is withdrawn.

In the past, it was fairly common to perform an invasive EP study to assess SA node function. Measurements of SN recovery time (SNRT) following rapid atrial pacing and SA conduction time using premature atrial stimuli paced into either a stable sinus rhythm or a paced atrial rhythm are described elsewhere.[1] We prefer to use noninvasive means to demonstrate SN dysfunction as they were shown to be at least as good if not better indicators than formal EP testing.[14] SNRTs were shown to significantly shorten due to the hypotension induced during rapid atrial pacing.[16] Likewise, SA node conduction times may also be affected during the atrial pacing used as a drive train prior to introduction of the premature stimulus.[17] Thus we will defer a formal discussion of these techniques here. The interested reader is referred to other sources.[1]

Indications for Treatment

The primary indication for treatment of this arrhythmia is symptomatic bradycardia. While this statement seems apparent, patients with asymptomatic sinus bradycardia are frequently referred for therapy. As mentioned earlier, symptoms in these patients may be subtle, ranging from sleep disturbances or exercise intolerance manifest by a sedentary lifestyle to syncope. Postoperative atrial surgery patients with documented near syncope or syncope with concomitant bradycardia are appropriate candidates for permanent pacemakers. Gillette et al[18] reported on 29 patients who underwent Mustard repair. Of these, 16 had symptoms of dizziness, near syncope, or syncope. The remaining patients had pacemakers implanted for concomitant antiarrhythmic therapy with a drug other than digitalis (10 patients) and low sleeping or awake heart rate without symptoms (3 patients). All 16 patients in the first group became asymptomatic after pacing. This was confirmed by others[19] and is now generally accepted as a class I indication for implantation of a pacemaker.[20] There is controversy about a second group of patients who received pacemakers in the study by Gillette. At the time of publication of that study, use of an antiarrhythmic medication other than digitalis with concomitant SN dysfunction was considered a class I indication. In the most recent recommendations,[20] however, this was changed to a class II indication (one where there is evidence to support either implantation or nonimplantation). Currently, we use sotalol or amiodarone for treatment of tachyarrhythmias coexisting with SN disease. In those patients who become symptomatic after initiating therapy, we then implant a pacemaker. This becomes problematic in the postoperative Fontan patient where transvenous access is unlikely due to recent modifications in the technique, ie, staged approach with a bidirectional Glenn anastomosis. Bradycardia in these patients may mediate the occurrence of tachycardias, and, in some cases where the bradycardia may not result in significant symptoms, pacing may be indicated to prevent the tachycardia. Silka et al[21] reported on 21 young patients with postoperative congenital heart disease in whom tachycardia developed in the setting of bradycardia. Dual-chambered or atrial-based pacing (DDD or AAI) resulted in a significant decrease in the number of episodes of both supraventricular tachycardias (SVTs) and ventricular tachycardias (VTs) [exclusive of atrial flutter (AF)]. Gillette et al[22] proposed the use of automatic atrial antitachycardia devices in many of these patients. The antibradycardia response of the pacemaker functions at a fixed rate regardless of the degree of chronotropic incompetence; there is no activity response mode available in these units. Of the 23 patients studied, 17 were either postoperative Fontan or transposition of the great arteries. The majority of patients were either completely controlled or significantly improved after pacemaker implantation. However, antitachycardia atrial pacing was associated with sudden death due to rapid ventricular responses. While this approach may address the tachycardia, therapy for the bradycardia is limited to the lower rate limit programmed in the device at any given time. Many of these patients spend the majority of their time chronotropically incompetent for everyday activity. Thus sensor-based pacing with varying lower rate limits for given levels of activity usually results in a significant improvement of lifestyle for the patient. The ideal prescription might be a device that has both automatic antitachycardia and rate-response features. Unfortunately, at this time, that device does not exist.

Patients with the LQTS and sinus bradycardia may develop exacerbation of their sinus bradycardia, especially once they are begun on β-blocker therapy. The concomitant use of β-blockers and pacemakers in this disease was shown to be effective in suppressing arrhythmia and improving symptoms.[23] Despite the fact that bradycardia may trigger polymorphic VT in these patients, pacing alone for sinus bradycardia without the use of β-blockers is not acceptable therapy and is contraindicated.[24]

Sudden episodes of sinus bradycardia may occur in patients with vasodepressor syncope. Periods of severe sinus bradycardia (heart rates <30 bpm) or asystole may occur and last for 5–15 or more seconds. Pacing alone is usually not completely effective in preventing symptoms as it will not address the vasodilatation that occurs simultaneously. Sra et al[25] showed that pharmacologic therapy is generally superior to pacing alone and should be the first choice in the management of these patients. However, some patients may exhibit a "malignant" form of syncope where the addition of pacing alleviates symptoms after trials with multiple drugs failed.[26,27]

Sinoatrial Exit Block

Exit block refers primarily to a disorder in impulse conduction rather than impulse formation. Thus for the SA node, impulse formation as a result of phase 4 depolarization of pacemaker cells is assumed to be normal. However, perinodal tissue, which may be injured or inexcitable, prevents normal conduction of the activation wavefront that would normally pro-

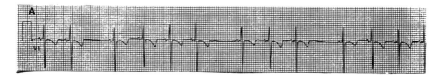

Figure 6. Type I SA node exit block (Wenckebach type). The third QRS starts the sequence. The PP interval between the third QRS and fourth QRS is 430 milliseconds. The following PP interval is 390 milliseconds, a decrement of 40 milliseconds. The following PP interval is 365 milliseconds, a decrement shorter than the previous cycle—25 milliseconds. This is followed by a pause of 1000 milliseconds, which is less than the two previous cycle lengths (CL) combined—1165 milliseconds.

ceed to depolarize the remaining atrial tissue.[28] As in type I and type II AVN block, the SN exhibits like properties. In type I AVN block (Wenckebach), the PR intervals prolong in a progressive fashion until there is failure to conduct. The first PR interval following a blocked P wave is the shortest PR interval in the sequence. The succeeding PR intervals are gradually prolonged, although the percent increase lessens in each successive beat. This results in a sequence of prolonging PR intervals while at the same time a shortening of the RR intervals. The same phenomenon occurs in type I SA block. Progressive delay in conduction of the pacemaker impulse from the SN results in a gradual shortening of the PP interval until there is failure to propagate out of the SN and no atrial activity occurs. Similar to AVN phenomena, the cycles recur in a repetitive sequence. This, along with shortening of the PP interval prior to the "long cycle" from the dropped beat differentiates this rhythm from sinus arrhythmia where the PP interval gradually prolongs prior to the pause. In type I SA block, the long cycle is less than the sum of the two preceding cycles as is the case in AVN Wenckebach (Figure 6).

Type II SA block (akin to type II AVN block) occurs when there is a sudden failure to propagate an impulse from the SA node to the rest of

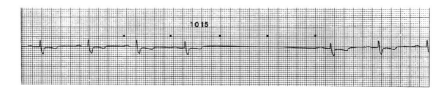

Figure 7. SN exit block. The basic CL is 1015 milliseconds. Following the fourth QRS, there is a pause. The time between the P wave of the fourth QRS and the P wave of the fifth QRS is an exact multiple of 1015 milliseconds—3045 milliseconds. Thus, there are two consecutive P waves that fail to exit the SA region and cause an atrial depolarization (3:1 exit block).

the atrium with little or no change in the preceding PP intervals. Examination of a long rhythm strip will usually demonstrate that the shortest PP interval, which corresponds to the true SN automaticity, is close to an exact multiple (ie, one half or one third) of the longest PP interval, which corresponds to 2:1 or 3:1 SA-atrial conduction (Figure 7).

Sinus Arrest

Sinus arrest occurs when there is a sudden absence of atrial activity due to failure of phase 4 depolarization occurring in the pacemaker cells of the SN. In sinus arrest, the longest PP interval is not a multiple of the shortest PP interval. Frequently, escape rhythms of atrial, junctional, or ventricular origin may occur in conjunction with the long pause. An atrial escape occurs when a P wave of different morphology occurs at a slower rate than the SN. Junctional escape occurs when there is a narrow QRS or QRS identical to the sinus-conducted QRS responsible for the rhythm. Ventricular escape occurs when a wide QRS follows the pause. In making the diagnosis of sinus arrest, it is important to exclude the presence of a premature atrial contraction that may be "hidden" in the T wave of the QRS prior to the pause. The PAC may reset the SA node and give the appearance of a sudden pause. Malignant vasodepressor syncope with asystole[29] must also be differentiated from sinus arrest. Head-up tilt (HUT) testing can be used to reproduce symptoms and, as mentioned earlier, can usually be treated medically. The indications for therapy would be identical for those of sinus bradycardia. If the rhythm

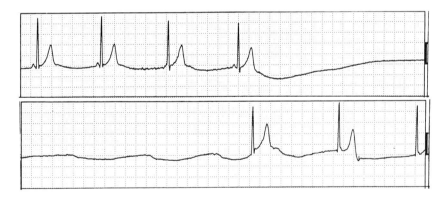

Figure 8. Sinus arrest. Continuous tracings on a female adolescent referred for evaluation of recurrent syncope. Sinus bradycardia with a junctional escape rhythm (note very short PR intervals in the second and third QRS complexes compared with the first and fourth) is followed by a 7.9-second pause. This occurred during micturition and resulted in syncope. Treatment with a β-blocker, fludrocortisone, and added salt to the diet eliminated the episodes.

is not due to a reversible condition (ie, hyperkalemia) or a treatable condition such as neurocardiogenic syncope, medical therapy and in rare cases, a pacemaker should be considered for symptoms of syncope or near syncope (Figure 8).

Disorders of Atrioventricular Conduction

First-Degree Atrioventricular Block

First-degree AV block is defined as prolongation of the PR interval beyond the norms for age. The normal interval changes with both age and heart rate, varying from 70 milliseconds to 170 milliseconds in the newborn to between 80 and 220 milliseconds in children 12–15 years of age[30] (Figure 9). Prolonged conduction within the atrium, AVN, or His-Purkinje system may manifest as first-degree block. It is found as either a normal variant[31] or in unoperated congenital heart disease including patent ductus arte-

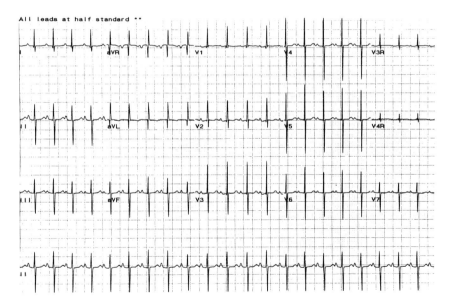

Figure 9. First-degree AV block. Recording from a 3-month-old referred for failure to thrive. Physical examination demonstrated the presence of a gallop rhythm. A chest radiograph showed cardiomegaly. The PR interval measures as long as 185 milliseconds, which is prolonged for age. RV hypertrophy and probable biventricular hypertrophy is also present. This is an example of an RA ectopic tachycardia that eventually responded to medical therapy with sotalol. First-degree AV block is unusual in an awake child of this age, and its presence, in the absence of other heart disease, should alert the physician to this possible diagnosis.

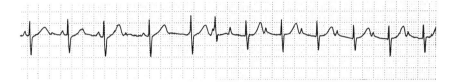

Figure 10. First-degree AV block. The tracing is from a 24-hour ambulatory monitor in a 9-year-old with SVT. The first four complexes have PR intervals of 125 milliseconds. Sinus slowing occurs between the third QRS and the fourth, followed by a junctional escape beat coincident with the onset of a P wave (note slight deformity in the upstroke of the QRS). This is followed by a PVC. Successive QRS complexes are conducted with a PR interval of 300 milliseconds. The patient subsequently underwent EP study where typical AVNRT was demonstrated. Thus, conduction in the first part of the tracing with a shorter PR interval was predominantly via the "fast pathway," while conduction in the later part of the tracing is via the "slow pathway." We assume that the PVC conducted retrograde into the fast pathway, with concealed conduction causing the fast pathway to be refractory, allowing subsequent antegrade conduction to proceed via the slow pathway.

riosus, Ebstein anomaly of the tricuspid valve, pulmonary stenosis, double outlet right ventricle (RV), ventricular septal defect (VSD), and coarctation of the aorta.[30] The P wave in the ECG may be broad as a result of atrial dilatation and affect measurement of the PR interval so that it is measured as prolonged; in these cases the delay in conduction is probably intraatrial rather than in the AVN itself. First-degree AV block can be seen as a result of drug therapy with several antiarrhythmic agents including digitalis, calcium channel blockers, β-blockers, and sotalol.[32] It is also seen in rheumatic fever, myocarditis, Duchenne muscular dystrophy, myotonic dystrophy, diphtheria, trichinosis, and mumps. Hyper- or hypokalemia, hyper- or hypocalcemia, hypomagnesemia, and hypoglycemia are among some of the metabolic abnormalities associated with first-degree AV block.[33] Rarely, a patient with AVN reentry tachycardia (AVNRT) may demonstrate two distinct alternating PR intervals—one short and one long—consistent with conduction over the fast or slow pathways, respectively. Conduction over slow pathway demonstrates first-degree AV block on the surface ECG[34] (Figure 10). Finally, increased vagal tone may be responsible for prolongation of the PR interval with either first-, second-, or higher-level block.[34] In general, this is a benign condition and there is no specific treatment.

Second-Degree Atrioventricular Block

There are two types of second-degree AV block: Mobitz type I, more commonly known as Wenckebach AV block, and Mobitz type II. In both cases there is failure to conduct some but not all atrial activity to the ventricles.

Type I Second-Degree Atrioventricular Block (Wenckebach)

Electrocardiogram Criteria: Typical Type I Block (Figure 11)

1. Progressive lengthening of the PR interval.
2. Progressively shorter increments in the successive PR intervals compared with the first PR interval prolongation.
3. Progressive shortening of the RR intervals once the PR prolongation takes place.
4. Failure to conduct an atrial event to the ventricle with an interceding RR interval equal to less than the sum of PP intervals.[30]

The "atypical" form (Figure 12), which may be seen with at least as much frequency as the "typical" form, differs in that the PR intervals in the final atrial event conducted may demonstrate a significantly longer increment than the previous beat, the first PR prolongation is not the longest, or the PR intervals in the middle of the cycle vary with unexpected shortening followed by failure to conduct.[35] Both of these forms are seen during 24-hour ambulatory monitoring of children during sleep periods

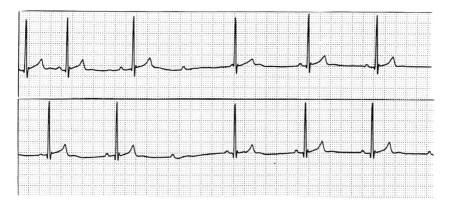

Figure 11. Type I and type II AV block. The strips are from the same patient, recorded during sleep 10 minutes apart. This patient is an asymptomatic 14-year-old male evaluated for chest pain. **Upper panel**: The third QRS demonstrates a PR interval of 220 milliseconds compared to the second QRS with a PR interval of 180 milliseconds. The third P wave is not conducted. A junctional escape beat coincides with the onset of the fourth P wave. The fifth and sixth QRS complexes have PR intervals of 150 and 180 milliseconds, respectively. Successive QRS complexes show progressively longer PR intervals prior to a dropped ventricular response. There is sinus arrhythmia present and thus the RR intervals do not shorten in this sequence. **Lower panel**: Ten minutes later, while still asleep, the third P wave is not conducted. The PR interval remains constant at 170 milliseconds. There is sinus arrhythmia present, accounting for the variation in CL seen between conducted QRS complexes.

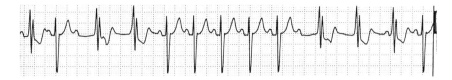

Figure 12. Atypical type I AV block with ventricular escape. The fifth and sixth QRSs in the tracing are narrow with PR intervals of 140 milliseconds. The next three complexes have a slightly longer PR interval of 160 milliseconds. Measurement of the RR intervals shows mild prolongation from 500 milliseconds to 525 milliseconds. The sixth P wave in this sequence is associated with a dropped ventricular response followed by an idioventricular escape rhythm for three beats prior to resumption of normal sinus rhythm.

where there is a predominance of vagal tone and is generally asymptomatic, requiring no intervention. Our experience has been that, even in patients who had congenital heart surgery, these episodes are unnoticed and incidentally found on routine ambulatory monitoring. In the event of associated symptoms of syncope, especially with exertion, further investigation is warranted. Permanent pacing may be indicated in selected patients with symptomatic type I AV block.[35]

Type II Second-Degree Atrioventricular Block

Electrocardiogram Criteria.

1. A relatively constant PP interval.
2. No progressive lengthening of the PR interval prior to an atrial event that suddenly fails to conduct.
3. The interceding RR interval is equal to the sum of two PP cycles.

This type of block is generally considered to indicate block in the His bundle or below.[30,35] In cases of fast atrial rates, higher grade block with 2:1, 3:1, or greater may be seen (Figure 13). Damage to the His bundle or below can be seen in patients after surgery for congenital heart defects and also in myocarditis. We saw this as a reversible phenomenon in children who develop rejection of their cardiac allograft after transplantation. Although relatively rare in children, this type of AV block warrants close scrutiny; if symptoms of near syncope or syncope occur a pacemaker is required.[33] Asymptomatic pediatric patients present somewhat of a dilemma. In adults the implantation of a permanent pacemaker is recommended because the block leads to Adams-Stokes attacks.[34] At this time, there are no large studies to support this recommendation in children, although it seems prudent to consider this in the postoperative patient.

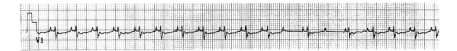

Figure 13. Mobitz type II AV block. The PP and RR intervals on this tracing are relatively constant at 440 milliseconds and the PR interval is constant at 120 milliseconds. QRS complexes 1–11 are conducted 1:1. The 12th P wave is not conducted and is followed by one sequence of apparent 2:1 AV block. Actually, the first and second QRS complexes following the dropped atrial impulse represent a junctional escape rhythm. Note the variable PR interval of these two beats and the nearly constant RR interval between the last conducted beat and the following two beats (800 and 840 milliseconds, respectively). Longer rhythm strips confirmed this finding.

Complete Atrioventricular Block

Complete AV block can be divided into two types: acquired and congenital. Each will be discussed individually as their etiologies and approach to treatment differ.

Acquired Atrioventricular Block

Etiology.   Damage to the His bundle or AVN resulting in AV block in children is most commonly associated with surgical correction of a congenital heart defect. This includes VSDs, either as isolated defects or as part of a more complex structural anomaly, ie, tetralogy of Fallot, AV septal defects, L-TGA with ventricular inversion, and VSD. In the case of ventricular inversion with VSD, the anterior displacement of the His bundle along the superior edge of the VSD places it at great risk to injury during closure of the defect. In addition, patients undergoing aortic valve replacement, or resection of a subaortic obstructive lesion, may suffer damage to the His bundle as it exits the AV septal region and enters the superior margin of the left ventricle (LV). Another significant cause of acquired AV block is myocarditis[36] (Figure 14). In most cases this is a temporary finding and usually resolves in less than 1 week, although some patients develop complete AV block. This is also true of rheumatic fever.[37]

In early reports the incidence found for surgical AV block was between 3% and 4% in patients with isolated VSD, tetralogy of Fallot, or AV canal-type defects,[38–40] although today that figure is more likely less than 3%, including newborn repairs.[41,42] Temporary or transient surgical AV block must be separated from permanent block. The former usually occurs intraoperatively or occasionally in the early postoperative period as a result of trauma to the AVN or His bundle. Resumption of normal sinus rhythm, if it is to resume, usually takes place in the first 2 weeks following surgery,[43] although cases were reported where normal sinus rhythm resumes up to 1

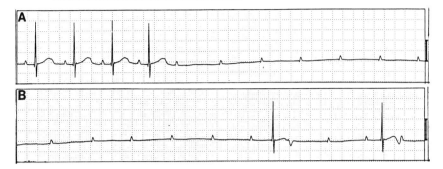

Figure 14. Acquired AV block. The tracings (**A** and **B**) are continuous from a 24-hour ambulatory monitor. These strips were recorded at 2:20 AM in a 7-year-old boy referred for evaluation of an irregular heart rate and a murmur. There was no history of syncope, although there was mild exercise intolerance. The first four beats are conducted with a PR interval of 200 milliseconds. There is paroxysmal AV block with a pause of just greater than 10 seconds. An endomyocardial biopsy was consistent with dilated cardiomyopathy. Polymerase chain reaction analysis was positive for adenovirus, the probable etiologic agent of a previously unrecognized myocarditis. The patient received a permanent transvenous pacemaker.

month after surgery.[44] Results at our institution reveal an increased incidence in permanent AV block in infants and children <10 kg in weight with transient AV block resolving at a mean of 2.3 days postoperatively.[42] Late-onset complete AV block following congenital heart surgery was associated with syncope or death.[45,46] Predisposing factors involved with these cases were the presence of transient postoperative complete block with return to sinus rhythm and the presence of complete right bundle-branch block (RBBB) with left anterior hemiblock. However, this pattern is frequently seen in postoperative tetralogy of Fallot patients (see below), few of whom progress to this result.

Evaluation and Treatment. The usual recommendation for postoperative heart block is to observe the patient for about 2 weeks prior to a decision for implantation of a permanent pacemaker.[43] If the patient has a stable junctional rhythm, we usually continue to observe the patient on a monitor with temporary pacing wires attached to a temporary demand pacemaker. It is important to evaluate the ability of the temporary pacemaker to actually pace the heart on a daily basis as deterioration in stimulation thresholds of the temporary pacing wires is common. In the absence of temporary wires, a transcutaneous pacing system should be utilized and placed on "standby," Infusion of isoproterenol may also be useful in situations where pacing either fails or is not available. We prefer to obtain 24-hour ambulatory monitors on these patients as they approach the end of their 10-day to 2-week waiting period. The rationale is that many of them

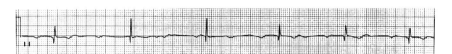

Figure 15. High-grade AV block. This record is from a patient who is 2 days post-operative from repair of an AV septal defect. The RR interval between the first and second as well as the second and third QRS is 1600 milliseconds. The following RR intervals are then 1480, 1360, and 1360 milliseconds. The PP interval varies between 630 and 720 milliseconds. Thus, the first three QRS complexes are due to AV block with a junctional escape rhythm. The fourth QRS is actually a sinus conducted beat with a PR interval of *320 milliseconds. The following two QRS complexes are also conducted with PR intervals of 350 milliseconds. Normal conduction resumed on the fifth postoperative day.

will have an accelerated junctional rhythm with sinus capture beats that can be missed unless a careful observer spends time evaluating the monitor (Figure 15). If AV conduction is seen, a longer period of waiting prior to implantation of a permanent pacemaker is justified.

In the late 1960s and early 1970s permanent pacemakers were somewhat cumbersome and not particularly easy to implant. Thus, it is not surprising that there are reports in the literature advocating not implanting a pacemaker in selected postoperative AV block patients.[44,47] However, this is clearly no longer the case, and no child with surgical AV block should be discharged from the hospital without a permanent pacemaker. While the mortality quoted by Lillihei et al[38] of 60% may overestimate the potential incidence, no death due to this complication should be acceptable. Pacemakers can be implanted by either the epicardial route through a limited subxiphoid incision in the operating room or transvenously in the catheterization laboratory. Small infants and patients without venous access (postoperative Fontan) are approached via the epicardial route, while most others receive transvenous devices. System longevity, which was a significant issue cited in the earlier studies, is not a major issue at this time given the advances in both lead technology and pacemaker programmability.

Congenital Atrioventricular Block

Electrocardiogram Criteria

1. Complete dissociation of the P wave and QRS.
2. Failure to conduct P waves that fall outside the T wave of the preceding QRS.
3. Atrial rate higher than the ventricular rate.

In the past the diagnosis of congenital AV block was made when a slow heart rate was noted in the newborn nursery or later. Currently, the diagnosis is often made by fetal echocardiography.[48] The incidence is thought to be around 1:20,000 births.[49] In 1964, Nakamura and Nadas[50] reported that up to 50% of such infants had definitive or probable congenital heart disease, with most of the remainder consisting of children born to mothers with collagen vascular disease as described by McCue et al[51] in 1977. Nearly one-half of mothers in one large study who gave birth to children with congenital AV block did not demonstrate clinical evidence of their immune disorder.[52] Such conditions included systemic lupus erythematosis, discoid lupus, Sjogren syndrome, leucoclastic vasculitis, Sicca symptoms, and undifferentiated autoimmune syndrome. Many of the mothers were diagnosed as a result of the finding of congenital AV block in the baby and some went on to develop symptoms a mean of 2.6 years later, although many remained asymptomatic. The antibodies responsible for this passive transplacental autoimmune injury were shown to be SSA/Ro and SSB/La. Subsequent pregnancies did not always result in a child with congenital AV block and, surprisingly, there were two sets of twins discordant for congenital block.

Other etiologies for congenital complete AV block include myocarditis, tumors that invade the AVN region such as mesothelioma, and patients with LQTS (Figure 4). Bharati and Lev[36] described pathological changes in autopsy specimens that include congenital fragmentation or displacement of the His bundle to the left side of the septum. The most common congenital heart defect associated with congenital AV block is l-TGA. Huhta et al[53] described the presence of this rhythm disturbance, particularly in those with intact ventricular septum. Theories of why those with intact septum have a higher incidence include increased mechanical stress on the septum and longer life span.[54]

Evaluation and Treatment. There were many published studies about the natural history of this disorder. However, in a recent study Michaelsson et al[55] prospectively analyzed the largest group of patients with congenital AV block ever studied. Previous data concerning patients with congenital AV block and LQTS[56] were validated; that is, there is a significant mortality associated with this combination that can probably be prevented by the implantation of a pacemaker. In a very early study from 1964, the authors found that sudden cardiac death occurred as a first symptom in five patients.[50] Exercise testing may be of limited value in evaluating the need for intervention. An earlier study[57] reported that complex ventricular ectopy was not uncommon in these patients and may indicate an increased risk of sudden death. However, in this study, although 64% of the patients with ventricular ectopy did experience a syncopal episode, another 15% of the 76 patients had syncope or presyncope but reasonable heart rates at rest and with exercise and without ventricular ectopy. Mitral regurgitation with significant myocardial dysfunction occurred in 15% of the patients in the study. The implantation of a pacemaker might have prevented ventricular dysfunction if it had been due to chronic dilatation of the LV in an attempt to augment stroke volume.

The initial evaluation of a newborn or child with complete AV block should include an echocardiogram to rule out the presence of any significant congenital heart defect. In addition, information about the size and function of the LV should be noted. Wall stress in asymptomatic young patients with congenital AV block is normal.[58] However, longer-term follow-up studies are needed to determine whether this becomes apparent at a later stage in life. A 24-hour ambulatory monitor should be performed in order to observe heart rates in the waking state or very long pauses in the escape rhythm (>3 seconds). The presence of a wide QRS escape rhythm is currently considered an indication for permanent pacing, but data from the Michaelsson study suggest that this may not be valid. In older children, exercise treadmill testing, although shown to have only limited predictive value, should still be considered to evaluate working capacity. While this may not screen patients at risk, it will still detect exercise intolerance in many of the patients who adapted to a sedentary lifestyle as a result of their heart rate limitations. Resting heart rate was shown to be a poor indicator of exercise response in these patients.[59] After pacing, considerable improvement in lifestyle is frequently seen in many of the patients who were previously not aware of symptoms of exercise intolerance. Current implantable devices are small and sophisticated. While there is surely a morbidity (and in rare cases, mortality) associated with pacemaker implantation, early intervention in the asymptomatic patient in the first decade of life should be considered. Although invasive EP studies were done to document the location of the block in these patients[60] EP studies are not routinely performed in these patients as there are no data to suggest that the level of block is predictive of symptoms or outcome.

Intraventricular Conduction Disorders

Right Bundle-Branch Block

Electrocardiogram Criteria

1. QRS duration >90 milliseconds in children <3 years.
2. QRS duration >100 milliseconds in older children.
3. QRS duration >120 milliseconds in adults.
4. Deep, slurred S waves in the left precordial leads, lead I, and often in lead aVL.
5. Initial R-wave component in the right chest leads is rapid, reflecting normal activation of the left bundle.
6. QRS complex in V_1, V_{3R}, V_{4R} may show rsr', rSr', RSr', RSR', or M-shaped pattern consistent with delayed activation of the RV.

Although some authors[30] proposed that LV hypertrophy (LVH) cannot be diagnosed in the presence of RBBB, others noted that this is still possible due to the fact that the initial depolarization forces, reflecting LV activation, are normal. However, the accuracy of voltage criteria for LVH still may make this a difficult diagnosis.[61,62] No studies to date demonstrated that the initial forces of the QRS preoperatively are identical to those postoperatively.

Clinical Correlation. RBBB is mostly an acquired condition as a result of surgery to correct or palliate congenital heart disease. This commonly occurs after repair of tetralogy of Fallot, AV septal defects, and VSDs.[63] Houyel et al[64] validated the hypothesis that a right atrial (RA) approach to closure of VSDs can reduce the incidence of RBBB but not complete AV block. In tetralogy of Fallot, complete RBBB (CRBBB) is probably due to the ventriculotomy rather than to direct injury to the central right bundle. Ziady et al[40] pointed out that infundibular resection for pulmonary valvotomy, without involving the ventricular septum, may produce RBBB. Undoubtedly, as Garson[30] noted, direct injury to the right bundle during repair of tetralogy of Fallot is responsible for up to half the incidence. Despite the current surgical approach, which involves closure of the VSD via the RA and infundibular resection without a lower ventriculotomy, we continue to see the majority of patients develop CRBBB postoperatively. Other etiologies for RBBB include any inflammatory injury to the myocardium such as in myocarditis or endocarditis, Kearns-Sayre syndrome,[65] Duchenne's muscular dystrophy, myotonic dystrophy, and isolated RBBB.[63] Familial cardiomyopathies with conduction system disease may also result in RBBB.[66,67] In addition to the RBBB seen in postoperative tetralogy of Fallot, left axis deviation or left anterior hemiblock is sometimes seen in combination (see below). Surgically induced RBBB is not thought to result in a poor prognosis and there is no good evidence that it results in hemodynamic compromise.[63] However, heritable forms of bundle-branch block, such as in Kearns-Sayre syndrome, may progress to sudden cardiac death. Therefore, the implantation of a permanent pacemaker is recommended in this group of patients.[20]

Left Bundle-Branch Block

Electrocardiogram Criteria

1. Prolongation of the QRS duration to >90 milliseconds in children <4 years of age.
2. QRS duration >100 milliseconds in children 4–16 years of age.
3. QRS duration >120 milliseconds in older patients.[30,62]
4. Absence of septal q waves in leads I, aVL, and V_6.
5. qS or rS pattern in V_1.
6. Notched (rsR′) or M-shaped pattern in V_6 similar to that seen in lead V_1 with RBBB (Figure 16).

Activation of the LV is delayed and occurs via transseptal propagation from the RV. ST segment depression and inversion of the T wave is seen

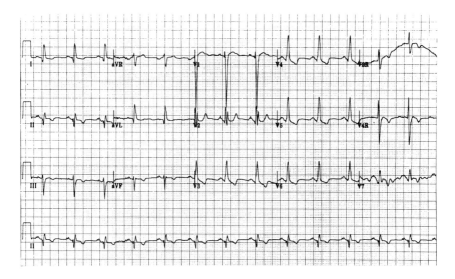

Figure 16. LBBB. This record is from an unoperated 28-year-old patient with dextrocardia, TGA, single atrium, and Eisenmenger's syndrome. Previous tracings from the patient 15 years ago did not show this pattern. It is presumed that high LV pressure associated with the irreversible pulmonary hypertension was responsible for this pattern.

in leads I, aVL, V_5, and V_6 with reciprocal changes in the right chest leads. Calculation of the frontal plane axis is performed using the major deflection, using the terminal part of the QRS if the initial and terminal parts are discordant. Left axis deviation, as in RBBB, can also be seen but has a high probability to progress to complete AV block.[30]

Clinical Correlation. The occurrence of left bundle-branch block (LBBB) is much less frequent than that of RBBB in children. The most common cause is a result of surgery in and around the aortic valve or subvalve region (Figure 17). As in RBBB, inflammation secondary to infections (endocarditis) or immunologic injury from myocarditis can result in LBBB. Additionally, the presence of a nodoventricular fiber (Mahaim) results in a LBBB pattern by virtue of "preexcitation" of the RV apex after the atrial depolarization began traversing the AVN but before entering the left bundle branch (Figure 18). Aberrant conduction during the initiation of SVT can result in the appearance of a LBBB tachycardia. If the tachycardia is not sustained, several initial beats can demonstrate this morphology.[68] Certain types of familial cardiomyopathy progressing from LBBB to complete AV block were also reported.[63] The presence of LBBB in the absence of other known heart disease should be thoroughly investigated. Exercise study and 24-hour ambulatory monitoring should be performed

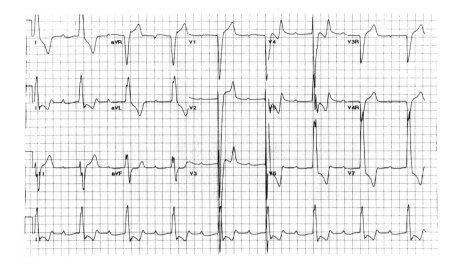

Figure 17. LBBB. This tracing is from a 16-year-old who recently underwent aortic valve replacement with an artificial valve. There is apparent sinus bradycardia at 50 bpm (1200 milliseconds) with a PR interval of 440 milliseconds and LBBB. Careful scrutiny of the tracing will reveal a deformity at the very end of the QRS that occurs exactly 600 milliseconds following the previous P wave. Thus there is actually 2:1 AV block with first-degree AV block and LBBB. During EP study prior to implantation of a permanent pacemaker, the PR interval delay was found to be secondary to HV prolongation (His-Purkinje system disease) rather than intranodal delay (LSRA-His was 90 milliseconds).

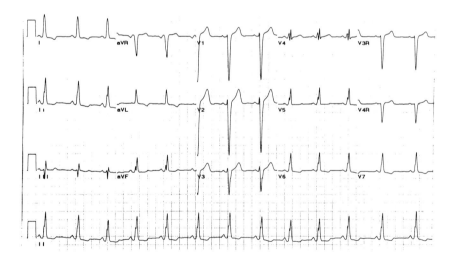

Figure 18. LBBB. This tracing is from a 14-year-old girl referred for "fast heart beats." Sinus rhythm with LBBB is seen. The PR interval is 120 milliseconds, normal for age. Treadmill exercise testing demonstrated gradual lengthening of the PR interval with continued LBBB at heart rates greater than 160 bpm. A diagnosis of a Mahaim fiber (nodoventricular) was suspected and confirmed at EP study.

to determine episodes of complete AV block. An echocardiogram to eval-uate myocardial function for the presence of occult cardiomyopathy is also appropriate. Pacemaker implantation should be performed in the presence of syncope or progressive AV block.

Left Anterior Hemiblock

Electrocardiogram Criteria

1. Duration of the QRS is only minimally affected (prolongation by <20 milliseconds).
2. The mean frontal plane axis of the QRS is more negative than −30° (negative in lead II).
3. Small q waves in leads I and especially in aVL.
4. Tall R waves in aVL as a result of unopposed terminal activation of the anterolateral wall of the LV.[30]

Normally, the LV is depolarized by two simultaneous wavefronts acti-vating the myocardium from below and moving upward to the left (left posterior fascicle) and another spreading in a superior to inferior orien-tation and to the left (anterior fascicle). Hemiblock is failure of conduction in one of the above-mentioned fascicles so that the simultaneous activation of the LV outlined above does not occur. The initial depolarization of the septum is not affected by this alteration. Left axis deviation that appears as

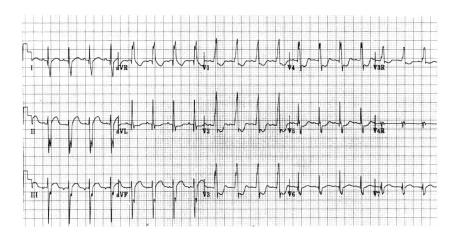

Figure 19. RBBB with left axis deviation (left anterior hemiblock). This record is from a 4-month-old infant with trisomy 21 who is postoperative repair of a complete AV canal defect. RBBB occurred as a result of the surgery. Left axis deviation was present in the initial ECG. Although there are q waves in leads I and aVL, this classic pattern may represent early activation of the left posterior fascicle. (See text for details.)

left anterior hemiblock occurs in atrial septal defect, primum/AV canal defect, tricuspid atresia, single atrium or single ventricle, double outlet RV, and in Noonan's syndrome. Left anterior hemiblock is also quite common in Chagas' or other forms of myocarditis, in the order of 50% to 80%.[69] It can also be seen in anomalous left coronary artery and as a normal variant.[30] Coexistent RBBB with left anterior hemiblock may occur after repair of tetralogy of Fallot and AV canal (Figure 19). Theories proposed for the occurrence of left anterior hemiblock in congenital heart disease include mechanical elongation and stretching of the anterior division of the left bundle branch, posterior displacement of the conduction system by the septal defect, anomalous development of the anterior division, interruption of the anterior division by anomalous insertion of the chordae tendineae of the mitral valve, and faster conduction through the posterior division by virtue of an early "take off" of the posterior division seen in some autopsy specimens.[69] No treatment is indicated for left anterior hemiblock regardless of whether it occurs in isolation or with complete RBBB.

Left Posterior Hemiblock

Electrocardiogram Criteria

1. Mild degree of right axis deviation with the frontal plane QRS axis falling between +90 and +180°.
2. Small q waves in leads II, III, and aVF because the initial forces are directed upward through the anterior fascicle.
3. Minimal prolongation of the QRS.

In left posterior hemiblock, the posteroinferior aspect of the LV is activated after the wavefront exits the anterosuperior aspect of the ventricle from the anterior fascicle. In the absence of RV hypertrophy, which can cause right axis deviation, the diagnosis can be made. It is very rare to see this pattern, although it was reported to occur in myocarditis and endocarditis and postoperatively.

Bifascicular Block

This category includes LBBB and RBBB with either left or right anterior hemiblock. As mentioned above, the most common occurrence of this pattern is RBBB with left anterior hemiblock occurring in postoperative tetralogy of Fallot. This occurs in between 8% and 23% of cases.[63] It can also be seen in myocarditis, endocarditis, and cardiomyopathy as well as in a progressive, heritable form resulting in complete AV block.[30,63] LBBB is considered a bifascicular block because it involves both the anterior and posterior fascicles of the left bundle. Except for Kearns-Sayre syndrome (see above), this disorder does not require any intervention.

References

1. Kugler JD. Sinus node dysfunction. In: Gillette PC, Garson AG Jr, eds. *Pediatric Arrhythmias, Electrophysiology and Pacing.* Philadelphia: WB Saunders Co; 1990:250–300.
2. Southall DP, Johnston F, Shinebourne EA, et al. 24 hour electrocardiographic study of heart rate and rhythm patterns in a population of healthy children. *Br Heart J* 1981;45:281–291.
3. Vincent GM. The heart rate of Romano-Ward syndrome patients. *Am Heart J* 1986;112:61–64.
4. Rosenbaum MB, Acunzo RS. Pseudo 2:1 atrioventricular block and T wave alternans in the long QT syndromes. *J Am Coll Cardiol* 1991;18:1363–1366.
5. Mehta AV, Chidambaram B, Garrett D. Familial symptomatic sinus bradycardia: Autosomal dominant inheritance. *Pediatr Cardiol* 1995;16:231–234.
6. Cowley CG, Tani LY, Judd VE, et al. Sinus node dysfunction in tuberous sclerosis. *Pediatr Cardiol* 1996;17:51–52.
7. Flinn CJ, Wolff GS, Cambell RM, et al. Natural history of supraventricular tachycardia in 182 children following the Mustard operation: A collaborative multicenter study. *J Am Coll Cardiol* 1983;1:613.
8. Byrum CJ, Bove EL, Sondheimer HM, et al. Sinus node shift after the Senning procedure compared with the Mustard procedure for transposition of the great arteries. *Am J Cardiol* 1987;60:346–350.
9. Deanfield J, Camm J, Macartney F, et al. Arrhythmia and late mortality after Mustard and Senning operation for transposition of the great arteries. An eight-year prospective study. *J Thorac Cardiovasc Surg* 1988;96:569–576.
10. Rhodes LA, Wernovsky G, Keane JF, et al. Arrhythmias and intracardiac conduction after the arterial switch operation. *J Thorac Cardiovasc Surg* 1995;109:303–310.
11. Kavey RE, Gaum WE, Byrum CJ, et al. Loss of sinus rhythm after total cavopulmonary connection. *Circulation* 1995;92:II304–II308.
12. Manning PB, Mayer JE Jr, Wernovsky G, et al. Staged operation to Fontan increases the incidence of sinoatrial node dysfunction. *J Thorac Cardiovasc Surg* 1996;111:833–839.
13. Meijboom F, Hess J, Szatmari A, et al. Long-term follow-up (9 to 20 years) after surgical closure of atrial septal defect at a young age. *Am J Cardiol* 1993;72:1431–1434.
14. Roos-Hesselink J, Perlroth MG, McGhie J, et al. Atrial arrhythmias in adults after repair of tetralogy of Fallot. Correlation with clinical, exercise, and echocardiographic findings. *Circulation* 1995;91:2214–2219.
15. Hesslein PS, Gutgesell HP, Gillette PC, et al. Exercise assessment of sinoatrial node function following the Mustard operation. *Am Heart J* 1982;103:351–357.
16. Nalos PC, Deng Z, Rosenthal ME, et al. Hemodynamic influences on sinus node recovery time: Effects of autonomic blockade. *J Am Coll Cardiol* 1986;7:1079–1086.
17. Benditt DG, Sakaguchi S, Goldstein MA, et al. Sinus node dysfunction: Pathophysiology, clinical features, evaluation and treatment. In: Zipes DP, Jalife J, eds. *Cardiac Electrophysiology From Cell to Bedside*, 2nd ed. Philadelphia: WB Saunders Co; 1995:1215–1247.
18. Gillette PC, Wampler DG, Shannon C, et al. Use of cardiac pacing after the Mustard operation for transposition of the great arteries. *J Am Coll Cardiol* 1986;7:138–141.

19. Albin G, Hayes DL, Holmes DR Jr. Sinus node dysfunction in pediatric and young adult patients: Treatment by implantation of a permanent pacemaker in 39 cases. *Mayo Clin Proc* 1985;60:667–672.
20. Dreifus LS, Fisch C, Griffin JC, et al. Guidelines for implantation of cardiac pacemakers and antiarrhythmia devices. A report of the American College of Cardiology/American Heart Association Task Force on Assessment of Diagnostic and Therapeutic Cardiovascular Procedures. (Committee on Pacemaker Implantation). *Circulation* 1991;84:455–467.
21. Silka MJ, Manwill JR, Kron J, et al. Bradycardia-mediated tachyarrhythmias in congenital heart disease and responses to chronic pacing at physiologic rates. *Am J Cardiol* 1990;65:488–493.
22. Gillette PC, Zeigler VL, Case CL, et al. Atrial antitachycardia pacing in children and young adults. *Am Heart J* 1991;122:844–849.
23. Eldar M, Griffin JC, VanHare GF, et al. Combined use of beta-adrenergic blocking agents and long-term cardiac pacing for patients with the long QT syndrome. *J Am Coll Cardiol* 1992;20:830–837.
24. Locati EH, Schwartz PJ. The idiopathic long QT syndrome: Therapeutic management. *Pacing Clin Electrophysiol* 1992;15:1374–1379.
25. Sra JS, Jazayeri MR, Avitall B, et al. Comparison of cardiac pacing with drug therapy in the treatment of neurocardiogenic (vasovagal) syncope with bradycardia or asystole. *N Engl J Med* 1993;328:1085–1090.
26. Grubb BP, Temesy-Armos P, Moore J, et al. Head-upright tilt-table testing in evaluation and management of the malignant vasovagal syndrome. *Am J Cardiol* 1992;69:904–908.
27. Kosinski DJ, Grubb BP, Elliott L, et al. Treatment of malignant neurocardiogenic syncope with dual chamber cardiac pacing and fluoxetine hydrochloride. *Pacing Clin Electrophysiol* 1995;18:1455–1457.
28. Fisch C. In: *Electrocardiography of Arrhythmias*. Philadelphia: Lea & Febiger; 1990:264–288.
29. Milstein S, Buetikofer J, Lesser J, et al. Cardiac asystole: A manifestation of neurally mediated hypotension-bradycardia. *J Am Coll Cardiol* 1989;14:1626–1632.
30. Garson A Jr. Arrhythmias. In: *The Electrocardiogram in Infants and Children: A Systematic Approach*. Philadelphia: Lea & Febiger; 1983:195–375.
31. Scott O, Williams GJ, Fiddler GI. Results of 24 hour ambulatory monitoring of electrocardiogram in 131 healthy boys aged 10 to 13 years. *Br Heart J* 1980;44:304–308.
32. Opie LH. In: *Drugs for the Heart*, 3rd ed. Philadelphia: WB Saunders Co; 1991:186–187.
33. Ross BD. First and second degree atrioventricular block. In: Gillette PC, Garson AG Jr, eds. *Pediatric Arrhythmias, Electrophysiology and Pacing*. Philadelphia: WB Saunders Co; 1990:301–305.
34. Prystowsky EN, Page RL. In: *Electrophysiology of the Sinoatrial and Atrioventricular Nodes*. New York: Alan R Liss; 1988:259–277.
35. Rardon DP, Miles WM, Mitrani RD, et al. In: Zipes DP, Jalife J, eds. *Cardiac Electrophysiology: From Cell to Bedside*, 2nd ed. Philadelphia: WB Saunders Co; 1995:935–942.
36. Bharati S, Lev M. Congenital abnormalities of the conduction system in sudden death in young adults. *J Am Coll Cardiol* 1986;8:1096–1104.
37. Thakur AK. Complete heart block as a first manifestation of acute rheumatic fever. *Indian H Journal* 1996;48:428–429.
38. Lillihei CW, Sellers RD, Bonnabeau RC, et al. Chronic postsurgical complete heart block. With particular reference to prognosis, management, and a new P-wave pacemaker. *J Thorac Cardiovasc Surg* 1963;46:436–456.

39. Fryda RJ, Kaplan S, Helmsworth JD. Postoperative complete heart block in children. *Br Heart J* 1971;33:456–462.
40. Ziady GM, Hallidie-Smith KA, Goodwin JF. Conduction disturbances after surgical closure of ventricular septal defect. *Br Heart J* 1972;34:1199–1204.
41. Weindling SN, Saul JP, Gamble WJ, et al. Duration of complete heart block after congenital heart surgery. *J Am Coll Cardiol* 1994;23:1A–484A.
42. Kertesz N, McQuinn T, Collins E, et al. Surgical atrioventricular block in 888 congenital heart operations: New implications for early implantation of a permanent pacemaker. *Pacing Clin Electrophysiol* 1996;19:613.
43. Driscoll DJ, Gillette PC, Hallman GL, et al. Management of surgical complete atrioventricular block in children. *Am J Cardiol* 1979;43:1175–1180.
44. Hofschire PJ, Nicoloff DM, Moller JH. Postoperative complete heart block in 64 children treated with and without cardiac pacing. *Am J Cardiol* 1977;39:559–562.
45. Moss AJ, Klyman G, Emmanouilides GC. Late onset complete heart block. Newly recognized sequela of cardiac surgery. *Am J Cardiol* 1972;30:884–887.
46. Nishimura RA, Callahan MJ, Holmes DR Jr, et al. Transient atrioventricular block after open-heart surgery for congenital heart disease. *Am J Cardiol* 1984;53:198–201.
47. Hurwitz RA, Riemenschneider TA, Moss AJ. Chronic postoperative heart block in children. *Am J Cardiol* 1968;21:185–189.
48. Schmidt KG, Ulmer HE, Silverman NH, et al. Perinatal outcome of fetal complete atrioventricular block: A multicenter experience. *J Am Coll Cardiol* 1991;91:1360–1366.
49. Michaelsson M, Engle MD. Congenital complete heart block: An international study of the natural history. *Cardiovasc Clin* 1972;4:85–101.
50. Nakamura FF, Nadas AS. Complete heart block in infants and children. *N Engl J Med* 1964;270:1261–1268.
51. McCue CM, Mantakas ME, Tinglestad JB, et al. Congenital heart block in newborns of mothers with connective tissue disease. *Circulation* 1977;56:82–90.
52. Waltuck J, Buyon JP. Autoantibody-associated congenital heart block: Outcome in mothers and children. *Ann Intern Med* 1994;120:544–551.
53. Huhta JC, Maloney JD, Ritter DG, et al. Complete atrioventricular block in patients with atrioventricular discordance. *Circulation* 1983;67:1374–1377.
54. Daliento L, Corrado D, Buja G, et al. Rhythm and conduction disturbances in isolated, congenitally corrected transposition of the great arteries. *Am J Cardiol* 1986;58:314–318.
55. Michaelsson M, Jonzon A, Riesenfeld T. Isolated congenital complete atrioventricular block in adult life. A prospective study. *Circulation* 1995;92:442–449.
56. Escher E, Michaelsson M. QT interval in congenital complete heart block. *Pediatr Cardiol* 1983;4:121–124.
57. Winkler RB, Freed MD, Nadas AS. Exercise-induced ventricular ectopy in children and young adults with complete heart block. *Am Heart J* 1980;99:87–92.
58. Kertesz NJ, Friedman R, Colan SD, et al. Preservation of enhanced left ventricular function and normal geometry in asymptomatic pediatric patients with congenital complete atrioventricular block. *Circulation* 1996;94:I-538.
59. Reybrouck T, Vanden Eynde B, Dumoulin M, et al. Cardiorespiratory response to exercise in congenital complete atrioventricular block. *Am J Cardiol* 1989;64:896–899.
60. Karpawich PP, Gillette PC, Garson A Jr, et al. Congenital complete atrioventricular block: Clinical and electrophysiologic predictors of need for pacemaker insertion. *Am J Cardiol* 1981;48:1098–1102.

61. Fisch, C. Electrocardiography and vectorcardiography. In: Braunwald E, ed. *Heart Disease. A Textbook of Cardiovascular Medicine,* 4th ed. Philadelphia: WB Saunders Co; 1992:116–160.
62. Rowlands DJ. *Clinical Electrocardiography.* London: Gower Medical Publishing; 1991.
63. Ewing L. Bundle branch and fascicular blocks. In: Gillette PC, Garson AG Jr, eds. *Pediatric Arrhythmias, Electrophysiology and Pacing.* Philadelphia: WB Saunders Co; 1990:317–327.
64. Houyel L, Vaksmann G, Fournier A, et al. Ventricular arrhythmias after correction of ventricular septal defects: Importance of surgical approach. *J Am Coll Cardiol* 1990;16:1224–1228.
65. Scheinman MM, Goldschlager NF, Peters RW. Bundle branch block. *Cardiovasc Clin* 1980;11:57–80.
66. Corrado D, Nava A, Buja G, et al. Familial cardiomyopathy underlies syndrome of right bundle branch block, ST segment elevation and sudden death. *J Am Coll Cardiol* 1996;27:443–448.
67. Brugada P, Brugada J. Right bundle branch block, persistent ST segment elevation and sudden cardiac death: A distinct clinical and electrocardiographic syndrome. A multicenter report. *J Am Coll Cardiol* 1992;20:1391–1396.
68. Cecchin F, Fenrich AL, Friedman RA, et al. Wide QRS tachycardia in infancy: Left bundle branch block is common during supraventricular tachycardia. 1994;15:254.
69. Rosenbaum MB, Elizari MV, Lazzari JO. In: *The Hemiblocks.* Oldsmar, Fla; Tampa Tracings; 1970:91–155.

Chapter 5

Supraventricular Tachycardia Mechanisms and Natural History

Barbara J. Deal, MD

For several decades, supraventricular tachycardia (SVT) in pediatric patients was labeled as "paroxysmal atrial tachycardia," or "PAT," without further discrimination of underlying mechanisms. Clinical electrophysiology (EP) studies and the ability to cure most forms of SVT with radiofrequency (RF) catheter ablation techniques advanced our understanding of the various distinct mechanisms of SVT. Because the clinical setting, natural history, and treatment vary with each type of SVT, a clear understanding of the classification of SVT is essential.

Reentrant mechanisms account for the vast majority of clinical episodes of SVT.[1] A reentrant rhythm, by definition, can be initiated and terminated with pacing, allowing the study of types of tachycardia and response to drug therapy using pacing techniques. The reentrant circuit involves two distinct pathways with unidirectional block in one limb, allowing an electrical impulse to traverse the second limb and "reenter" the blocked pathway from the other direction. The classical example of reentrant SVT is atrioventricular (AV) reciprocating tachycardia, utilizing the AV node (AVN) as one limb and an accessory connection (AC) as the other pathway of the reentrant circuit. Automatic rhythms demonstrate enhanced abnormal automaticity or firing of a relatively discrete focus and account for less than 10% of clinical episodes of SVT. An automatic rhythm cannot be initiated and terminated with pacing techniques, although the automatic focus may be suppressed by more rapid

From Deal B, Wolff G, Gelband H, (eds.). *Current Concepts in Diagnosis and Management of Arrhythmias in Infants and Children.* Armonk, NY: Futura Publishing Co., Inc.; © 1998.

_____ Table 1 _____

Classification of SVT

AV reentrant tachycardia
    Orthodromic reciprocating
    Permanent form of junctional reciprocating
    Antidromic reciprocating
AVNRT
    Typical: slow-fast
    Atypical: fast-slow
Primary atrial tachycardia
    Atrial flutter
    Atrial reentrant
    Atrial fibrillation
    Automatic atrial
    Multifocal atrial

pacing rates. Triggered activity was identified as the mechanism underlying a small percentage of atrial tachycardias.[2]

Based on a combination of anatomic and EP considerations, Table 1 presents a simplified classification scheme for SVT. AV reentrant tachycardia utilizes an AC as an essential part of the tachycardia circuit, with the AVN usually participating as the other limb; tachycardia cannot continue if block occurs in any part of this circuit. AVN reentry tachycardia (AVNRT) involves a functional and anatomic dissociation of conduction within the AVN, allowing impulses to reenter the node retrogradely as depolarization proceeds simultaneously to the ventricles. Primary atrial tachycardia includes all forms of SVT where the electrical disturbance takes place within atrial tissue, and the AVN and ventricles are "bystanders," or not necessary for tachycardia to continue. A typical example of primary atrial tachycardia is atrial flutter (AF), where tachycardia persists in the setting of AV block.

The relative incidence of the various types of SVT varies with age (Table 2). In a large series of 704 adult patients undergoing EP studies, AVNRT

_____ Table 2 _____

Relative Incidence of Types of SVT (%)

Study	Population	AV Nodal	AV Reentrant	Primary Atrial
Josephson and Wellens[1]	Adult	51	34	15
Wu et al[3]	Adult	72	13	15
Gillette[4]	Pediatric	24	33	42
Ko et al[5]	Pediatric	13	73	14
Naheed et al[6]	Fetal	—	73	27

accounted for 51% of SVT as reported by Josephson and Wellens.[1] In that series, AV reentry tachycardia was present in 34% and atrial tachycardia accounted for 15% of SVT mechanisms. Similarly, Wu and colleagues,[3] in a study of 69 adult patients excluding those with evidence of preexcitation, reported a slightly higher incidence of AVNRT (72%), with AV reentry in 13% and atrial reentry tachycardia in 15%. Patients with AC-mediated tachycardia tended to be younger, have faster heart rates in tachycardia, and to have no associated organic heart disease. Atrial tachycardia was often associated with organic heart disease. These authors concluded that older age and associated organic heart disease suggested an acquired anatomic basis for most atrial and some AVNRT, with stretch, fibrosis, and longitudinal dissociation of conduction providing part of the arrhythmia substrate; the low prevalence of organic heart disease and younger age at presentation in patients with AV reentrant SVT is consistent with a congenital anatomic basis for tachycardia.

Gillette[4] first reported on mechanisms of SVT in childhood in 1976, studying 35 patients aged 1 week to 18 years. Almost half of their population had either congenital heart disease or cardiomyopathy. In that series, a higher incidence of atrial tachycardia was identified, 42%, likely reflecting the frequently associated heart disease. AV reentry was present in 33%, and AVN tachycardia was present in 24% of patients in their series. Ko and associates[5] reported the results of transesophageal studies in 135 children with SVT presenting at a median age of 0.5 years, excluding patients with operated congenital heart disease or myopathy. SVT using ACs was present in 73% of patients, with atrial tachycardia in 14% and AVN reentry in 13%. SVT using an AC was present in over 80% of neonates. Primary atrial tachycardia had a relatively even distribution across all age groups, while AVNRT rarely appeared before age 2 years. Recently, Naheed and coworkers[6] reported the mechanisms of tachycardia in 30 fetuses, evaluated by echo-Doppler in utero and transesophageal pacing studies in the neonatal period. AV reentrant tachycardia was the predominant mechanism of SVT in the fetus, present in 73%, with the remainder having AF. AVNRT was not identified in their series.

These studies convincingly demonstrate an age-related incidence of tachycardia mechanisms, with SVT due to an AC the predominant mechanism in the fetus and young child, and AVNRT typically appearing about age 5–10 years, increasing in frequency to become the predominant mechanisms among adults. Primary atrial tachycardia accounts for 10% to 15% of SVT at all ages.

Atrioventricular Reentrant Tachycardia

Tachycardia utilizing an AC as one limb of the reentrant circuit is the most frequent type of SVT encountered in infancy and early childhood. Wolff-Parkinson-White (WPW) syndrome is diagnosed when the AC is apparent during sinus rhythm, resulting in a slurred upstroke of

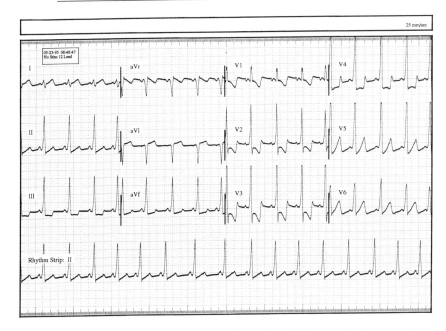

Figure 1. Preexcitation in 2-year-old boy. Note short PR interval with slurred up-stroke to QRS, especially in leads I and V_1, with negative delta wave in AV_L. QRS duration is slightly prolonged for age.

the QRS (the delta wave) and a shortened PR interval (due to preexcitation of the ventricle via the AC) (Figure 1). The incidence of WPW syndrome in the general adult population is 0.15% to 0.3% and among children with congenital heart disease is 0.3% to 1.0%.[7,8] However, at least 50% of children with SVT utilizing an AC have no apparent preexcitation during sinus rhythm and are described as having "concealed" ACs. In almost 90% of AV reentrant tachycardia, conduction proceeds antegradely via the AVN to the ventricles and returns retrogradely via the AC; this is termed orthodromic reciprocating tachycardia (ORT), (orthodromic refers to conduction in the "same direction" as normal AVN conduction). A variant of ORT is the permanent form of junctional reciprocating tachycardia (PJRT), first described by Coumel[9] in 1967. The AC is typically located in the posteroseptal region of the heart, with very slow conduction resulting in a slower but incessant form of SVT, which may produce cardiomyopathy if unrecognized. In less than 10% of patients with reciprocating tachycardia, tachycardia proceeds from the atria over an AC to the ventricles and returns via the AVN, known as antidromic reciprocating tachycardia (opposite direction).[10] Subtle variants of preexcitation, including atriofascicular (Mahaim) connections, are reviewed comprehensively by Gallagher et al.[11] Primary atrial tachycardia, such as AF or fibrillation, may be conducted to the ventricles over an AC; if AC conduction is rapid, ventricular fibrillation may result.[12,13]

Electrocardiogram Criteria

1. ORT (Figure 2)
   a. Typically regular, narrow QRS morphology, although rate-related bundle branch block may occur in as many as 15% to 30% of episodes.
   b. SVT rates 150–300 beats per minute (bpm) (neonates, average rate 280 bpm).
   c. Retrograde P waves following QRS, with RP interval greater than 70 milliseconds.
   d. Terminates in presence of AV block.

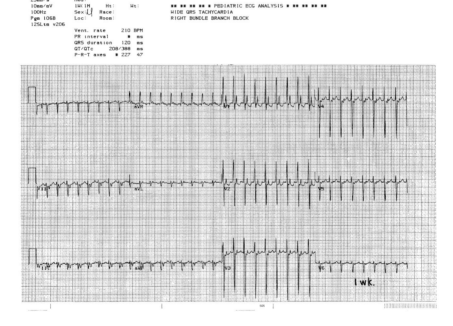

Figure 2. ORT in 1-week-old infant with regular narrow QRS tachycardia at 210 bpm. Note retrograde sharp P waves following QRS complex, best seen in leads II, III, AV$_F$, V$_1$, and V$_2$. RP interval is approximately 80 milliseconds.

2. PJRT (Figure 3).
   a. A variant of ORT, with a slowly conducting AC resulting in incessant tachycardia.
   b. Predominantly regular narrow QRS morphology.
   c. SVT rates 130–220 bpm; catecholamine sensitivity results in rate variability with exertion or stress.
   d. Retrograde P waves with long RP interval, usually greater than 150 milliseconds (PR less than RP interval).
   e. Typically inverted retrograde P waves in leads II, III, and AVF.
   f. Terminates in presence of AV block.
   g. Spontaneous reinitiation with sinus acceleration.
3. Antidromic reciprocating tachycardia (Figure 4).
   a. Wide QRS tachycardia.
   b. Preexcited QRS morphology identical to preexcitation pattern during sinus rhythm.
   c. 1:1 AV relation.
   d. Terminates in presence of AV block.

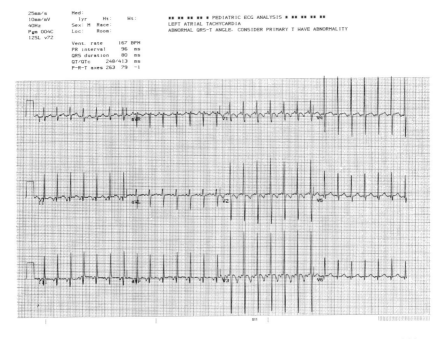

Figure 3. Permanent form of junctional reciprocating tachycardia in 1-year-old boy with regular narrow QRS tachycardia at 170 bpm. Retrograde P waves are seen as inverted P waves in leads II, III, AV$_F$ with long RP interval (280 milliseconds).

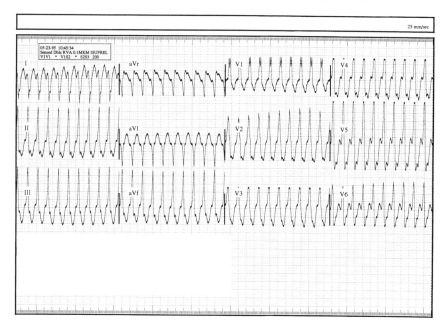

Figure 4. Antidromic tachycardia in same patient as Figure 1. Note similarity of QRS complexes during tachycardia to those present in sinus rhythm. There is 1:1 AV conduction with P waves visible in lead II.

Clinical Correlation

More than half of first episodes of SVT are due to an AC present in childhood and are more common among males.[14] Associated structural heart disease is present in approximately 20% of patients, most commonly Ebstein's anomaly of the tricuspid valve.[15] A hereditary contribution to the development of ACs is suggested by the rare occurrence of familial preexcitation.[16] The mean heart rate for SVT in infancy is 280 bpm, ranging from 215–350 bpm.[15,17] In a multicenter study of 321 infants with SVT and preexcitation, the QRS was narrow during SVT in 98% of electrocardiograms (ECGs) available for review (ORT).[18] Atrial fibrillation is extremely rare in infancy, noted in only 0.4% of infants in the multicenter study. AF, although not common, is present in 1% to 4% of infants with preexcitation.

Up to 50% of infants will present with evidence of congestive heart failure, including tachycardia, pallor, irritability, and poor feeding.[8,15,19] Unexplained hypothermia with poor perfusion, usually interpreted as sepsis but with negative cultures, may occur. In the older infant, irritability associated with vomiting and sometimes diarrhea is not uncommon. In approximately 20% of infants, SVT is detected during routine examination without symptoms.[15,17,19]

In the older child, the heart rate during tachycardia ranges from 160–280 bpm, with shorter durations of tachycardia, due to both spontaneous termination and earlier medical intervention. Orthodromic tachycardia with a narrow QRS morphology remains the most common mechanism, although antidromic tachycardia occurs in 5% of patients.[10] Frequently, the complaint is of palpitations or chest or abdominal pain. Syncope, particularly with exertion, may occur infrequently, but the presence of congestive heart failure beyond infancy is extremely uncommon.[19] The development of heart failure suggests a slower, incessant tachycardia of long duration, as seen with the permanent form of junctional reciprocating tachycardia.

The peak age for occurrence of SVT presenting in childhood is the first 2 months of life, with almost 40% of first episodes of SVT taking place in this period.[20] The frequency of SVT decreases markedly through infancy, with at least two thirds of infants no longer having SVT at 1 year of age.[8,15,19,21,22] Following the occurrence of SVT in infancy, approximately 40% to 70% of patients followed long term will have recurrences of tachycardia.[15,20,22] Age-related peaks both in the occurrence and recurrence of tachycardia episodes appear in the 5- to 8- and 10- to 13-year-old age groups.[20,22] In addition, tachycardia episodes presenting in these older age groups tend to be persistent throughout childhood.[20] The disappearance of preexcitation during sinus rhythm is not predictive of subsequent recurrences of SVT.[15,20] Possible explanations for this pattern include changes in the conduction characteristics of both the AVN and the AC, together with changes in the initiating events for tachycardia.[23,24] Both conduction and refractory periods of the AC prolong with age.[23,25,26] Dunnigan et al[24] found that atrial extrasystoles and sinus acceleration were common initiating events in infants, compared to atrial and ventricular extrasystoles and sinus pauses with junctional escapes in the older child.

The risk of atrial or ventricular fibrillation increases in the second decade, with a small percentage of patients, particularly adolescent males, presenting with cardiac arrest as the initial arrhythmia.[12,13,27–29] The risk of cardiac arrest due to preexcitation is estimated to be ~1.5 of 1000 patient years.[30] The mechanism is ventricular fibrillation following the rapid conduction of atrial fibrillation to the ventricles over an AC (Figure 5A and 5B). In a study of 31 patients with WPW syndrome and ventricular fibrillation, Klein and associates[12] identified risk including atrial fibrillation and reciprocating tachycardia, multiple ACs, and a shortest preexcited RR interval during atrial fibrillation less than 250 milliseconds. In this series, ventricular fibrillation was the initial manifestation of WPW syndrome in 10% of their patients, occurring in three children less than 16 years old. Montoya and colleagues[13] reported a similar series of 23 patients with a mean age of 31 ± 12 years, with risk factors including male gender, per-

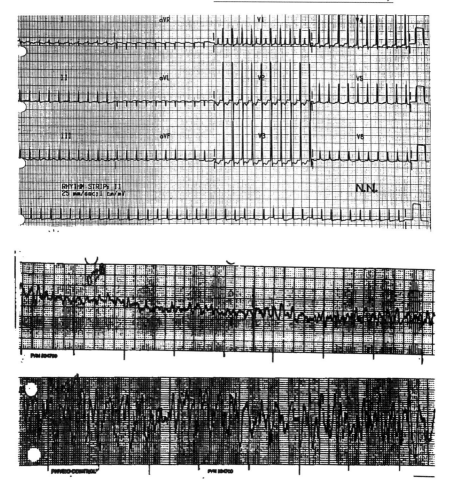

Figure 5. A: ECG during first clinical recurrence of SVT in 1-month-old male with known WPW treated with digoxin. Regular narrow QRS tachycardia at 250 bpm with retrograde P waves seen in V_1; RP interval about 120 milliseconds. **B**: Rhythm strip in same patient, obtained within minutes of ECG shown above. Ventricular fibrillation developed spontaneously prior to any intervention. Presumably ORT triggered atrial fibrillation, with rapid antegrade conduction via AC to ventricles, resulting in ventricular fibrillation.

manent preexcitation, a shortest preexcited RR interval during atrial fibrillation less than 220 milliseconds, and multiple ACs. Timmermans and coworkers[28] reviewed 15 patients with WPW and a history of cardiac arrest: ventricular fibrillation was the first manifestation of WPW in 53% and was more common among males and patients with septal ACs. In a series of 10 children with WPW and cardiac arrest reported by Bromberg,[29] ventricular fibrillation was the initial arrhythmia in 2 patients. A shortest preexcited RR interval <220 milliseconds during atrial fibrillation was highly sensitive but not specific for patients with cardiac arrest.[29] A retrospective study by the Pediatric Electrophysiology Society[27] identified 42 children with a cardiac arrest due to WPW syndrome between 1969 and 1993. The median age at cardiac arrest was 10 years and ranged from 1 day to 21 years. Structural heart disease was present in 31% of patients, and 64% of patients were males. Mortality was 36%, with significant neurological damage in 33% of survivors. The cardiac arrest was the initial documented arrhythmia in 48% of patients, although 25% of these patients were known to have preexcitation on ECG. In the 15 patients with an initial cardiac arrest and no known WPW syndrome, 47% (7/15) had prior symptoms of palpitations or syncope without further evaluation. Thus, it appears that young patients with WPW syndrome may have a relatively higher risk of cardiac arrest as the initial presentation in almost 50% of this series. Clearly, the overall risk of sudden death remains low, but problems remain in identifying asymptomatic WPW syndrome patients and defining risk in patients known to have preexcitation.

Atrioventricular Nodal Reentrant Tachycardia

As the name implies, AVNRT is a reentrant rhythm within the AVN, with two functionally and probably anatomically distinct AVN pathways.[31,32] The "compact AVN" lies at the apex of the triangle of Koch and penetrates the central fibrous body to become the bundle of His. Current thinking, supported by the results of catheter ablation techniques, supports the presence of additional transitional AVN cells, with "fast pathway" input located in the anterior atrial septum, superior to the compact node, and "slow pathway" fibers located inferior and posterior to the compact node, near the os of the coronary sinus (CS). Conduction during normal sinus rhythm occurs predominantly over the "fast" pathway, with a normal PR interval. Due to a discrepancy in refractory periods, a premature impulse may block in the fast pathway and conduct over the slow pathway. If sufficient delay is present, allowing the fast pathway to recover function, this impulse may reenter the fast pathway in a retrograde fashion, allowing circus-movement tachycardia. This is the most common type of AVN reentry, labeled the "slow-fast" form, accounting for almost 90% of clinical episodes of AVNRT.[1] Atypical AVN reentry results from antegrade conduction over the fast pathway, with retrograde conduction via the slow pathway (fast-slow), resulting in a long RP interval. Catheter ablation in the region of the CS os is successful in modifying slow pathway function and eliminating tachycardia.[33]

Electrocardiogram Criteria

1. "Typical" AVN reentry (slow-fast) (Figure 6).
   a. Regular, narrow QRS tachycardia at rates from 150–300 bpm (mean, 170 bpm in older patients).
   b. Retrograde P waves within QRS or at terminal end of QRS; RP interval <70 milliseconds.
   c. Retrograde P waves may simulate an S wave in leads II, III, AVF, and an r′ in lead V_1.
   d. SVT may persist with 2:1 AV conduction, although rare.
2. "Atypical" AVN reentry (fast-slow).
   a. Narrow QRS tachycardia.
   b. Retrograde P waves with long RP interval and short PR interval.
   c. Negative P waves in leads II, III, AVF, and V_4–V_6.

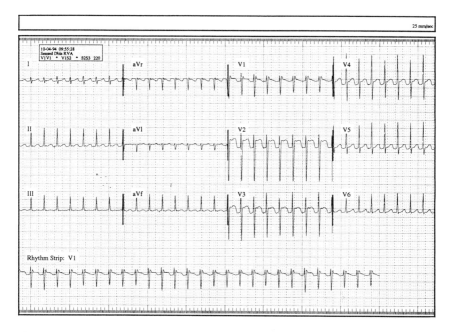

Figure 6. AVN reentry SVT in 5-year-old girl with regular, narrow QRS tachycardia. Retrograde P waves are not easily seen, but may be recognized at the end of the QRS in leads II, III, AV_F, with RP interval of 40 milliseconds. Note rsr′ pattern in lead V_1 often seen in AVNRT.

Clinical Correlation

AVNRT is not associated with structural heart disease and is slightly more common among females.[1] In the older child, episodes of AVNRT are paroxysmal and may be terminated frequently with vagal maneuvers. Although it is an uncommon arrhythmia among toddlers, in this age group episodes may occur frequently throughout the day without significant cardiac symptoms. Continuous ambulatory monitoring may show numerous bursts of tachycardia, with either right or left bundle branch aberrancy at the onset of episodes, mimicking ventricular tachycardia. The observation of rapid pounding in the neck is common with this arrhythmia and may be a useful clinical marker.[34]

As discussed above, AVNRT has a striking age-related incidence, suggesting developmental changes in AV conduction are important in its genesis. AVN reentry was not diagnosed in a series of 30 fetuses with SVT evaluated postnatally by Naheed et al[26] and was present during infancy in only 3 of 137 patients (2.2%) reported by Ko et al.[5] By age 6–10 years, AVN reentry accounts for 31% of SVT mechanisms[5] and more than 50% of SVT in adult patients.[13] Dual AVN physiology was reported in 35% to 46% of children,[35,36] and up to 85% of adults.[1]

Therapeutic options for AVNRT includes vagal maneuvers, digoxin, β-blockers, calcium channel blockers, and catheter modification of the slow pathway of the AVN.

Primary Atrial Tachycardia

As described above, the electrical disturbance in primary atrial tachycardia is confined to atrial tissue, with tachycardia persisting in the presence of AV block. These tachycardias are relatively uncommon, accounting for up to 15% of SVT, but occur at all ages. The EP mechanisms are diverse, including reentrant, automatic, and triggered activity.

Atrial Flutter

Typical AF (type I) is a regular, reentrant rhythm originating in the right atrium (RA). Fixed anatomic obstacles, particularly the inferior vena caval orifice and the os of the CS, in addition to functionally slowed (anisotropic) conduction contribute to the reentrant circuit. Current studies of typical AF describe a counterclockwise activation circuit proceeding from the posteroinferior RA, up the atrial septum, and then coursing inferiorly via the crista terminalis.[37] Anatomically guided ablation in the area of the posteroinferior RA successfully terminated AF.[38]

Electrocardiogram Criteria: Atrial Flutter (Figure 7)

1. Rapid, regular, sawtooth flutter waves (monomorphic negative or biphasic P waves visible in leads II, III, and AVF).

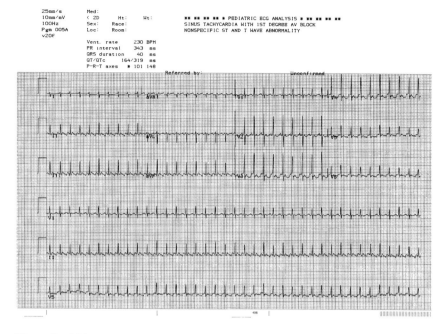

25mm/s
10mm/mV
100Hz
Pgm 005A
v20F

Med:
< 2D   Ht: Wt:
Sex: Race:
Loc: Room:

** ** ** ** * PEDIATRIC ECG ANALYSIS * ** ** ** **
SINUS TACHYCARDIA WITH 1ST DEGREE AV BLOCK
NONSPECIFIC ST AND T WAVE ABNORMALITY

Vent. rate   230 BPM
PR interval   343 ms
QRS duration   40 ms
QT/QTc   164/319 ms
P-R-T axes   * 101 148

Figure 7. AF in a neonate. Sawtooth flutter waves are best seen in leads II, III, and AVF. The atrial rate is 460 bpm with 2:1 AV conduction.

2. Atrial rates between 250 and 480 bpm.
3. Variable AV conduction, usually 2:1

Atypical AF (type II) has similar atrial rates, but clockwise activation proceeding caudally from the superior RA along the atrial septum, resulting in positive P waves in the inferior leads.

Clinical Correlation

AF has a bimodal distribution in childhood, appearing in the neonate without structural heart disease, and in the older child or adolescent in the setting of structural heart disease.[39-42]

Neonatal AF is often recognized in utero or at birth, with congestive heart failure developing probably due to delay in recognition of the arrhythmia.[40] Associated structural heart disease is uncommon, although recent studies identified a significant association with accessory AV connections.[6,43,44] Naheed and colleagues[6] induced SVT with conduction over an AC in five of seven infants presenting with in utero AF. This suggests that the immature fetal atrium may be particularly vulnerable to the development of flutter resulting from rapid ventriculoatrial conduction. Conversion to sinus rhythm may be effectively achieved with low-energy direct-current cardioversion, transesophageal pacing, or digoxin.[39–41] Late recurrences of AF are uncommon,[39,40] making chronic prophylactic therapy unnecessary in most cases.

AF associated with structural heart disease accounts for almost 95% of flutter beyond infancy. The highest risk groups are patients following Mustard, Senning, or Fontan procedures, repair of secundum atrial septal defect, repair of tetralogy of Fallot, mitral valve disease (rheumatic or surgical), and dilated cardiomyopathy. Distinction should be made between patients with typical AF with sawtooth flutter waves and the slower form of atrial reentrant tachycardia often seen following atrial surgery; the latter patients have a distinct ECG appearance and are discussed below. Flutter associated with heart disease tends to recur and is difficult to control medically[42,45–49]; the goal of therapy is to eliminate tachycardia and not merely to control the ventricular response. A multicenter collaborative study[42] of postoperative pediatric patients with AF demonstrated cardiac mortality in 20% of patients in whom drug therapy did not eliminate the arrhythmia versus 5% of patients with effective drug therapy, emphasizing the need for appropriate antiarrhythmic therapy. The development of flutter often indicates significant hemodynamic abnormalities. Resolution of flutter is achieved in more than half of patients following surgery to improve hemodynamics.[46,50] Besides sudden death, cardiac thrombosis and stroke are risks associated with AF in this population.[46–49]

Atrial Reentry Tachycardia

Atrial reentry tachycardia is a relatively rare arrhythmia, accounting for less than 8% of SVT in adults.[51] As the name implies, it is thought to be a reentrant rhythm localized to atrial tissue, although triggered activity is important in some cases.[52–54] Tachycardia may be reproducibly initiated and terminated with pacing and persists in the presence of AV block. In the setting of structural heart disease, the distinction between atrial reentry tachycardia and AF is largely based on the slower atrial rates in atrial reentry and the presence of discrete or low amplitude P waves versus typical sawtooth flutter waves.[55]

Electrocardiogram Criteria: Atrial Reentry (Figure 8A)

1. P wave, usually distinct from sinus P wave, precedes QRS complex
2. Atrial rates typically less than 250 bpm.
3. PR interval usually prolonged, related to rate of SVT.
4. SVT persists with AV block, allowing identification of P waves.
5. Variable RR intervals may occur due to varying AV conduction.

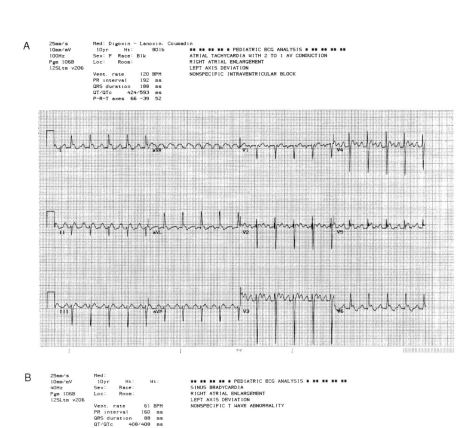

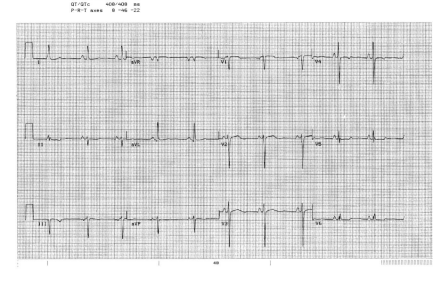

Figure 8. A: Atrial reentry tachycardia in 10-year-old girl status post-Fontan procedure. Note large discrete P waves with a short isoelectric phase between P waves, best seen in leads II and AVF. Atrial rate is 240 bpm with 2:1 AV conduction. **B**: Same patient, ECG following conversion of atrial tachycardia. Note sinus bradycardia with different P-wave morphology. Left axis deviation and decreased right ventricular voltage typical of tricuspid atresia.

6. Although usually narrow QRS complexes, wide QRS tachycardia may occur due to rate-related bundle branch block or preexisting heart disease.

Clinical Correlation

Atrial reentry tachycardia is most common in the setting of structural heart disease, particularly postoperative patients and those with cardiomyopathy, although it may occasionally occur in the otherwise normal heart.[5-48,56,57] In the postoperative patient, this arrhythmia is often diagnosed as AF, although the atrial rate is usually less than 250 bpm, and flutter waves are not present. The ECG features of atrial tachycardia in the postoperative congenital heart disease population were summarized by Muller[55] into three groups. The most common ECG appearance (37%) showed no clearly visible P waves, with atrial rates of 170–290 bpm. The second most common presentation showed clearly detectable P waves with an isoelectric baseline between P waves, with atrial rates of 158–375 bpm. Only 30% of postoperative patients demonstrated typical

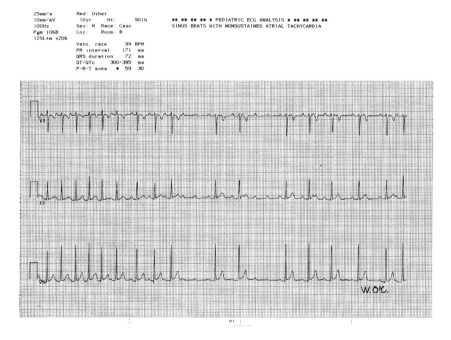

Figure 9. Atrial reentry tachycardia in 10-year-old boy with no structural heart disease. Note discrete P waves with morphology similar to sinus P waves. Atrial rate is 190 bpm with variable AV conduction.

flutter waves in leads II, III, and AVF, with atrial rates of 230–375 bpm. As AV conduction is typically 2:1 or greater, this arrhythmia should be suspected when a heart rate greater than 100 bpm is detected during a routine examination of the postoperative Mustard, Senning, or Fontan patient (Figure 8A). Undetected, it will result in the development of congestive heart failure, thrombosis, neurologic events, or sudden death.[45,46,49] Extensive atrial suture lines, elevated atrial pressure, and anatomic obstacles within the atrium (superior and inferior vena caval orifices, tricuspid valve leaflet, CS os) are thought to be etiologic.[45–48] Medical management is frustrating, even with the use of type III antiarrhythmic agents, but occasionally success is achieved.[49] The prevention of bradycardia by atrial pacing may significantly decrease the frequency of SVT.[58] Atrial antitachycardia pacemakers, catheter ablation, and surgical reoperation, including cryoablation in the posteroinferior RA, are other current treatment options.[50,59–62]

In the patient without structural heart disease, episodes of atrial reentry tachycardia are paroxysmal and often refractory to multiple medications (Figure 9). Adenosine-sensitive atrial tachycardia is described,[2] and these authors believe this response indicates triggered activity. When atrial activation indicates origin near the sinus node, with P waves similar to sinus P waves, this arrhythmia is called sinoatrial reentry.[63,64] RF catheter ablation and surgical resections were used successfully to eliminate this arrhythmia.[65–67]

Atrial Fibrillation

Atrial fibrillation is much less common than AF and also occurs much less frequently in children versus adults. Atrial fibrillation has a prevalence of less than 0.4% in patients under the age of 40 years, increasing to 5% to 9% between the ages 60 to 90 years.[68,69] The mechanism of atrial fibrillation is thought to be multiple reentrant wavelets, circulating concurrently,[70] perpetuated by dilated atria, shortened atrial refractoriness, and inhomogeneous conduction and refractoriness.

Electrocardiogram Criteria: Atrial Fibrillation (Figure 10)

1. Absence of discrete atrial activity.
2. Disorganized atrial activity at rates greater than 350 bpm, resulting in coarse or fine fibrillatory waves, best seen in V_1 and V_2.
3. "Irregularly irregular" ventricular response, due to variable AV conduction.

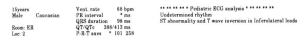

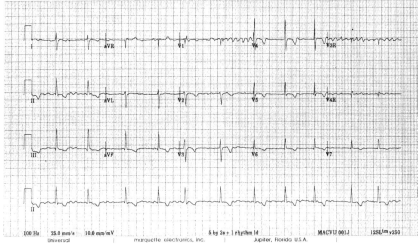

Figure 10. Atrial fibrillation in 15-year-old boy status post-Fontan procedure. Note disorganized atrial activity with coarse fibrillation seen in leads II and V_1. The RR interval is irregular.

Clinical Correlation

Atrial fibrillation in childhood occurs in the setting of structural heart disease, thyrotoxicosis, in association with SVT due to an AC and, rarely, in familial forms or associated with high vagal tone.[71-73] As reported by Radford and Izukawa,[71] associated structural heart disease most commonly includes cardiomyopathy (hypertrophic, dilated, and secondary to hemochromatosis of thalassemia), rheumatic mitral disease, Ebstein's anomaly, and postoperative Mustard, atrial septal defect, and tetralogy of Fallot. Cerebral embolic phenomena with significant sequelae occurred in 8.5% of patients in this series.[71] As with AF, the development of atrial fibrillation often signals hemodynamic deterioration, prompting a reevaluation of potentially correctable residual abnormalities. Atrial fibrillation associated with hypertrophic cardiomyopathy is associated with sudden death in addition to the risk of stroke.[74] Lone atrial fibrillation, occurring in the absence of identifiable heart disease or predisposing factors, is exceedingly uncommon in childhood, and was present in only one patient in Radford's series.[71,75,76] The occurrence of familial atrial fibrillation was described, as was fibrillation precipitated by vagal tone resulting in sinus bradycardia.[73]

The development of atrial fibrillation during an episode of reciprocating SVT is estimated to occur in at least 12% of adult patients[77] and may be somewhat less in childhood. In the presence of an AC capable of rapid antegrade conduction, atrial fibrillation may be conducted rapidly to the ventricles and precipitate ventricular fibrillation.[12,78,79] This arrhythmia is one presumed mechanism of cardiac arrest in patients with WPW syndrome and forms the basis for the recommendation to avoid digoxin in the presence of preexcitation. Digoxin, although slowing conduction at the AVN, is capable of enhancing antegrade conduction across an AC, increasing the risk of ventricular fibrillation developing from atrial fibrillation or flutter.[78]

Automatic Atrial Tachycardia

Automatic atrial tachycardia is a chronic form of incessant tachycardia due to inappropriately rapid firing of an ectopic atrial focus.[80-82] Although accounting for only 4% to 6% of SVT, it is an important cause of cardiomyopathy.[83-89]

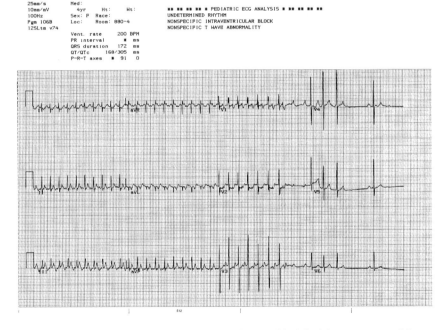

Figure 11. Automatic atrial tachycardia in 4-year-old girl without structural heart disease. Note discrete P waves with abnormal morphology and notching and long PR interval. Atrial rate is initially 240 bpm, with cool down prior to termination. Atrial tachycardia persists in presence of AV block.

Electrocardiogram Criteria: Automatic Atrial Tachycardia (Figure 11)

1. Distinctly visible P waves with abnormal morphology (notching) or axis compared with sinus P waves.
2. Prolonged PR interval, particularly with faster rates.
3. Atrial rates 130–280 bpm.
4. Atrial rate variability, with "warm up" at initiation and "cool down" prior to termination.
5. Atrial tachycardia persists with AV block.
6. Rate-related bundle branch block during fastest rates may occur.
7. QRS complexes may be normal, but may show left ventricular hypertrophy and strain with ventricular dysfunction.

Clinical Correlation

Automatic atrial tachycardia is usually identified in patients with structurally normal hearts and is present in all age groups. Heart rates in tachycardia range from 130–300 bpm and may exhibit striking catecholamine sensitivity, with rapid increases in heart rate with stress or exertion. Recognition of abnormal P-wave morphology is critical to the diagnosis, as many foci are located in the RA and may have a normal P-wave axis.[86–88,90–92] More than one ectopic focus is present in up to 20% to 30% of patients.[88,92,93]

Tachycardia-induced cardiomyopathy is often the presenting symptom of automatic atrial tachycardia, with tachycardia mistakenly thought to represent sinus tachycardia secondary to congestive failure[83–85,87–89] (Figure 12). The development of heart failure is related to both the heart rate and the duration of tachycardia; most patients with congestive heart failure have heart rates >140 bpm.[83,86–88,90,91] Multiple authors report the reversibility of heart failure with control of the arrhythmia, indicating tachycardia is the etiology of myocardial dysfunction.[83–85,88] In a review of patients listed for heart transplantation with the diagnosis of "idiopathic dilated cardiomyopathy," Zimmerman and associates[89] identified automatic atrial tachycardia in 27% of patients; an average heart rate at presentation >150 bpm was highly sensitive and specific for identifying this arrhythmia. Thus, patients with chronic atrial tachycardia should be evaluated for evidence of ventricular dysfunction, and patients with idiopathic cardiomyopathy require careful scrutiny of the atrial rhythm.[83–85,87,89]

Pharmacologic therapy for automatic atrial tachycardia is difficult, with little effect of digoxin or type IA antiarrhythmic agents such as procainamide or quinidine.[80,86,91] Amiodarone, particularly in combination with β-blocking agents, was effective in 63% of patients in one series[88]; sotalol, flecainide, and propafenone are also effective.[90,94] The presence of multiple

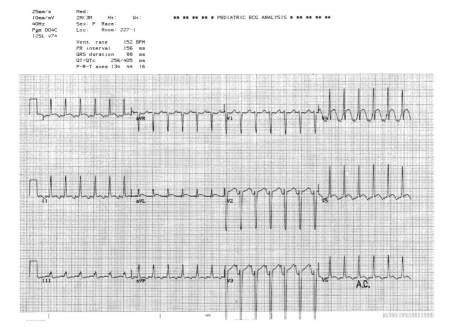

Figure 12. Automatic atrial tachycardia in 2-month-old infant presenting with shock and severe congestive failure. The abnormal P wave with notching best seen in leads I, II, AV$_F$, and V$_6$ distinguish this rhythm from sinus tachycardia. Decreased RV voltage, left ventricular hypertrophy, and ST elevation in V$_3$–V$_5$ noted.

foci complicates either pharmacologic or ablative therapy. Spontaneous resolution of atrial tachycardia following achievement of sinus rhythm with medications is reported in 33% to 95% of patients.[86,88,90,91,94] RF catheter ablation is highly effective in approximately 80% of patients,[92,93,95] with surgery reserved for refractory cases.[96]

Multifocal Atrial Tachycardia

Multifocal atrial tachycardia is a rare arrhythmia, identified in 0.36% of hospitalized adults, and typically occurs in elderly patients with chronic pulmonary disease, diabetes, or other acute illnesses.[97,98] The incidence in childhood is much lower, predominantly occurring in infants.[99–101] The EP mechanism is not known, with some evidence favoring triggered activity.[102]

Electrocardiogram Criteria: Multifocal Atrial Tachycardia (Figure 13)

1. Irregular atrial rate >100 bpm.
2. At least three different, distinct, nonsinus P-wave morphologies.

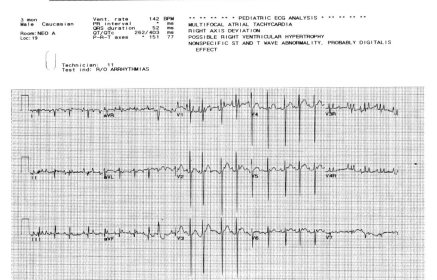

3 mon
Male Caucasian

Room: NEO A
Loc: 19

Vent. rate   142 BPM
PR interval   * ms
QRS duration   52 ms
QT/QTc   262/403 ms
P-R-T axes   * 151 77

** ** ** ** * PEDIATRIC ECG ANALYSIS * ** ** ** **
MULTIFOCAL ATRIAL TACHYCARDIA
RIGHT AXIS DEVIATION
POSSIBLE RIGHT VENTRICULAR HYPERTROPHY
NONSPECIFIC ST AND T WAVE ABNORMALITY, PROBABLY DIGITALIS
EFFECT

Technician: 11
Test ind: R/O ARRHYTHMIAS

Figure 13. Multifocal atrial tachycardia in 3-month-old infant. Irregular "chaotic" atrial activity with several different P-wave morphologies noted.

3. Isoelectric baseline between P waves.
4. Varying PP, PR, and RR intervals.

Clinical Correlation

Close to 75% of pediatric patients with multifocal atrial tachycardia present in infancy, usually in the neonatal period.[99–101,103] Structural heart disease is identified in approximately half of patients, notably hypertrophic cardiomyopathy.[91,101] Pulmonary disease, dysmorphism, and neurologic abnormalities are frequently associated.[100,101,103] About one third of patients have no other identifiable abnormality. Treatment is directed at any precipitating cause, such as hypoxia, with antiarrhythmic therapy reserved for patients with incessant arrhythmias, significant symptoms, or high ventricular rates.[101] Antiarrhythmic therapy is very difficult, with success reported with magnesium, β-blockade, amiodarone, and propafenone[100,101,104]; digoxin is not effective and may be harmful.[99] There is a high incidence of spontaneous resolution of this arrhythmia, favoring nonintervention whenever possible.[99–101] Although sudden death was reported in infants with chaotic atrial rhythm, it is not likely that this arrhythmia was etiologic in their deaths.[99,101–103]

References

1. Josephson ME, Wellens HJJ: Differential diagnosis of supraventricular tachycardia. *Cardiol Clin* 1990;8:411–442.
2. Engelstein ED, Lippman N, Stein KM, et al. Mechanism-specific effects of adenosine on atrial tachycardia. *Circulation* 1994;89:2645–2654.
3. Wu D, Denes P, Amat-y-Leon F, et al. Clinical, electrocardiographic and electrophysiologic observations in patients with paroxysmal supraventricular tachycardia. *Am J Cardiol* 1978;41:1045–1051.
4. Gillette PC. The mechanisms of supraventricular tachycardia in children. *Circulation* 1976;54:133–139.
5. Ko JK, Deal BJ, Strasburger JF, et al. Supraventricular tachycardia mechanisms and their age distribution in pediatric patients. *Am J Cardiol* 1992;69:1028–1032.
6. Naheed ZJ, Strasburger JF, Deal BJ, et al. Fetal tachycardia: mechanisms and predictors of hydrops fetalis. *J Am Coll Cardiol* 1996;27:1736–1740.
7. Chung KY, Walsh TJ, Massie E. Wolff-Parkinson-White syndrome. *Am Heart J* 1965;69:116–133.
8. Swiderski J, Lees MH, Nadas AS. The Wolff-Parkinson-White syndrome in infancy and childhood. *N Engl J Med* 1962;267:968–974.
9. Coumel P, Cabrol C, Fabiato A, et al. Tachycardie permanente par rhythme réciproque. *Arch Mal Coeur* 1967;60:1830–1864.
10. Bardy GH, Packer DL, German LD, et al. Preexcited reciprocating tachycardia in patients with Wolff-Parkinson-White syndrome: incidence and mechanisms. *Circulation* 1984;70:377–391.
11. Gallagher JJ, Selle JG, Sealy WC, et al. Variants of pre-excitation: update 1989. In: Zipes DB, Jalife J, eds. *Cardiac Electrophysiology from Cell to Bedside.* Philadelphia: WB Saunders Co; 1990:480–490.
12. Klein GJ, Bashore TM, Sellers TD, et al. Ventricular fibrillation in the Wolff-Parkinson-White syndrome. *N Engl J Med* 1979;301:1080–1085.
13. Montoya PT, Brugada P, Smeets J, et al. Ventricular fibrillation in the Wolff-Parkinson-White syndrome. *Eur Heart J* 1991;12:144–150.
14. Rodriguez L-M, de Chillou C, Schläpfer J, et al. Age at onset and gender of patients with different types of supraventricular tachycardias. *Am J Cardiol* 1992;70:1213–1215.
15. Deal BJ, Keane JF, Gillette PC, et al. Wolff-Parkinson-White syndrome and supraventricular tachycardia during infancy: management and follow-up. *J Am Coll Cardiol* 1985;5:130–135.
16. Vidaillet HJ Jr, Pressley JC, Henke E, et al. Familial occurrence of accessory atrioventricular pathways (preexcitation syndrome). *N Engl J Med* 1987;317:65–69.
17. Sreeram N, Wren C. Supraventricular tachycardia in infants: response to initial treatment. *Arch Dis Child* 1990;65:127–129.
18. Byrum CJ, Kavey RE, Deal BJ, et al. Wolff-Parkinson-White syndrome and supraventricular tachycardia presenting in infancy: a multi-center investigation. In: *Proceedings of the Second World Congress of Pediatric Cardiology.* New York: Springer-Verlag; 1985.
19. Nadas AS, Daeschner CW, Roth A, et al. Paroxysmal tachycardia in infants and children. *Pediatrics* 1952;9:167–181.
20. Perry JC, Garson A Jr. Supraventricular tachycardia due to Wolff-Parkinson-White syndrome in children: early disappearance and late recurrence. *J Am Coll Cardiol* 1990;16:1215–1220.

21. Giardina ACV, Ehlers KH, Engle MA. Wolff-Parkinson-White syndrome in infants and children. A long-term follow-up study. *Br Heart J* 1972;34:839–846.
22. Lundberg A. Paroxysmal atrial tachycardia in infancy: long-term follow-up study of 49 subjects. *Pediatrics* 1982;70:638–642.
23. Benson DW Jr, Dunnigan A, Benditt DG. Follow-up evaluation of infant paroxysmal atrial tachycardia: transesophageal study. *Circulation* 1987;75:542–549.
24. Dunnigan A, Benditt DG, Benson DW Jr. Modes of onset ("initiating events") for paroxysmal atrial tachycardia in infants and children. *Am J Cardiol* 1986;57:1280–1287.
25. Chang R-KR, Wetzel GT, Shannon KM, et al. Age- and anesthesia-related changes in accessory pathway conduction in children with Wolff-Parkinson-White syndrome. *Am J Cardiol* 1995;76:1074–1076.
26. Naheed ZJ, Diamandakis VM, Benson DW Jr, et al. Age-related conduction characteristics of Wolff-Parkinson-White syndrome in pediatric patients. *Pediatr Cardiol* 1995;16:251.
27. Deal BJ, Dick M, Beerman L, et al. Cardiac arrest in young patients with Wolff-Parkinson-White syndrome. *Pacing Clin Electrophysiol* 1995;18:815.
28. Timmermans C, Smeets JLRM, Rodriguez LM, et al. Aborted sudden death in the Wolff-Parkinson-White syndrome. *Am J Cardiol* 1995;76:492–494.
29. Bromberg BI, Lindsay BD, Cain ME, et al. Impact of clinical history and electrophysiologic characterization of accessory pathways on management strategies to reduce sudden death among children with Wolff-Parkinson-White syndrome. *J Am Coll Cardiol* 1996;27:690–695.
30. Munger TM, Packer DL, Hammill SC, et al. A population study of the natural history of Wolff-Parkinson-White syndrome in Olmsted County, Minnesota, 1953–1989. *Circulation* 1993;87:866–873.
31. Akhtar M, Jazayeri MR, Sra J, et al. Atrioventricular nodal reentry. Clinical, electrophysiological, and therapeutic considerations. *Circulation* 1993;88:282–295.
32. Sung RJ, Lauer MR, Chun H. Atrioventricular node reentry: current concepts and new perspectives. *Pacing Clin Electrophysiol* 1994;17:1413–1430.
33. Jackman WM, Beckman KJ, McClelland JH, et al. Treatment of supraventricular tachycardia due to atrioventricular nodal reentry, by radiofrequency catheter ablation of slow-pathway conduction. *N Engl J Med* 1992;327:313–318.
34. Gürsoy S, Steurer G, Brugada J, et al. Brief report: the hemodynamic mechanism of pounding in the neck in atrioventricular nodal reentrant tachycardia. *N Engl J Med* 1992;327:772–774.
35. Thapar MK, Gillette PC. Dual atrioventricular nodal pathways: a common electrophysiologic response in children. *Circulation* 1979;60:1369–1374.
36. Casta A, Wolff GS, Mehta AV, et al. Dual atrioventricular nodal pathways: a benign finding in arrhythmia-free children with heart disease. *Am J Cardiol* 1980;46:1013–1018.
37. Olshansky B, Wilber DJ, Hariman RJ. Atrial flutter: update on the mechanism and treatment. *Pacing Clin Electrophysiol* 1992;15:2308–2335.
38. Saoudi N, Atallah G, Kirkorian G, et al. Catheter ablation of the atrial myocardium in human type I atrial flutter. *Circulation* 1990;81:762–771.
39. Rowland TW, Mathew R, Chameides L, et al. Idiopathic atrial flutter in infancy: a review of eight cases. *Pediatrics* 1978;61:52–56.
40. Martin TC, Hernandez A. Atrial flutter in infancy. *Pediatrics* 1982;100:239–242.
41. Dunnigan A, Benson DW Jr, Benditt DG. Atrial flutter in infancy: diagnosis, clinical features, and treatment. *Pediatrics* 1985;75:725–729.
42. Garson A Jr, Bink-Boelkens M, Hesslein PS, et al. Atrial flutter in the young: a collaborative study of 380 cases. *J Am Coll Cardiol* 1985;6:871–878.

43. Johnson WH Jr, Dunnigan A, Fehr P, et al. Association of atrial flutter with orthodromic reciprocating fetal tachycardia. *Am J Cardiol* 1987;59:374–375.
44. Till J, Wren C. Atrial flutter in the fetus and young infant: an association with accessory connections. *Br Heart J* 1992;67:80–83.
45. Weber HS, Hellenbrand WE, Kleinman CS, et al. Predictors of rhythm disturbances and subsequent morbidity after the Fontan operation. *Am J Cardiol* 1989;64:762–767.
46. Peters NS, Somerville J. Arrhythmias after the Fontan procedure. *Br Heart J* 1992;68:199–204.
47. Gelatt M, Hamilton RM, McCrindle BW, et al. Risk factors for atrial tachyarrhythmias after the Fontan operation. *J Am Coll Cardiol* 1994;24:1735–1741.
48. Cecchin F, Johnsrude CL, Perry JC, et al. Effect of age and surgical technique on symptomatic arrhythmias after the Fontan procedure. *Am J Cardiol* 1995;76:386–391.
49. Balaji S, Johnson TB, Sade RM, et al. Management of atrial flutter after the Fontan procedure. *J Am Coll Cardiol* 1994;23:1209–1215.
50. Kao JM, Alejos JC, Grant PW, et al. Conversion of atriopulmonary to cavopulmonary anastomosis in management of late arrhythmias and atrial thrombosis. *Ann Thorac Surg* 1994;58:1510–1514.
51. Wellens HJJ, Brugada P. Mechanisms of supraventricular tachycardia. *Am J Cardiol* 1988;62:10D–15D.
52. Wu D, Amat-y-Leon F, Denes P, et al. Demonstration of sustained sinus and atrial re-entry as a mechanism of paroxysmal supraventricular tachycardia. *Circulation* 1975;51:234–243.
53. Haines DE, DiMarco JP. Sustained intraatrial reentrant tachycardia: clinical, electrocardiographic and electrophysiologic characteristics and long-term follow-up. *J Am Coll Cardiol* 1990;15:1345–1354.
54. Chen S-A, Chiang C-E, Yang C-J, et al. Sustained atrial tachycardia in adult patients. Electrophysiological characteristics, pharmacological response, possible mechanisms, and effects of radiofrequency ablation. *Circulation* 1994;90:1262–1278.
55. Müller GI, Deal BJ, Strasburger JF, et al. Electrocardiographic features of atrial tachycardias after operation for congenital heart disease. *Am J Cardiol* 1993;71:122–124.
56. Beerman LB, Neches WH, Fricker FJ, et al. Arrhythmias in transposition of the great arteries after the Mustard operation. *Am J Cardiol* 1983;51:1530–1534.
57. Vetter VL, Tanner CS, Horowitz LN. Inducible atrial flutter after the Mustard repair of complete transposition of the great arteries. *Am J Cardiol* 1988;61:428–435.
58. Silka MJ, Manwill JR, Kron J, et al. Bradycardia-mediated tachyarrhythmias in congenital heart disease and responses to chronic pacing at physiologic rates. *Am J Cardiol* 1990;65:488–493.
59. Fukushige J, Porter CJ, Hayes DL, et al. Antitachycardia pacemaker treatment of postoperative arrhythmias in pediatric patients. *Pacing Clin Electrophysiol* 1991;14:546–556.
60. Triedman JK, Saul JP, Weindling SN, et al. Radiofrequency ablation of intraatrial reentrant tachycardia after surgical palliation of congenital heart disease. *Circulation* 1995;91:707–714.
61. Kalman JM, VanHare GR, Olgin JE, et al. Ablation of 'incisional' reentrant atrial tachycardia complicating surgery for congenital heart disease. Use of entrainment to define a critical isthmus of conduction. *Circulation* 1996;93:502–512.

62. VanHare GF, Lesh MD, Ross BA, et al. Mapping and radiofrequency ablation of intraatrial reentrant tachycardia after the Senning or Mustard procedure for transposition of the great arteries. *Am J Cardiol* 1996;77:985–991.

63. Gomes JA, Hariman RJ, Kang PS, et al. Sustained symptomatic sinus node reentrant tachycardia: incidence, clinical significance, electrophysiologic observations and the effects of antiarrhythmic agents. *J Am Coll Cardiol* 1985;5:45–57.

64. Gomes JA, Mehta D, Langan MN. Sinus node reentrant tachycardia. *Pacing Clin Electrophysiol* 1995;18:1045–1057.

65. Kay GN, Chong F, Epstein AE, et al. Radiofrequency ablation for treatment of primary atrial tachycardias. *J Am Coll Cardiol* 1993;21:901–909.

66. Sanders WE, Sorrentino RA, Greenfield RA, et al. Catheter ablation of sinoatrial node reentrant tachycardia. *J Am Coll Cardiol* 1994;23:926–934.

67. Wyndham CRC, Arnsdorf MF, Levitsky S, et al. Successful surgical excision of focal paroxysmal atrial tachycardia. Observations in vivo and in vitro. *Circulation* 1980;62:1365–1372.

68. Ostrander LD Jr, Brandt RL, Kjelsberg MO, et al. Electrocardiographic findings among the adult population of a total natural community, Tecumseh, Michigan. *Circulation* 1965;31:888–898.

69. Camm AJ, Evans KE, Ward DE, et al. The rhythm of the heart in active elderly subjects. *Am Heart J* 1980;99:598–603.

70. Waldo AL. Mechanisms of atrial fibrillation, atrial flutter, and ectopic atrial tachycardia—a brief review. *Circulation* 1987;75:37–40.

71. Radford DJ, Izukawa T. Atrial fibrillation in children. *Pediatrics* 1977;59:250–256.

72. Belhassen B, Pauzner D, Blieden L, et al. Intrauterine and postnatal atrial fibrillation in the Wolff-Parkinson-White syndrome. *Circulation* 1982;66:1124–1128.

73. Phair WB. Familial atrial fibrillation. *Can Med Assoc J* 1963;89:1274–1276.

74. Stafford WJ, Trohman RG, Bilsker M, et al. Cardiac arrest in an adolescent with atrial fibrillation and hypertrophic cardiomyopathy. *J Am Coll Cardiol* 1986;7:701–704.

75. Brand FN, Abbott RD, Kannel WB, et al. Characteristics and prognosis of lone atrial fibrillation. 30-year follow-up in the Framingham Study. *JAMA* 1985;254:3449–3453.

76. Kopecky SL, Gersh BJ, McGoon MD, et al. The natural history of lone atrial fibrillation. A population-based study over three decades. *N Engl J Med* 1987;317:669–674.

77. Hamer ME, Wilkinson WE, Clair WK, et al. Incidence of symptomatic atrial fibrillation in patients with paroxysmal supraventricular tachycardia. *J Am Coll Cardiol* 1995;25:984–988.

78. Sellers TD Jr, Bashore TM, Gallagher JJ. Digitalis in the pre-excitation syndrome. Analysis during atrial fibrillation. *Circulation* 1977;56:260–267.

79. Byrum CJ, Wahl RA, Behrendt DM, et al. Ventricular fibrillation associated with use of digitalis in a newborn infant with Wolff-Parkinson-White syndrome. *J Pediatr* 1982;101:400–403.

80. Keane JF, Plauth WJ Jr, Nadas AS. Chronic ectopic tachycardia of infancy and childhood. *Am Heart J* 1972;84:748–757.

81. Scheinman MM, Basu D, Hollenberg M. Electrophysiologic studies in patients with persistent atrial tachycardia. *Circulation* 1974;50:266–273.

82. Gillette PC, Garson A Jr. Electrophysiologic and pharmacologic characteristics of automatic ectopic atrial tachycardia. *Circulation* 1977;56:571–575.

83. Kugler JD, Baisch SD, Cheatham JP, et al. Improvement of left ventricular dysfunction after control of persistent tachycardia. *J Pediatr* 1984;105:543–548.
84. Gillette PC, Smith RT, Garson A Jr, et al. Chronic supraventricular tachycardia. A curable cause of congestive cardiomyopathy. *JAMA* 1985;253:391–392.
85. Packer DL, Bardy GH, Worley SJ, et al. Tachycardia-induced cardiomyopathy: reversible form of left ventricular dysfunction. *Am J Cardiol* 1986;57:563–570.
86. Koike K, Hesslein PS, Finlay CD, et al. Atrial automatic tachycardia in children. *Am J Cardiol* 1988;61:1127–1130.
87. Gelb BD, Garson A Jr. Noninvasive discrimination of right atrial ectopic tachycardia from sinus tachycardia in "dilated cardiomyopathy." *Am Heart J* 1990;120:886–891.
88. Naheed ZJ, Strasburger JF, Benson DW Jr, et al. Natural history and management strategies of automatic atrial tachycardia in children. *Am J Cardiol* 1995;75:405–407.
89. Zimmerman FJ, Pahl E, Rocchini AP, et al. High incidence of incessant supraventricular tachycardia in pediatric patients referred for cardiac transplantation. *Pacing Clin Electrophysiol* 1996;19:663.
90. Von Bernuth G, Engelhardt W, Kramer HH, et al. Atrial automatic tachycardia in infancy and childhood. *Eur Heart J* 1982;13:1410–1415.
91. Mehta AV, Sanchez GR, Sacks EJ, et al. Ectopic automatic atrial tachycardia in children: clinical characteristics, management and follow-up. *J Am Coll Cardiol* 1988;11:379–385.
92. Tracy CM, Swartz JF, Fletcher RD, et al. Radiofrequency catheter ablation of ectopic atrial tachycardia using paced activation sequence mapping. *J Am Coll Cardiol* 1993;21:910–917.
93. Goldberger J, Kall J, Ehlert F, et al. Effectiveness of radiofrequency catheter ablation for treatment of atrial tachycardia. *Am J Cardiol* 1993;72:787–793.
94. Bauersfeld U, Gow RM, Hamilton RM, et al. Treatment of atrial ectopic tachycardia in infants <6 months old. *Am Heart J* 1995;129:1145–1148.
95. Walsh EP, Saul JP, Hulse JE, et al. Transcatheter ablation of ectopic atrial tachycardia in young patients using radiofrequency current. *Circulation* 1992;86:1138–1146.
96. Anderson KP, Stinson EB, Mason JW. Surgical exclusion of focal paroxysmal atrial tachycardia. *Am J Cardiol* 1982;49:869–874.
97. Habibzadeh MA. Multifocal atrial tachycardia: a 66 month follow-up of 50 patients. *Heart Lung* 1980;9:328–335.
98. Kastor JA. Multifocal atrial tachycardia. *N Engl J Med* 1990;322:1713–1717.
99. Bisset GS III, Seigel SF, Gaum WE, et al. Chaotic atrial tachycardia in childhood. *Am Heart J* 1981;101:268–272.
100. Liberthson RR, Colan SD. Multifocal or chaotic atrial rhythm: report of nine infants, delineation of clinical course and management, and review of the literature. *Pediatr Cardiol* 1982;2:179–184.
101. Dodo H, Gow RM, Hamilton RM, et al. Chaotic atrial rhythm in children. *Am Heart J* 1995;129:990–995.
102. Levine JH, Michael JR, Guarnieri T. Treatment of multifocal atrial tachycardia with verapamil. *N Engl J Med* 1985;312:21–25.
103. Yeager SB, Hougen TJ, Levy AM. Sudden death in infants with chaotic atrial rhythm. *Am J Dis Child* 1984;138:689–692.
104. Fish FA, Mehta AV, Johns JA. Characteristics and management of chaotic atrial tachycardia of infancy. *Am J Cardiol* 1996;78:1052–1055.

onds. A VA interval that is longer than 150 milliseconds suggests an AC that conducts slower than most; this is commonly seen in the permanent form of junctional reciprocating tachycardia (PJRT). In PJRT, the reentrant loop involves the AVN as the antegrade limb and the slowly conducting AC as the retrograde limb. The longer VA interval manifests on the surface ECG as a prolonged RP interval, measured from the onset of the QRS to the onset of the P wave. Although most types of SVT are paroxysmal, PJRT is frequently incessant (thus the name).[14]

Features of the EP findings from a patient with a right-sided AC are shown in Figure 3. A paced drivetrain (S_1-S_1 = 400 milliseconds) is delivered to the atrium followed by a single atrial extrastimulus. The atrial im-

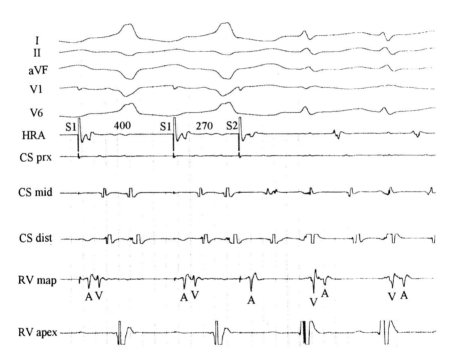

Figure 3. The RV mapping electrogram is near the AC. When it is placed along the AV groove both atrial (A) and ventricular (V) depolarization potentials can be recorded. The closer the mapping catheter is to the AC, the shorter the recorded AV interval, with ultimate fusion of these intervals. At the RV mapping site the recorded electrogram shows a short AV interval (beats 1–2), with the ventricular depolarization occurring 50 milliseconds before the beginning of the delta wave. When the AV reentrant tachycardia is initiated, a short retrograde VA interval is recorded in the RV mapping site. The above findings prove that the AC is located in the right side of the heart near the mapping catheter site (Figure 4). From top to bottom: ECG I, II, aVF, V1, V6, high right atrium (HRA), proximal coronary sinus (CS prx), mid-CS (CS mid), distal CS (CS dist), RV mapping (RV map), and RV apex electrograms.

pulses during the drivetrain conduct to the ventricles via the AC (note the short PR interval and delta wave on the surface ECG). The premature beat from the extrastimulus (S_2, delivered 270 milliseconds after the last beat of the drivetrain) conducts to the ventricles via the AVN (note the longer PR and narrow QRS complex on the surface ECG). This premature atrial impulse is the longest atrial coupling interval to block in the AC and defines the antegrade effective refractory period of the AC. When the antegrade AC becomes refractory, the impulse is conducted to the ventricles via the AVN (long PR), and the impulse approaches the AC from a retrograde direction. By this time, the AC is no longer refractory and is therefore available for retrograde conduction of the impulse. This beat then "reenters" the atrium and can initiate sustained reentry SVT. Of note, ECG recordings and 24-hour cardioscans in patients with SVT often show that well-timed premature atrial complexes often initiate clinical tachycardia.

Once SVT is induced, a "mapping" catheter can be repositioned along the AV annulus using fluoroscopy (Figure 4) and used with the appearance of recorded intracardiac electrograms to determine the location of the AC. When the catheter is placed along the AV groove, both atrial (A) and ventricular (V) depolarizations are recorded. Localization of a manifest AC during sinus rhythm is based on (1) fusion of the local AV electrograms, with inscription of an AC electrogram potential and (2) a local ventricular electrogram preceding the onset of the surface delta wave. A concealed AC is localized based on the earliest retrograde VA activation recorded during either ventricular pacing or ORT.

A left lateral AC is shown in Figure 5. During sinus rhythm with preexcitation, AV fusion is noted near the site of the AC. The earliest ventricular depolarization occurs in the distal CS electrogram, establishing that the AC is located at the left lateral AV region (Figure 6). During ORT, earliest retrograde atrial activation is likewise recorded on the distal CS electrode pair.

Various medications are commonly used during an EP study to facilitate induction, clarify the mechanism, or initiate or terminate SVT. In some sedated patients, induction of AV reentry tachycardia requires an intravenous infusion of isoproterenol during pacing protocols. These patients generally require a dose of at least 0.02 μg/kg per minute, or enough to increase the baseline sinus rate by about 20%. Intravenous adenosine, by blocking conduction in the AVN, may facilitate identification of an AC. When adenosine is administered during sinus (or paced atrial) rhythm, an AC that was otherwise quite subtle or absent on resting ECG may show maximal preexcitation due to AVN blockade. When adenosine is administered during ORT, tachycardia usually terminates in the antegrade limb of the reentry circuit—the AVN. In this case, the last recorded activity of the SVT circuit is the retrograde atrial activation via the AC, evidenced by a P wave on the surface ECG or local atrial electrogram on intracardiac recordings.

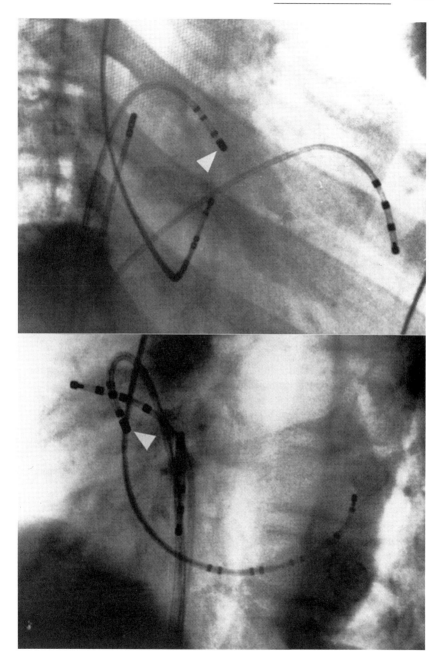

Figure 4. Right anterior oblique view (**upper panel**) and left anterior oblique view (**lower panel**) of the position of mapping catheter (arrowhead) for the right anterior-lateral accessory pathway.

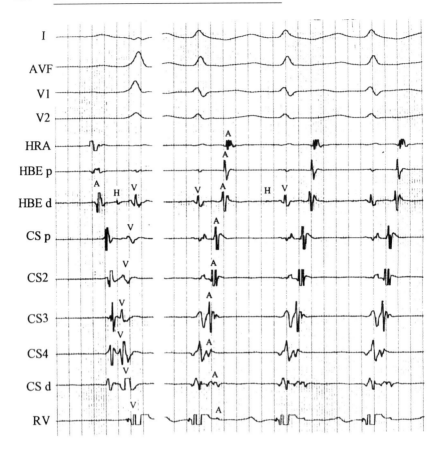

Figure 5. During sinus rhythm with preexcitation (**left panel**) the earliest ventricular depolarization occurs in the CS4 electrogram, which is located in the distal CS (see Figure 6). During ORT (**right panel**), the earliest retrograde atrial activation is also recorded at CS4 electrogram.

As alluded to above, the EP study may be used to identify patients with preexcitation who are at risk for syncope or sudden death. Patients with preexcitation at highest risk for cardiac arrest are those with a shortest preexcited RR interval less than 220 milliseconds during atrial fibrillation.[15] The shortest preexcited RR intervals represent antegrade conduction of atrial impulses of very high frequency to the ventricles via the AC. The preexcited RR interval depends on the EP characteristics of the AC, AVN, and ventricular myocardium, and on the patient's autonomic tone.[16] Figure 7 shows ECG tracings in a patient with a left-sided AC and antegrade conduction at a paced CL of 250 milliseconds. The shortest RR interval during induced atrial fibrillation was 200 milliseconds, placing this patient in the high-risk group.[17] Importantly, patients with preexcitation appear to have

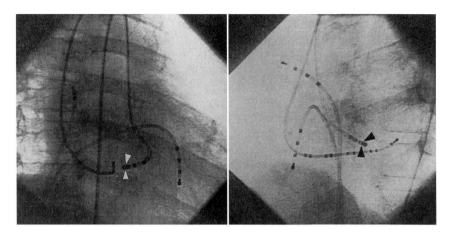

Figure 6. Right anterior oblique view (**left panel**) and left anterior oblique view (**right panel**) of the position of mapping catheter (arrowhead) for a left lateral accessory pathway.

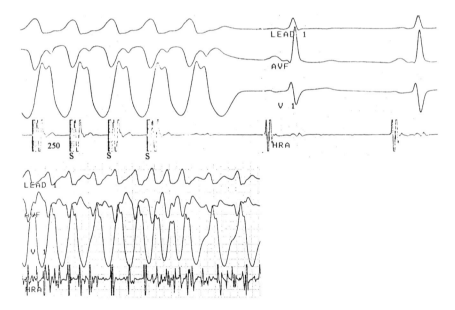

Figure 7. Upper panel: Rapid atrial pacing (**left-hand side**) at a pacing CL of 250 milliseconds results in 1:1 accessory pathway conduction (paper speed 100 mm per second). When pacing is discontinued the sinus beats (**right-hand side**) conduct to the ventricle via the AVN (with a normal PR and a narrow QRS). **Lower panel**: When atrial fibrillation is induced by rapid atrial pacing (actual pacing is not shown, paper speed 50 mm per second) all conducted beats are preexcited (with wide QRS) and the shortest preexcited RR interval is 200 milliseconds (ie, the patient is in the high-risk group).

a higher incidence of spontaneous and inducible atrial fibrillation than the general population.[17-19]

Atrioventricular Nodal Reentrant Tachycardia

Electrophysiological Characteristics of Atrioventricular Nodal Reentrant Tachycardia

1. Initiation and termination by extrastimulation or rapid pacing.
2. Normal antegrade and retrograde AV conduction.
3. Earliest retrograde activation at the His junction.
4. SVT may persist with AV block (uncommon).
5. Presence of dual AVN physiology.
6. Exclusion of an AC in the SVT circuit.

The development of AVN reentry tachycardia (AVNRT) results from functional dissociation of conduction over (anatomically) distinct AVN pathways. Normal antegrade AVN conduction during sinus rhythm proceeds predominantly over the so-called "fast pathway," located in the atrial septum anterior and superior to the compact AVN. The "slow pathway" of the AVN lies posterior and inferior to the compact node and courses on the atrial side of the tricuspid annulus near the CS os. A premature atrial impulse may find the fast pathway fibers refractory and conduct to the compact node via the posterior slow fibers with a longer PR interval. The anatomic and functional differences between the fast and slow fibers form the basis for "dual AVN physiology" and the substrate for the common and uncommon forms of AVNRT. In the common form of AVNRT, antegrade conduction shifts to the slower, posteriorly located fibers, and conduction returns to the atrium over the fast pathway (slow-fast form). In the uncommon form of AVNRT, the circuit is reversed (fast-slow form).

The conduction properties of the AVN differ importantly from those of atrial and ventricular tissue and typical ACs. Extrastimuli delivered to the atrium, ventricle, or AC conduct rapidly without significant delay. Extrastimuli delivered to the AVN show a significant conduction delay that becomes more pronounced at progressively shorter extrastimulus intervals (S_1–S_2). Conduction times through the normal AVN following atrial extrastimulation (termed "A_2-H_2" interval) display a smooth "decremental" property, with gradual prolongation of AVN conduction time over a range of atrial extrastimulation.[20] The presence of dual AVN pathways imposes discontinuity on the AVN conduction curve, due to an abrupt shift in conduction from the fast to the slow AVN fibers. The presence of dual AVN physiology can be recognized by sudden prolongation of AVN conduction time (A_2H_2) of >50 milliseconds with a small (10 milliseconds) decrement of the premature atrial extrastimulus (A_1-A_2).[21-24] However, dual AVN pathways are inferred if pacing-induced AVN reentry beats or AVNRT are demonstrated, even with a gradual prolongation of AVN conduction without abrupt jumps (a smooth continuous A_2-H_2 curve).[21,25] It is important to note that the presence of dual AVN physiology does not necessarily mean a patient has (or will have) AVNRT. Although 35% of children have evidence of dual AVN pathways, AVNRT accounts for less than 20% of SVT in children and usually occurs in older children.[26,27]

Common Form of Atrioventricular Nodal Reentrant Tachycardia

The common form of AVNRT is illustrated in Figure 8, with antegrade conduction over the slow pathway and retrograde conduction via the fast AVN pathway. Atrial activation via the anterior fast pathway is recorded by the HBE catheter, and slow pathway activation is recorded by the proximal electrodes of the CS catheter, near the os of the CS. The fast AVN pathway effective refractory period is defined as the longest atrial coupling interval

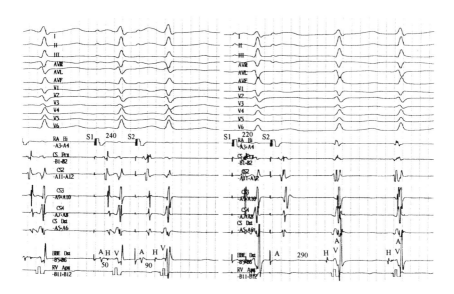

Figure 8. Atrial extrastimulation protocol demonstrates dual AVN pathways and a common form of AVNRT. **Left**: When atrial extrastimulation is delivered with an S_1S_1 450 milliseconds and an S_1S_2 240 milliseconds, both the S_1 and S_2 beats conduct to the ventricle via the fast AVN route with an A_1H_1 of 50 milliseconds and an A_2H_2 of 90 milliseconds. **Right**: When the S_1S_2 is decreased to 220 milliseconds (**right panel**) the A_2H_2 suddenly increases to 290 milliseconds (ie, via the slow AVN input route) and SVT is initiated.

(A_1A_2) at which AVN conduction is blocked or shifts from a fast to a slow pathway. When the fast AVN pathway becomes refractory, the impulse conducts to the ventricle via the slow pathway, freeing the fast pathway for retrograde conduction and the initiation of AVNRT. Note that retrograde VA conduction during tachycardia is very fast, resulting in a VA interval less than 60 milliseconds recorded in the HBE or less than 95 milliseconds recorded in the HRA.[28] The short VA time correlates with the surface ECG findings during AVNRT, with P waves "buried" in the QRS complex.

The ventricle is a requisite component of AV reentrant SVT (using an AC), and tachycardia cannot continue when there is AV or VA conduction block. In contrast, the ventricle is not a necessary part of the circuit in AVN reentry. Figure 9 shows pacing-induced narrow QRS tachycardia (CL 310 msec) with 2:1 AV block. Demonstration of AV or VA block during tachycardia is conclusive evidence that the tachycardia is not AV reentrant tachycardia utilizing an AC as a limb of the reentrant loop.

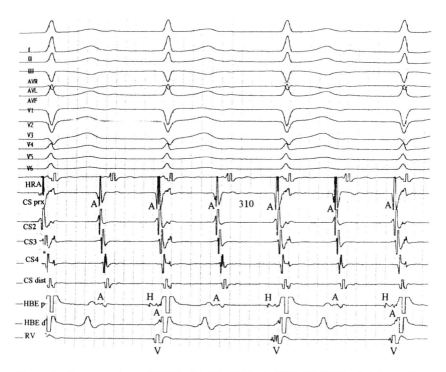

Figure 9. Common-form AVNRT with 2:1 AV block. With 2:1 AV block, it is possible to recognize A from V in the retrogradely conducted beat. Antegrade conduction has a long AH interval of 250 milliseconds (antegrade slow pathway) and retrograde conduction has a short HA interval of 30 milliseconds (or a negative VA interval; retrograde via the fast AVN pathway).

Uncommon Form of Atrioventricular Nodal Reentrant Tachycardia

The fast-slow form of AVRNT is illustrated in Figure 10. During ventricular pacing, retrograde activation is via the slow AVN pathway in the right posteroseptal region. When ventricular pacing is discontinued, the normal antegrade nodal pathway is available and initiates the uncommon form of AVNRT (antegrade fast and retrograde slow AVN pathway conduction). Because of the slow retrograde conduction, the AV (PR) and VA (RP) intervals are almost equal.

Occasionally, EP studies in patients with AC-mediated tachycardia reveal dual AVN physiology and inducible AVNRT. Alternatively, a patient with AVNRT may have an AC that does not participate in SVT, but rather acts as a "bystander" to conduct impulses that originate from the reentry circuit. It is not uncommon for a new tachycardia mechanism to become manifest after a previous tachycardia was eliminated by radiofrequency (RF) catheter ablation. After a "successful" ablation, repeat stimulation is often done with isoproterenol challenge to test efficacy of the procedure and to attempt to bring out a second SVT that was not initially apparent.

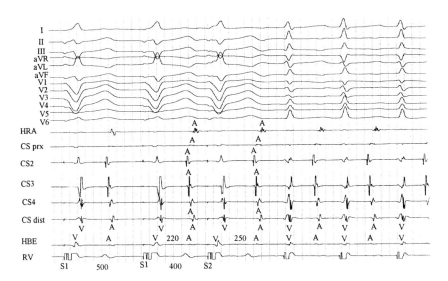

Figure 10. Right ventricular pacing (with retrograde slow AVN pathway conduction) induces an uncommon form of AVNRT. During the ventricular extrastimulation with S_1S_1 500 milliseconds and S_1S_2 400 milliseconds, all retrograde VA conduction is via the slow AVN pathway characterized by a long VA conduction time and decremental conduction properties. Earliest retrograde atrial depolarization of this slow AVN pathway is located at the right posteroseptal region (CS2 at the CS ostium).

Atrial Flutter

Electrophysiological Characteristics of Atrial Flutter

1. Rapid, regular atrial depolarization, rates 240–433 bpm.
2. Initiation and termination by rapid atrial pacing or extrastimuli.
3. Unaffected by variable AV conduction.

Atrial flutter is an atrial tachycardia with rates ranging from 240–433 bpm and beat-to-beat consistency of atrial CL (variation <20 milliseconds).[29] The ventricular response of atrial flutter may vary from 1:1 to 4:1. The mechanism is due to intraatrial reentry that can occur because of natural obstacles such as the venae cavae, tricuspid annulus, and CS and anisotropic conduction (where conduction velocity is "direction-dependent") through the atria.[30-36] Although atrial flutter has many similarities to intraatrial reentry tachycardia that is often seen in patients with postoperative congenital heart disease (see below), many pediatric electrophysiologists refer to them as separate entities.

In adults, atrial flutter is classified as type I or type II. Type I is more common and is characterized by negative P waves in ECG leads II, III, and aVF with a sawtooth appearance and a slower atrial rate of 240–340 bpm. Type II atrial flutter has positive P waves in the inferior leads with a faster atrial rate of 340–433 bpm. While type I flutter can be converted by atrial pacing, type II flutter is difficult to terminate.[29] With atrial pacing, type I flutter is sometimes converted to type II flutter or atrial fibrillation. While type I flutter typically has a reentrant wave front in the RA that is counterclockwise (viewed in the AP position),[37,38] type II atrial flutter has a variety of reentrant patterns.[39,40]

Electrophysiologically, both types of atrial flutter exhibit uniformity of interval, morphology, and amplitude of the atrial electrograms. Figure 11 shows the intracardiac electrograms during atrial flutter, where the CL is 180–190 milliseconds (or 316–333 bpm) and there is 2:1 AV conduction via the AVN. In this example, the atrial activation sequence (best seen on the atrial beats between the QRS complexes) shows that the impulses course in the following sequence: SVC-RA junction, RA anteroseptal, RA posteroseptal, RA posterior, and IVC-RA junction. This pattern describes a clockwise wave front as occurs in type II atrial flutter.

During atrial stimulation protocols, unsuspected sustained or nonsustained atrial flutter is occasionally induced in patients without a prior history of flutter or structural heart disease. In this setting, inducible atrial flutter is likely to be a nonspecific finding and does not require treatment.

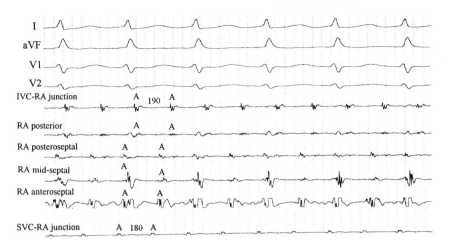

Figure 11. Atrial flutter with 2:1 AV block and clockwise rotating atrial flutter wave. IVC: inferior vena cava; SVC: superior vena cava.

Atrial Reentrant and Sinoatrial Tachycardia

Electrophysiological Characteristics of Atrial Reentrant Supraventricular Tachycardia

1. Regular atrial depolarizations.
2. Initiation and termination with atrial extrastimulation or rapid pacing.
3. Unaffected by variable AV conduction.
4. Atrial activation sequence distinct from sinus rhythm.

Atrial reentry tachycardia occurs commonly in patients who previously underwent extensive atrial surgery (eg, closure of atrial septal defect, Mustard operation, Fontan procedure). This tachycardia was also referred to as postoperative atrial flutter, atrial muscle reentry tachycardia, intraatrial reentry tachycardia, and incisional atrial tachycardia.[41-46] The mechanism of atrial reentry tachycardia is similar to atrial flutter that occurs more commonly in adults. In atrial reentry tachycardia, potential reentry circuits exist around natural obstacles (orifices of SVC and IVC, tricuspid annulus, and os of the CS) as well as surgical obstacles such as atriotomy scars, patches, and anastomoses.[36,45,46] Multiple areas of slow conduction that are critical for initiating and maintaining reentry tachycardia exist around areas of prior surgery.[46]

An EP study of atrial reentry tachycardia generally begins with initiating and terminating tachycardia with atrial pacing protocols; this can be done from either a transesophageal or intracardiac approach. Termination of atrial tachycardia with pacing is an important prerequisite before implanting an antitachycardia device in a patient with medically refractory tachycardia. Occasionally, an intravenous infusion of isoproterenol may be required to induce atrial reentry tachycardia in a sedated patient.

The EP study may also determine the location of individual atrial reentrant circuits. Recent studies of patients undergoing intracardiac EP mapping of tachycardia for ablation using RF catheter or surgical techniques showed that an individual patient may have multiple different atrial circuits.[44] During each episode of tachycardia, only one circuit predominates. To define the precise location of the active reentry circuit, two or more multipolar catheters are usually placed in the RA, and tachycardia is induced with standard pacing protocols. As the reentrant wave front passes each pair of electrodes, local atrial activation can be recorded. Figure 12 demonstrates atrial reentrant tachycardia (atrial CL 280 milliseconds) with a counterclockwise reentrant loop traveling from the SVC-RA junction to the lateral RA then inferior RA. The timing of atrial electrograms during atrial tachycardia can be considered together with known anatomic obstacles (natural and surgical) and the fluoroscopic location of each electrode pair to determine which atrial sites contribute to the reentry circuit.[45,46] Entrainment pacing techniques, where the tachycardia CL is transiently increased to a somewhat faster paced CL, were shown to more precisely

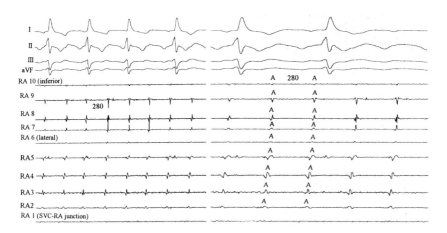

Figure 12. Intraatrial reentrant tachycardia with an atrial CL of 280 milliseconds (214 bpm). **Right panel**: paper speed 100 mm per second. **Left panel**: paper speed 50 mm per second. With a 20-pole halo catheter placed in the right atrium, the simultaneously recorded multiple atrial electrograms demonstrate a counterclockwise loop atrial reentrant wave front traveling from the SVC-RA junction to the RA lateral wall and then to the RA inferior wall.

define various components of the reentry circuit necessary for successful catheter or surgical ablation.[46]

Sinoatrial (SA) reentrant tachycardias have an underlying mechanism similar to that of atrial reentrant tachycardias, but the atrial rate is slower (<240 bpm) and usually in the range of 120–200 bpm. Vagal maneuvers may slow SA reentrant tachycardia, but the tachycardia per se is independent of conduction through the AVN. SA reentrant tachycardia is characterized by sudden onset and termination, relatively constant atrial CL, and the same atrial activation sequence (and surface P-wave morphology) as that of sinus rhythm. This arrhythmia is rare in children, and isolated atrial reentrant beats may be a nonspecific response to atrial programmed stimulation in patients with other forms of SVT.

Atrial Fibrillation

Electrophysiological Characteristics of Atrial Fibrillation

1. Absence of discrete regular atrial activity.
2. Variable RR intervals or random AV conduction.
3. Irregular baseline between QRS complexes.

Atrial fibrillation is rare in children without underlying heart disease, but may occur in a patient with atrial enlargement from mitral regurgitation (eg, cardiomyopathy or rheumatic heart disease)[47] or coexist with atrial reentrant tachycardia in a patient with postoperative congenital heart disease. The mechanism of atrial fibrillation involves multiple reentry circuits revolving around functional (not anatomic) obstacles that are defined by the conduction and refractory properties of the involved atrial tissue.[48] Atrial fibrillation may then be seen as consisting of many small disorganized reentry wavelets coexisting throughout the atrium. Intracardiac EP recordings of atrial fibrillation are demonstrated in Figure 13. The atrial electrograms show irregularities of polarity, morphology, and interbeat interval. Not uncommonly, various areas of the atria show different degrees of organization.

Atrial fibrillation is uniformly unresponsive to conversion attempts with atrial pacing protocols, although it may be induced during attempted conversion of atrial reentrant tachycardia.[49,50] Fortunately, induced atrial fibrillation in most patients is usually nonsustained and well tolerated. However, the incidence of spontaneous and inducible atrial fibrillation is increased in patients with preexcitation syndromes, in which case atrial fibrillation may not be tolerated.

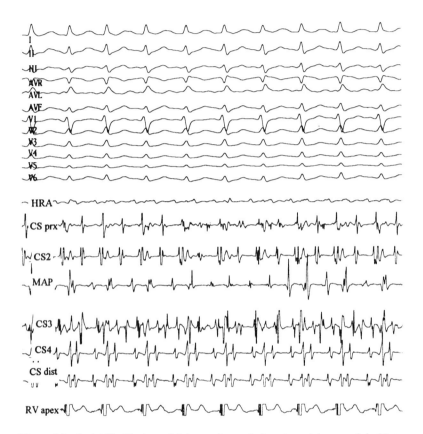

Figure 13. Atrial fibrillation with irregular and chaotic atrial potentials. Note that different atrial sites may record different types of fibrillation potentials: while in CS4 and distal CS electrograms (placed in the left lateral AV groove) there are discrete atrial potentials separated by isoelectric baselines, in the proximal CS (placed at the CS ostium) and CS3 electrograms (placed in the left posterior AV groove) at times the atrial potentials are discrete without isoelectric baselines. This may be due to organization in some areas and not in others (multiple reentry loops). MAP: mapping electrogram.

Automatic Atrial Tachycardia

Electrophysiological Characteristics of Automatic Atrial Tachycardia

1. P-wave morphology and/or axis differs from sinus.
2. Inability to initiate or terminate with atrial pacing or extrastimulation.
3. Resetting or transient suppression by atrial extrastimulation without termination.
4. Atrial rate warms up and cools down.
5. Unaffected by variable AV conduction.

Automatic atrial tachycardia is more common in children than in adults and is frequently refractory to medical treatment.[51,52] It is usually incessant and can cause tachycardia-induced cardiomyopathy if not treated. The mechanism appears to be due to abnormal automaticity from a discrete atrial focus that lies somewhere other than the SN. Studies of catheter ablation of automatic atrial tachycardia showed that foci typically are found at the base of the right or left atrial appendage, along the crista terminalis, or near the orifice of a pulmonary vein.[53]

The P-wave morphology of automatic atrial tachycardia is different from sinus P waves and reflects the location of the abnormal atrial focus. ECG recordings of runs of automatic atrial tachycardia often show warming up (the rate increasing gradually) on initiation and cooling down on termination. Tachycardia rates are variable (usually between 120–300 bpm) and are often influenced by autonomic tone. Because the AVN is not involved in the tachycardia, atrial impulses may or may not conduct through the AVN. The surface ECG occasionally shows intermittent AV block of the P waves. Additionally, the PR interval of conducted beats may lengthen significantly at faster atrial rates. This ECG finding distinguishes automatic atrial tachycardia from sinus tachycardia, when the SNs and AVNs are under similar autonomic influence. Because automatic atrial tachycardia is not due to a reentry mechanism, it can neither be induced nor terminated with atrial pacing techniques. Rapid atrial pacing may, however, cause transient suppression of this tachycardia, termed ''overdrive suppression.''

Precise localization of the focus of automatic atrial tachycardia (Figure 14), using mapping techniques, is done prior to catheter ablation. When the mapping catheter is placed at the site of the ectopic focus, the local atrial electrogram generally precedes the surface P wave by 20–60 milliseconds.[53]

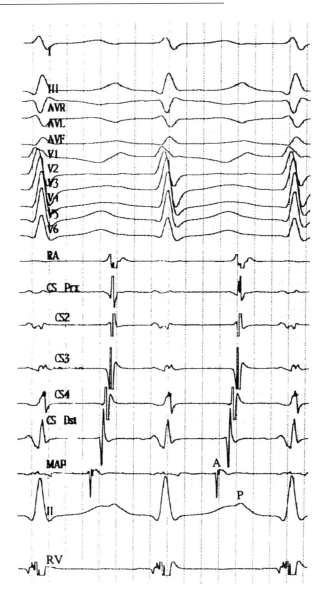

Figure 14. Automatic atrial tachycardia with a CL of 370 milliseconds (162 bpm). Note that the MAP placed at the site of tachycardia (in the left atrium anterior to the left auricular appendage) records an atrial potential 50 milliseconds earlier than the surface ECG P wave of lead II. Paper speed = 100 mm/second.

Junctional Ectopic Tachycardia

Electrophysiological Characteristics of Junctional Ectopic Tachycardia

1. Lack of conversion by overdrive atrial or ventricular pacing.
2. Overdrive suppression by atrial or ventricular pacing, followed by a warm up period.
3. VA dissociation with ventricular rate faster than atrial rate or VA association with retrograde atrial activation via the AVN.

Junctional ectopic tachycardia (JET) occurs rarely as a congenital arrhythmia, and is encountered more frequently after cardiac surgery [eg, ventricular septal defect (VSD) closure in an infant].[54,55] The congenital form is usually refractory to drugs and can cause tachycardia-induced cardiomyopathy.[54] Postoperative JET often produces poor hemodynamic status but generally subsides in a few days; however, untreated patients have a high mortality.[55] JET originates from the compact AVN or peri-AVN tis-

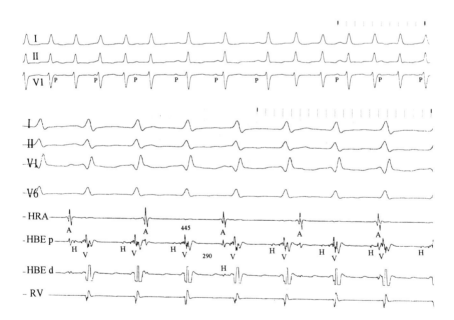

Figure 15. Upper panel: (surface ECG, paper speed 500 mm per second) JET with a P-QRS dissociation. The tachycardia shifts into sinus rhythm for a few beats then restarts with a warm-up phenomenon. **Lower panel**: (paper speed 100 mm per second) VA dissociation in the intracardiac recordings with an atrial CL of 445 milliseconds and junctional tachycardia CL of 290 milliseconds. Note His bundle depolarization potential precedes each ventricular depolarization complex.

sues and is felt to be due to abnormally enhanced automaticity. Tachycardia rates vary with autonomic tone, core body temperature, and administration of sympathomimetic agents; rates exhibit warm-up and cool-down behavior similar to that seen in automatic atrial tachycardia.

The EP diagnosis of JET is confirmed by surface ECG tracings showing rapid, usually narrow QRS tachycardia dissociated from a slower atrial rhythm (Figure 15). Occasionally, 1:1 VA conduction occurs during JET, when retrograde atrial activation occurs via the AVN. Intracardiac EP study of postoperative JET is not commonly performed. When surface P waves are small and difficult to appreciate on the ECG of a postoperative patient who may have JET, recordings on transesophageal lead or temporary pacing wires can facilitate diagnosis.

Treatment

The treatment of SVT is divided into two parts: acute termination of an episode of tachycardia and prevention of recurrences. The acute treatment begins with documentation of the arrhythmia with a 12-lead ECG, assessment of hemodynamic status, and recognition of the arrhythmia mechanism. Chronic therapy is based on the SVT mechanism, the patient's age, symptoms during tachycardia, and frequency of episodes as well as access to medical care and sophistication of the patient's caretaker.[56]

The decision to initiate chronic therapy in infants is based on symptoms, response to therapy, and frequency of episodes. Infants with single or rare episodes of SVT, terminated easily with ice, without significant compromise, and with competent caretakers, may do well without chronic medication. Approximately 30% to 40% of infants with SVT fit this category, which is similar to the percentage of infants who have no recurrences on oral digoxin.[58,59] In contrast, infants with SVT resulting in hemodynamic compromise, or infants with a wide QRS tachycardia, will require aggressive pharmacologic treatment to prevent recurrences. Transesophageal pacing is used in some centers to identify the mechanism of SVT and response to isoproterenol, assess the risk of rapid conduction over an AC, and test the efficacy of drug therapy.[58]

The use of digoxin in infants with manifest preexcitation is associated with a 1% to 5% risk of sudden death.[57] The mechanism of cardiac arrest is presumably due to rapid conduction of atrial fibrillation over the AC, producing ventricular fibrillation. Most centers currently use propranolol as initial therapy in this population. Although it is not an absolute contraindication,[59] verapamil probably should be avoided in infancy because of the possibility of hypotension.[60]

In approximately 10% of infants, SVT is refractory to therapy with digoxin or propranolol. Flecainide, sotalol, propafenone, and amiodarone were successfully used in these patients, sometimes in combination with propranolol or procainamide.[61–77] Amiodarone with flecainide was a successful combination in extremely difficult cases.[78] These infants need inpatient monitoring until sinus rhythm is maintained, with careful monitoring of serum drug levels, especially flecainide, as proarrhythmia is of concern. Medical therapy will allow some infants to outgrow their tachycardia, as the natural history of SVT in infancy favors resolution. In patients continuing to require medications, catheter ablation may be safely performed at age 2–3 years.[79,80] Experimental data showing late enlargement of RF lesions in infant lambs[81] discouraged the use of ablation in infants, except for rare life-threatening situations.[82]

In older children with manifest preexcitation, digoxin and calcium channel blockers should be avoided because of the possibility of enhancing conduction over the AC[57]; β-blockers and types I and III agents may be used.[68,77] In a small percentage of children and young adults, the initial presentation of WPW may be cardiac arrest.[83,84] For this reason, in symptomatic patients with WPW over about age 5 years, ablation is generally recommended.

The optimal management of asymptomatic children with WPW is controversial. As noted above, rarely their first symptom may be cardiac arrest. Risk stratification using treadmill testing or transesophageal pacing with isoproterenol may be performed.[85,86] Using that approach, patients without inducible SVT or atrial fibrillation and with long refractory periods of the AC may be observed. Other patients, particularly those in competitive athletics, may prefer ablation therapy (see Chapters 10 and 12.)

For children with AV reentrant tachycardia without manifest preexcitation (concealed ACs), and for patients with AVNRT, treatment is not necessary if episodes are short, infrequent, and not associated with hemodynamic compromise. For the symptomatic older child, ablative therapy or pharmacologic therapy are both acceptable; β-blockers, calcium channel blockers, type I and type III agents may be effective.

Atrial Flutter

Neonates with atrial flutter may be converted with transesophageal pacing or electrical cardioversion and usually do not require chronic therapy.[87] Older patients with atrial flutter should be treated with the primary goal of maintaining sinus rhythm. Prior to conversion of flutter, evaluation for the presence of intracardiac thrombi should be performed with transthoracic or transesophageal echocardiogram due to the risk of embolization with any type of cardioversion.[88] A course of anticoagulation therapy before and/or after conversion of atrial flutter is recommended, especially in those at risk for thrombosis (after Fontan or Mustard operation).[89,90] After acute conversion with atrial pacing, direct current cardioversion, or ibutilide,[89–91] type IA or type III medications may maintain sinus rhythm.

If this is not possible, then AV blocking agents should be utilized to control the ventricular response. Type IA (eg, procainamide or quinidine) or IC (eg, flecainide) antiarrhythmic agents will increase the atrial refractory period and may result in sinus rhythm. In these situations it may be advisable also to use AVN blocking medication (digoxin, propranolol, or verapamil) to slow the ventricular response because the tachycardia is often resistant or recurrent. In patients with resistant flutter, type III agents (eg, sotalol or amiodarone) may be considered. If sick sinus syndrome is coexistent, a pacemaker may be required.

In postoperative patients, the perioperative development of atrial reentrant tachycardia may be an acute response to surgery, and antiarrhythmic therapy may be withdrawn after 3–6 months. The later development of atrial tachycardia may herald significant residual defects which should be evaluated, particularly in Fontan patients. We recommend catheterization in patients with recurrent episodes of tachycardia to detect hemodynamic abnormalities that may be unrecognized by echocardiogram. Mortality due to arrhythmia in this population may be as high as 20%.[92] The presence of significant underlying bradycardia may predispose to the development of tachycardia. Procainamide or sotalol may be effective in minimizing recurrences; alternatively, rare episodes that are hemodynamically well tolerated may be managed with transesophageal conversion.[93,94] The long-term use of amiodarone in this setting is not routinely recommended, due to the anticipated side effects.

RF catheter ablation in this setting currently has success rates of 30% to 50%, with a high incidence of recurrence.[44,45] Recent reports of surgical conversion of Fontan patients with refractory arrhythmias to a total cavopulmonary anastomosis show improvement in symptoms, but recurrence of tachycardia is high.[95,96,96A] The addition of intraoperative cryoablation of the arrhythmia circuit and antitachycardia pacing appears to significantly improve the outcome, with withdrawal of antiarrhythmic medications possible in most patients.[97,97A]

Automatic Atrial Tachycardia

The decision to treat ectopic atrial tachycardia depends upon the rate, duration, and hemodynamic effects of tachycardia. Occasionally, the rate is within the same range of the sinus rate and then requires no treatment. This subset of patients requires surveillance because of the changing nature of this arrhythmia; most patients will require treatment. The most successful pharmacologic agents utilized include β-blockers, amiodarone, and sotalol.[98,99] If sinus rhythm is achieved, spontaneous resolution after medical therapy is reported to occur in up to 75% of patients.[99] Ablative therapy is very effective and may be used as initial therapy or for drug-resistant ectopic atrial tachycardia or for recurrence after drug withdrawal.[53,100,101] The presence of more than one ectopic focus reduces the success of therapy with either medication or ablation. While ablative therapy is relatively contraindicated in infants, it may be necessary for refractory tachycardia and severe symptoms.

Atrial Fibrillation

The goals of treatment in patients with atrial fibrillation include termination of acute episodes, control of ventricular rate, and prevention or reduction of recurrences.[90] Transthoracic and/or transesophageal echocardiogram should be obtained prior to attempted cardioversion to identify thrombosis in the atrium or ventricle.[102,103] Anticoagulation for 3–4 weeks by heparin and/or warfarin for the prevention of thromboembolic events before initiating antiarrhythmic agents or DC cardioversion is recommended.[104] Anticoagulation therapy should be continued for at least 3–4 weeks after conversion to sinus rhythm.[105] Synchronized direct current cardioversion is performed using 1 J/kg initially.[89] Class IA or class III agents are usually prescribed for maintaining sinus rhythm after cardioversion. The ventricular rate should be controlled by using digoxin, calcium channel blockers, or β-blockers. However, in the case of atrial fibrillation with WPW syndrome, administration of digoxin or a calcium channel blocker is avoided due to the possibility of enhancing 1:1 AV conduction via the accessory pathway, thereby triggering ventricular fibrillation. As with atrial reentrant tachycardia, the development of atrial fibrillation in patients with structural heart disease may indicate hemodynamic deterioration, and further evaluation may be necessary to determine surgical options.

Junctional Ectopic Tachycardia

Not all patients with JET require treatment. If the rate is near or slightly higher than the sinus rate, the patient needs no therapy; for high rates drug therapy may be indicated. The incidence of postoperative JET appears to be related to the surgical technique and hemodynamic results. The initial approach is to withdraw chronotropic agents, correct electrolyte imbalance, and maintain adequate fluid volume; cooling the patient and digoxin are also used with variable success.[106] The type IC agent, propafenone, was used with some success.[107,108] Currently, intravenous amiodarone has gained favor in the postoperative setting.[109-111] In the postoperative setting paired ventricular pacing can effectively slow the ventricular rate and increase the cardiac output. This is performed with a ventricular pacing protocol of a single S_1 coupled to a single S_2, in which the S_1-S_2 interval is programmed to be slightly longer than the ventricular effective refractory period; thus the S_2 captures the ventricle without producing an effective ventricular contraction.[112] In the congenital form, successful ablative therapy without producing heart block was reported.[113]

37. Cosio FG, López-Gil M, Goicolea A, et al. Radiofrequency ablation of the inferior vena cava-tricuspid valve isthmus in common atrial flutter. *Am J Cardiol* 1993;71:705–709.
38. Olshansky B, Okumura K, Hess PG, et al. Demonstration of an area of slow conduction in human atrial flutter. *J Am Coll Cardiol* 1990;16:1639–1648.
39. Cohen SI, Koh D, Lau SH, et al. P loops during common and uncommon atrial flutter in man. *Br Heart J* 1977;39:173–180.
40. Watson RM, Josephson ME. Atrial flutter. I. Electrophysiologic substrates and modes of initiation and termination. *Am J Cardiol* 1980;45:732–741.
41. Gomes JA, Mehta D, Langan MN. Sinus node reentrant tachycardia. *Pacing Clin Eletcrophysiol* 1995;18:1045–1057.
42. Gomes JA, Hariman RJ, Kang PS, et al. Sustained symptomatic sinus node reentrant tachycardia: incidence, clinical significance, electrophysiologic observations and the effects of antiarrhythmic agents. *J Am Coll Cardiol* 1985;5:45–57.
43. Sanders WE Jr, Sorrentino RA, Greenfield RA, et al. Catheter ablation of sinoatrial node reentrant tachycardia. *J Am Coll Cardiol* 1994;23:926–934.
44. Triedman JK, Saul JP, Weindling SN, et al. Radiofrequency ablation of intra-atrial reentrant tachycardia after surgical palliation of congenital heart disease. *Circulation* 1995;91:707–714.
45. Van Hare GF, Lesh MD, Ross BA, et al. Mapping and radiofrequency ablation of intraatrial reentrant tachycardia after the Senning or Mustard procedure for transposition of the great arteries. *Am J Cardiol* 1996;77:985–991.
46. Kalman JM, Van Hare GF, Olgin JE, et al. Ablation of 'incisional' reentrant atrial tachycardia complicating surgery for congenital heart disease: use of entrainment to define a critical isthmus of conduction. *Circulation* 1996;93:502–512.
47. Camm AJ, Obel OA. Epidemiology and mechanism of atrial fibrillation and atrial flutter. *Am J Cardiol* 1996;78:3–11.
48. Wells JL Jr, Karp RB, Kouchoukos NT, et al. Characterization of atrial fibrillation in man: studies following open heart surgery. *Pacing Clin Electrophysiol* 1978;1:426–438.
49. Haines DE, DiMarco JP. Sustained intraatrial reentrant tachycardia: clinical, electrocardiographic and electrophysiologic characteristics and long-term follow-up. *J Am Coll Cardiol* 1990;15:1345–1354.
50. Chen S-A, Chiang C-E, Yang C-J, et al. Sustained atrial tachycardia in adult patients. Electrophysiologic characteristics, pharmacological response, possible mechanisms, and effects of radiofrequency ablation. *Circulation* 1994;90:1262–1278.
51. Gillette PC, Garson A Jr: electrophysiologic and pharmacologic characteristics of automatic ectopic atrial tachycardia. *Circulation* 1977;56:571–575.
52. Mehta AV, Sanchez GR, Sacks EJ, et al. Ectopic automatic atrial tachycardia in children: clinical characteristics, management and follow-up. *J Am Coll Cardiol* 1988;11:379–385.
53. Walsh EP, Saul JP, Hulse JE, et al. Transcatheter ablation of ectopic atrial tachycardia in young patients using radiofrequency current. *Circulation* 1992;86:1138–1146.
54. Villain E, Vetter VL, Garcia JM, et al. Evolving concepts in the management of congenital junctional ectopic tachycardia. A multicenter study. *Circulation* 1990;81:1544–1549.
55. Grant JW, Serwer GA, Armstrong BE, et al. Junctional tachycardia in infants and children after open heart surgery for congenital heart disease. *Am J Cardiol* 1987;59:1216–1218.

56. Benson DW Jr, Deal BJ. Primary treatment of supraventricular tachycardia in infants and children. *Prog Pediatr Cardiol* 1995;4:209–214.
57. Benson DW Jr, Dunnigan A, Benditt DG, et al. Prediction of digoxin treatment failure in infants with supraventricular tachycardia: role of transesophageal pacing. *Pediatrics* 1985;75:288–293.
58. Wu MH, Chang YC, Lin JL, et al. Probability of supraventricular tachycardia recurrence in pediatric patients. *Cardiology* 1994;85:284–289.
59. Deal BJ, Keane JF, Gillette PC, et al. Wolff-Parkinson-White syndrome and supraventricular tachycardia during infancy: management and follow-up. *J Am Coll Cardiol* 1985;5:130–135.
60. Epstein ML, Kiel EA, Victorica BE. Cardiac decompensation following verapamil therapy in infants with supraventricular tachycardia. *Pediatrics* 1985;75:737–740.
61. Till JA, Shinebourne EA. Supraventricular tachycardia: diagnosis and current acute management. *Arch Dis Child* 1991;66:647–652.
62. Musto B, D'Onofrio A, Cavallaro C, et al. Electrophysiologic effects and clinical efficacy of flecainide in children with recurrent paroxysmal supraventricular tachycardia. *Am J Cardiol* 1988;62:229–233.
63. Zeigler V, Gillette PC, Ross BA, et al. Flecainide for supraventricular and ventricular arrhythmias in children and young adults. *Am J Cardiol* 1988;62:818–820.
64. Till JA, Shinebourne EA, Rowland E, et al. Paediatric use of flecainide in supraventricular tachycardia: clinical efficacy and pharmacokinetics. *Br Heart J* 1989;62:133–139.
65. Perry JC, McQuinn RL, Smith RT Jr, et al. Flecainide acetate for resistant arrhythmias in the young: efficacy and pharmacokinetics. *J Am Coll Cardiol* 1989;14:185–191.
66. Fish FA, Gillette PC, Benson DW Jr: proarrhythmia, cardiac arrest and death in young patients receiving encainide and flecainide. The Pediatric Electrophysiology Group. *J Am Coll Cardiol* 1991;18:356–365.
67. Tipple M, Sandor G. Efficacy and safety of oral sotalol in early infancy. *Pacing Clin Electrophysiol* 1991;14:2062–2065.
68. Maragnès P, Tipple M, Fournier A. Effectiveness of oral sotalol for treatment of pediatric arrhythmias. *Am J Cardiol* 1992;69:751–754.
69. Pfammatter JP, Paul T, Lehmann C, et al. Efficacy and proarrhythmia of oral sotalol in pediatric patients. *J Am Coll Cardiol* 1995;26:1002–1007.
70. Musto B, D'Onofrio A, Cavallaro C, et al. Electrophysiological effects and clinical efficacy of propafenone in children with recurrent paroxysmal supraventricular tachycardia. *Circulation* 1988;78:863–869.
71. Guccione P, Drago F, DiDonato RM, et al. Oral propafenone therapy for children with arrhythmias: efficacy and adverse effects in midterm follow-up. *Am Heart J* 1991;122:1022–1027.
72. Reimer A, Paul T, Kallfelz H-C. Efficacy and safety of intravenous and oral propafenone in pediatric cardiac dysrhythmias. *Am J Cardiol* 1991;68:741–744.
73. Beaufort-Krol GCM, Bink-Boelkens MTE: oral propafenone as treatment for incessant supraventricular and ventricular tachycardia in children. *Am J Cardiol* 1993;72:1213–1214.
74. Janousek J, Paul T, Reimer A, et al. Usefulness of *propafenone* for supraventricular arrhythmias in infants and children. *Am J Cardiol* 1993;72:294–300.
75. Shuler CO, Case CL, Gillette PC. Efficacy and safety of amiodarone in infants. *Am Heart J* 1993;125:1430–1432.
76. Coumel P, Fidelle J. Amiodarone in the treatment of cardiac arrhythmias in children: one hundred thirty-five cases. *Am Heart J* 1980;100:1063–1069.

77. Pongiglione G, Strasburger JF, Deal BJ, et al. Use of amiodarone for short-term and adjuvant therapy in young patients. *Am J Cardiol* 1991;68:603–608.
78. Fenrich AL Jr, Perry JC, Friedman RA. Flecainide and amiodarone: combined therapy for refractory tachyarrhythmias in infancy. *J Am Coll Cardiol* 1995; 68:1195–1198.
79. Case CL, Gillette PC, Oslizlok PC, et al. Radiofrequency catheter ablation of incessant, medically resistant supraventricular tachycardia in infants and small children. *J Am Coll Cardiol* 1992;20:1405–1410.
80. Erickson CC, Walsh EP, Triedman JK, et al. Efficacy and safety of radiofrequency ablation in infants and young children <18 months of age. *Am J Cardiol* 1994;74:944–947.
81. Saul JP, Hulse JE, Papagiannis J, et al. Late enlargement of radiofrequency lesions in infant lambs. Implications for ablation procedures in small children. *Circulation* 1994;90:492–499.
82. Kugler JD. Radiofrequency catheter ablation for supraventricular tachycardia. Should it be used in infants and small children? *Circulation* 1994;90:639–641.
83. Deal BJ, Dick M, Beerman L, et al. Cardiac arrest in young patients with Wolff-Parkinson-White syndrome (abstract). *Pacing Clin Electrophysiol* 1995;18:815.
84. Timmermans C, Smeets JLRM, Rodriguez L-M, et al. Aborted sudden death in the Wolff-Parkinson-White syndrome. *Am J Cardiol* 1995;76:492–494.
85. Dunnigan A, Benson DW Jr, Benditt DG. Atrial flutter in infancy: diagnosis, clinical features, and treatment. *Pediatrics* 1985;75:725–749.
86. Strasberg B, Ashley WW, Wyndham CR, et al. Treadmill exercise testing in the Wolff-Parkinson-White syndrome. *Am J Cardiol* 1980;45:742–748.
87. Critelli G, Grassi G, Perticone F, et al. Transesophageal pacing for prognostic evaluation of preexcitation syndrome and assessment of protective therapy. *Am J Cardiol* 1983;51:513–518.
88. Bikkina M, Alpert MA, Mulekar M, et al. Prevalence of intraatrial thrombus in patients with atrial flutter. *Am J Cardiol* 1995;576:186–189.
89. Kerber RE. Transthoracic cardioversion of atrial fibrillation and flutter: standard techniques and new advances. *Am J Cardiol* 1996;78(suppl 8A):22–26.
90. Anderson JL. Acute treatment of atrial fibrillation and flutter. *Am J Cardiol* 1996;78:17–21.
91. Kowey PR, VanderLugt JT, Luderer JR. Safety and risk/benefit analysis of ibutilide for acute conversion of atrial fibrillation/flutter. *Am J Cardiol* 1996;78:46–52.
92. Garson A Jr, Bink-Boelkens M, Hesslein PS, et al. Atrial flutter in the young: a collaborative study of 380 cases. *J Am Coll Cardiol* 1985;6:871–878.
93. Butto F, Dunnigan A, Overholt ED, et al. Transesophageal study of recurrent atrial tachycardia after atrial baffle procedures for complete transposition of the great arteries. *Am J Cardiol* 1986;57:1356–1362.
94. Kantharia BK, Mookherjee S. Clinical utility and the predictors of outcome of overdrive transesophageal atrial pacing in the treatment of atrial flutter. *Am J Cardiol* 1995;76:144–147.
95. Kreutzer J, Keane JF, Lock JE, et al. Conversion of modified Fontan procedure to lateral atrial tunnel cavopulmonary anastomosis. *J Thorac Cardiovasc Surg* 1996;111:1169–1176.
96. Kao JM, Alejos JC, Grant PW, et al. Conversion of atriopulmonary to cavopulmonary anastomosis in management of late arrhythmias and atrial thrombosis. *Ann Thorac Surg* 1994;58:1510–1514.
96A. Triedman JK, Bergau DM, Saul JP, et al. Efficacy of radiofrequency ablation for control of intraatrial reentrant tachycardia in patients with congenital heart disease. J Am Coll Cardiol 1997;30:1032–1038.

97. Deal BJ, Mavroudis C, Backer CL, et al. Surgical cryoablation of arrhythmia circuit in Fontan patients (abstract). *Circulation* 1995;94(suppl I):1020.

97A. Mavroudis C, Backer CL, Deal BJ, et al. Fontan conversion to cavopulmonary connection and cryoablation of arrhythmia circuit. J Thorac Cardiovasc Surg 1998; 115: in press.

98. von Bernuth G, Engelhardt W, Kramer HH, et al. Atrial automatic tachycardia in infancy and childhood. *Eur Heart J* 1992;13:1410–1415.

99. Naheed ZJ, Strasburger JF, Benson DW Jr, et al. Natural history and management strategies of automatic atrial tachycardia in children. *Am J Cardiol* 1995;75:405–407.

100. Tracy CM, Swartz JF, Fletcher RD, et al. Radiofrequency catheter ablation of ectopic atrial tachycardia using paced activation sequence mapping. *J Am Coll Cardiol* 1993;21:910–917.

101. Dhala AA, Case CL, Gillette PC. Evolving treatment strategies for managing atrial ectopic tachycardia in children. *Am J Cardiol* 1994;74:283–286.

102. Feltes TF, Friedman RA. Transesophageal echocardiographic detection of atrial thrombi in patients with nonfibrillation atrial tachyarrhythmias and congenital heart disease. *J Am Coll Cardiol* 1994;24:1365–1370.

103. Grimm RA, Stewart WJ, Black IW, et al. Should all patients undergo transesophageal echocardiography before electrical cardioversion of atrial fibrillation? *J Am Coll Cardiol* 1994;23:533–541.

104. Collins LJ, Silverman DI, Douglas PS, et al. Cardioversion of nonrheumatic atrial fibrillation. Reduced thromboembolic complications with 4 weeks of precardioversion anticoagulation are related to atrial thrombus resolution. *Circulation* 1995;92:160–163.

105. Manning WJ, Silverman DI, Keighley CS, et al. Transesophageal echocardiographically facilitated early cardioversion from atrial fibrillation using short-term anticoagulation: final results of a prospective 4.5-year study. *J Am Coll Cardiol* 1995;25:1354–1361.

106. Bash SE, Shah JJ, Albers WH, et al. Hypothermia for the treatment of post-surgical greatly accelerated junctional ectopic tachycardia. *J Am Coll Cardiol* 1987;10:1095–1099.

107. Garson A Jr, Moak JP, Smith RT Jr, et al. Usefulness of intravenous propafenone for control of postoperative junctional ectopic tachycardia. *Am J Cardiol* 1987;59:1422–1424.

108. Paul T, Reimer A, Janousek J, et al. Efficacy and safety of propafenone in congenital junctional ectopic tachycardia. *J Am Coll Cardiol* 1992;20:911–914.

109. Figa FH, Gow RM, Hamilton RM, et al. Clinical efficacy and safety of intravenous amiodarone in infants and children. *Am J Cardiol* 1994;74:573–577.

110. Raja P, Hawker RE, Chaikitpinyo A, et al. Amiodarone management of junctional ectopic tachycardia after cardiac surgery in children. *Br Heart J* 1994;72:261–265.

111. Perry JC, Fenrich AL, Hulse JE, et al. Pediatric use of intravenous amiodarone: efficacy and safety in critically ill patients from a multicenter protocol. *J Am Coll Cardiol* 1996;27:1246–1250.

112. Waldo AL, Krongrad E, Kupersmith J, et al. Ventricular paired pacing to control rapid ventricular heart rate following open heart surgery. Observations on ectopic automaticity. Report of a case in a four-month-old patient. *Circulation* 1976;53:176–181.

113. Young ML, Mehta MB, Martinez RM, et al. Combined alpha-adrenergic blockade and radiofrequency ablation to treat junctional ectopic tachycardia successfully without atrioventricular block. *Am J Cardiol* 1993;71:883–885.

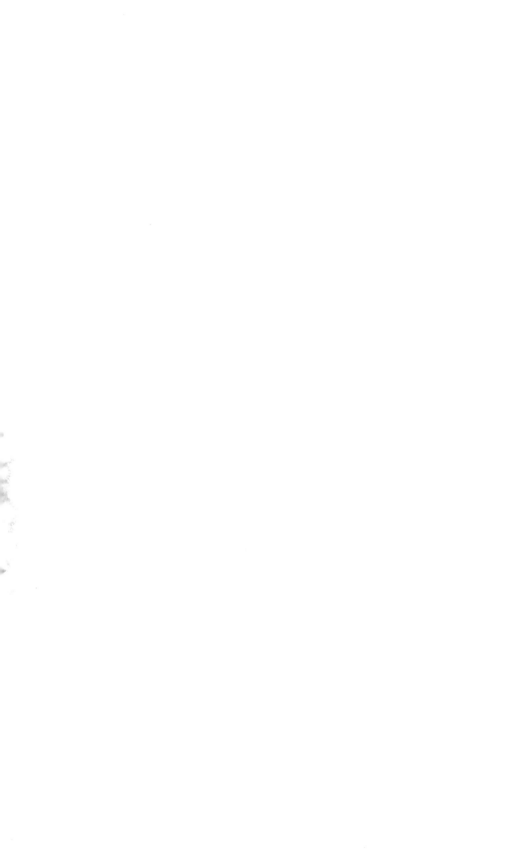

Chapter 7

Ventricular Tachycardia

Macdonald Dick II, MD
and Mark W. Russell, MD

Definition and Mechanisms

Ventricular tachycardia (VT) may be defined as an abnormally accelerated cardiac rhythm, at a rate ≥ 120 beats per minute (bpm) or 25% bpm faster than the sinus rate (Figure 1). This arrhythmia is due to abnormal ventricular impulse generation and/or conduction arising within the peripheral Purkinje network or, less frequently, within the more central trifascicular system (His bundle and bundle branches) or the ventricular myocardium.[1,2] The cells of the His bundle branch Purkinje system exhibit normal automaticity (slow diastolic depolarization, albeit at very slow rates ≤ 50 bpm) and comprise the slower escape mechanisms in the hierarchy of the cardiac impulse. In contrast, myocytes from the working myocardium exhibit automaticity and spontaneous discharge only under abnormal conditions, such as hypoxia, variances in concentrations of extracellular and intracellular ions (eg, potassium) critical for excitation, various membrane active medications (particularly antiarrhythmic drugs), or structural changes in the ion channels [congenital long QT syndrome (LQTS)]. Furthermore, the ion channels in the sarcolemma of the myocyte are, in part, composed of proteins that are encoded by specific genes on at least four different chromosomes (11, 3, 4, and 7); mutations in these genes encode defective channels that result in the long QT phenotypes and the characteristic torsades de pointes VT (Figure 2).[3] Alterations in ion channel density or structure may play a role in the threshold of vulnerability for VT

From Deal B, Wolff G, Gelband H, (eds.). *Current Concepts in Diagnosis and Management of Arrhythmias in Infants and Children.* Armonk, NY: Futura Publishing Co., Inc.; © 1998.

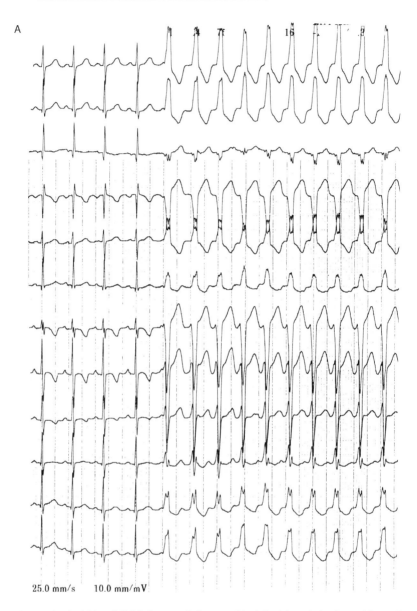

25.0 mm/s   10.0 mm/mV

Figure 1. A: 12-lead ECG from a 2.5-year-old girl with palpitations. Normal sinus rhythm is on the left side of the tracing; in the middle and right side of the tracing onset of wide QRS tachycardia at rate of 180–190 bpm (25% faster than the sinus rate) can be seen. The patient was otherwise asymptomatic and had a normal echocardiogram. The morphology of the wide QRS tachycardia is that of LBBB with an inferior frontal plane axis, indicating probable origin from the RVOT.

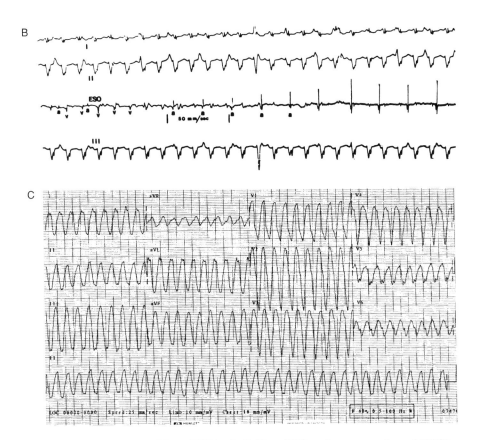

Figure 1. (*continued*) **B**: Three ECG leads (I, II, and III) and a transesophageal (ESO) bipolar electrogram demonstrating wide QRS tachycardia recorded from a 2-day-old infant are shown. On the left-hand side of the figure, the atrial electrograms (a) and the ventricular electrograms (v) waves recorded through the transesophageal electrode catheter are of near equal amplitude, but do not appear to be at the same rate. As the transesophageal catheter is slowly withdrawn, the atrial (a) electrogram becomes more evident (right side of the figure) due to both an increased amplitude and a slower rate than the ventricular rate (wide QRS complex). These tracings clearly demonstrate AV dissociation confirming VT, and, by this example, illustrate the diagnostic value of transesophageal recordings. (see Figure 3D). **C**: Twelve-lead ECG from a 27-year-old woman with palpitations and syncope. She had undergone repair of the tetralogy of Fallot 20 years prior to this event. The ECG demonstrated wide QRS tachycardia which required DC cardioversion. Programmed ventricular extra stimulation during EP study demonstrated VT (see Figure 3D).

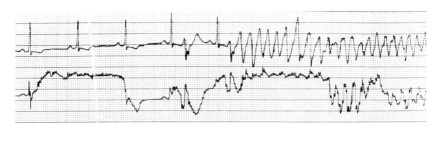

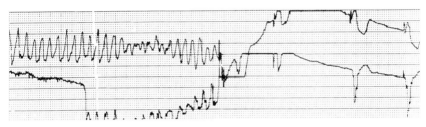

Figure 2. Onset of torsades de points in a 13-year-old girl with a normal QT interval. The torsades is terminated by discharge from an implantable cardiodefibrillator. Note the undulating shape of the QRS complex (both in amplitude and polarity) as if it were spiraling around a center core.

seen in patients in a number of diverse clinical settings (ischemia, infarct, cardiomyopathy, and following surgery for congenital cardiac malformations).

The current hypotheses regarding the mechanisms of human VT are (1) reentry, mediated by unidirectional block and slow conduction through or around localized areas of ventricular myocardium, and/or (2) abnormal automaticity, related to an alteration in phase 4 slow diastolic depolarization, occurring within diseased myocardium, and (3) triggered activity (early or late after depolarizations) occurring in diseased human cardiac tissue.[4-11] Triggered activity was detected in diseased human cardiac tissue by microelectrode techniques, and criteria were advanced in an effort to apply its observed cellular electrophysiological (EP) characteristics to clinical arrhythmias; accelerated junctional tachycardia and possibly accelerated ventricular rhythm may represent clinical forms of this mechanism.[12,13] Presented in this chapter are the electrocardiographic (ECG) characteristics, incidence, prognosis, and recent EP and therapeutic advances of VT in the young.

Electrocardiogram

The chief ECG feature of VT is an accelerated heart rate, usually $\geq 150–250$ bpm, with a wide QRS complex (Table 1). The ECG features

_____ Table 1 _____

Electrocardiographic Features of Ventricular Tachycardia

Electrocardiographic Finding	Comment
Atrioventricular dissociation	Virtually diagnostic
Capture and fusion beats	Normalizes the QRS complex
QRS morphology and duration	Wide QRS (120 ms except in infants;[3] 140 ms in older patients); abnormal T wave
	QRS complex different shape than sinus QRS complex
Torsades de pointes	Spiraling, undulating QRS waveform twisting around a point moving in time; associated with the long QT syndromes

that confirm VT are atrioventricular (AV) dissociation (Figure 1) in the absence of retrograde conduction (as often occurs at fast ventricular rates) and fusion or capture beats as a result of ventricular capture by a sinus beat (or a second focus) during the VT. There are five other different rhythms that produce wide QRS tachycardia, all of which can be misinterpreted as VT (Figure 3).[14] The first rhythm, accelerated ventricular rhythm (Figure 4), is a distinctive form of VT; it meets all the ECG and EP criteria for VT, but is usually only somewhat faster than the sinus rate and is not associated with hemodynamic instability.[15-17] The other four forms of wide QRS tachycardia that mimic VT are supraventricular rhythms: (1) supraventricular

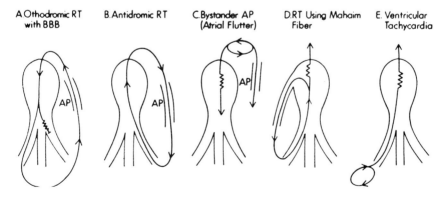

Figure 3. Depiction of the five mechanisms of wide QRS tachycardia (see text). Reproduced with permission from reference 14.

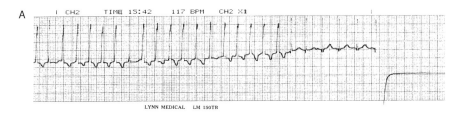

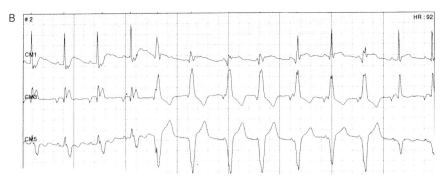

Figure 4. A: ECG tracing demonstrating wide QRS tachycardia in a 4-month-old girl; she had intermittent wide QRS tachycardia since birth but had no symptoms. She did not respond to propranolol, disopyramide, or phenytoin. This tachycardia demonstrates AV dissociation and fusion beats. However, the rate is only 25% (an increase from 150 bpm to 167 bpm) faster than the narrow QRS sinus rhythm and thus is an accelerated ventricular rhythm rather than VT. The tachycardia resolved by 2 years of age, but she continues to exhibit ventricular premature beats at 13 years. **B**: ECG tracing demonstrating accelerated AV rhythm in a 13-year-old boy with Ebstein's anomaly of the tricuspid valve shortly after closure of his ASD and reconstruction of his tricuspid valve. Note the initial sinus rhythm at 94 bpm with a wide QRS complex of right bundle block (right side of tracing). A spontaneous wide QRS rhythm of a slightly faster rate of 100 bpm then develops. Note the AV dissociation and fusion beats, indicating the ventricular origin of the rhythm. The accelerated ventricular rhythm spontaneously resolved without specific treatment.

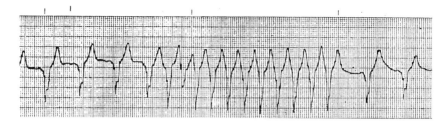

Figure 5. Run of wide QRS tachycardia in an 18-year-old man 10 years following the Rastelli operation for transposition of the great arteries, VSD, and pulmonary stenosis. Note the wide QRS morphology of the tachycardia is identical to that during sinus rhythm immediately preceding it.

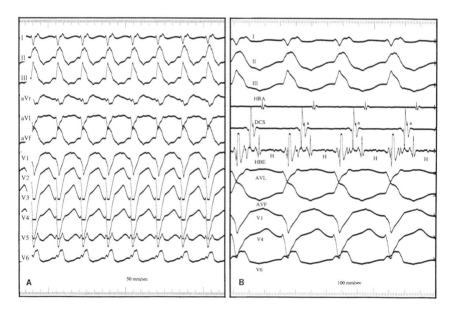

Figure 6. **A**: 12-lead ECG demonstrating wide QRS tachycardia [cycle length (CL) = 325 milliseconds] with LBBB configuration in a 14-year-old boy. **B**: At EP study, the His bundle potential (H) was recorded prior to the wide QRS complex; also a small "a" wave was noted at the terminal portion of the DCS electrogram activated prior to atrial activation on the His bundle electrogram (HBE). These findings indicate that the wide QRS tachycardia resulted from rate-related LBBB during SVT supported retrogradely through a concealed left posterior accessory pathway (see Figure 3A). a—atrial electrogram, DCS—distal coronary sinus, H—His bundle electrogram, HBE—His bundle tracing, and HRA—high right atrial (RA) tracing.

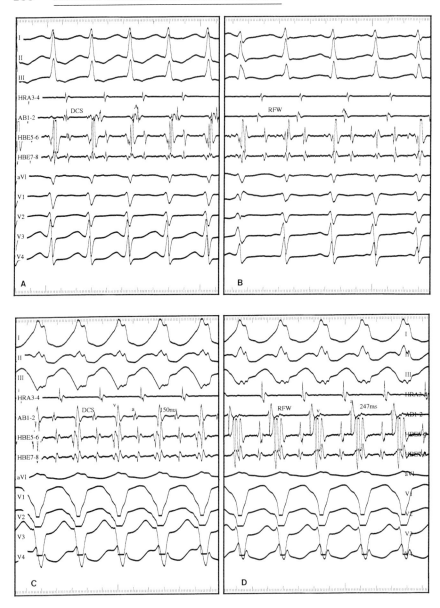

Figure 7. **A** and **B** were recorded from a 5-year-old boy during EP study for wide QRS tachycardia. **A** and **B** demonstrate narrow QRS tachycardia; in **A** the tachycardia is supported retrogradely through a left-sided accessory pathway as demonstrated by the earliest atrial (A) electrogram recorded through the distal coronary sinus (DCS) bipolar electrodes; in contrast, in **B**, the tachycardia is supported retrogradely by a right sided accessory pathway as indicted by the earliest atrial electrogram (A) recorded through bipolar electrodes located at the right free wall (RFW) of the RA near the AV ring. Paper speed = 100 mm/s.

Figure 7. (*continued*) **C** and **D** demonstrate a wide QRS tachycardia in the same patient as in **A** and **B**. In **C** the tachycardia is supported retrogradely through the left-sided accessory pathway (where the VA interval is shortest, 150 milliseconds). In **D** the atrial (a) electrogram recorded through the bipolar electrodes at the RFW exhibits the longest VA interval (247 milliseconds) but a very short AV interval (the a electrogram is transcribed just before the QRS complex). The tracings in **C** and **D** indicate anomalous antegrade conduction across the right-sided accessory pathway and retrograde conduction through the left sided pathway. Thus this wide QRS tachycardia is due to an anomalous right-sided accessory AV pathway conducting antegradely, so-called antidromic reciprocating tachycardia (as well as the left-sided accessory pathway conducting retrogradely). The patient underwent successful ablation of both pathways. Paper speed = 100 mm/s (see Figure 3B).

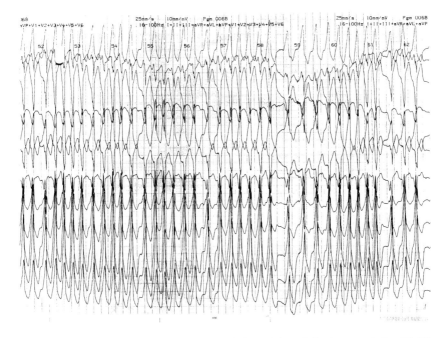

Figure 8. 12-lead ECG from a 16-year-old boy with palpitations and the Wolff-Parkinson-White (WPW) syndrome. Note the wide QRS tachycardia with variable and frequent very short (160 milliseconds) RR intervals, suggesting atrial fibrillation with rapid anomalous antegrade conduction across the accessory pathway. ECG leads are listed (lead I through V6) at the top of the page corresponding to the tracings arrayed from top to bottom. This patient underwent successful ablation of right-sided pathway (see Figure 3C).

tachycardia (SVT) in the presence of preexisting bundle-branch block (Figure 5); 2) SVT with rate-related (phase 3) bundle-branch block (Figure 6); 3) SVT with fast antegrade conduction across accessory connection(s) (AC) during antidromic AV reentry tachycardia (Figure 7); and (4) atrial flutter (AF) or fibrillation with antegrade conduction across an AC (Figure 8). Fortunately, both preexisting disease in the conduction system (except for the postoperative group) and clinically significant fast conducting AC are infrequent in children.

Clinical Electrophysiological Studies

The advent of intracardiac His bundle recording, programmed extrastimulation of the heart, and endocardial mapping contributed greatly to the understanding of VT and led to new therapeutic approaches, including acute drug testing, surgical endocardial excision, and, more recently, radiofrequency ablation (RFA) of either a segment of the reentry circuit or abnormal automatic focus. In 1972 Wellens and associates,[6,7] using programmed stimulation of the heart in patients with sustained VT, developed the clinical EP criteria for reentry within the ventricles. These criteria included reproducible initiation and termination of the tachycardia by critically timed premature stimuli delivered to the ventricles as well as the demonstration of incremental intraventricular conduction delay during programmed ventricular extrastimulation (Figure 9). In contrast to the significance of sustained monomorphic VT in response to ventricular extrastimuli, the importance of a nonsustained ventricular response is uncertain. Programmed extrastimulation and endocardial mapping support reentry as the most common mechanism of VT. Paced mapping and continuous diastolic electrical activity (fragmented electrograms) in conjunction with concealed entrainment facilitates precise mapping of the reentrant circuit.[18,19] The stimulation techniques used to detect reentry are especially useful in the management of postoperative pediatric patients with life-threatening sustained monomorphic VT as well as in selected patients with symptomatic complex ventricular arrhythmias.[20] Other mechanisms such as abnormal automaticity, triggered activity, and anisotropic conduction are also important. However, the classification and treatment of VT will remain largely empirical, dependent on the ECG features, the clinical EP mechanisms of the tachycardia, and the patient's clinical setting[21,22] until there is clarification of the cellular, subcellular, and molecular definition of the channels, receptors, and pumps involved in myocardial excitation.

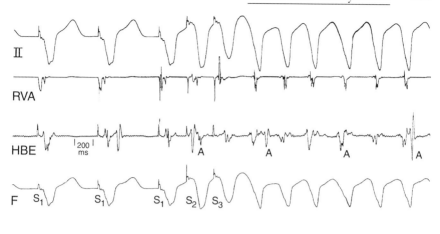

A

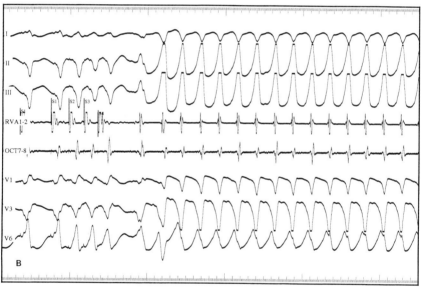

Figure 9. Programmed ventricular extrastimulation in a 13-year-old girl 4 years after repair of pulmonary atresia and VSD (**A**) and in a 10-year-old boy with transposition of the great arteries, VSD, and pulmonary atresia 6 years after the Rastelli procedure (**B**). Both tracings demonstrate monomorphic VT induced by extrastimulation. Identical clinical wide QRS tachycardia resulted in palpitations and faintness in both patients as well as syncope in the girl. The girl remained inducible on procainamide, disopyramide, mexiletine, and propafenone. She underwent conduit revision and cryotherapy of the arrhythmogenic focus at the egress of the conduit, successfully ablating the tachycardia. The boy responded to amiodarone.

Incidence

The incidence of VT in the young is unknown. VT accounts for 6% of all tachyarrhythmias ($n = 631$) seen at our institution, almost one half of these patients having heart disease; in contrast, SVT (all forms) comprises the other 94%. Data that include both single ventricular premature beats as well as repetitive beats indicate that the incidence of ventricular arrhythmias in the young ranges from 0.5% in newborns and infants to 18% to 50% in older children,[1,23] depending upon the method of detection, presence, and severity of underlying heart disease and the form of ascertainment (random vs. selected).[24-31] Although the incidence of VT in young individuals is unknown, young athletes may have an incidence of nonsustained VT, including accelerated ventricular rhythm (a run of three or more ventricular beats) as high as 10%.[32]

Clinical Characteristics

Accelerated Ventricular Rhythm

Accelerated ventricular rhythm was suggested as an alternative term for VT when the wide QRS tachycardia is ≤120 bpm or at a rate only slightly faster than the sinus rate; it was reported in infants as well as in older children and adolescents (Figure 4). The QRS duration in the infant is usually twice that of the normally conducted beats but may not reach the duration (>120 milliseconds) seen in older patients. It is differentiated from VT by its slower rate, absence of symptoms, and normal cardiac structure and function. The mechanism is heterogeneous; the tachycardia in some patients appears to be reentry and, in others, abnormal automaticity or triggered activity.[15-17] The significance of this arrhythmia is its proper recognition so that unnecessary and potentially toxic medications are not administered.

VT in the newborn and infant is rare. VT in the infant (Figure 4), which was shown in some patients to be based on reentry,[33] is usually self-terminating and tends to decrease with increasing age. Several investigators defined this form of VT as similar if not synonymous with accelerated ventricular rhythm (Figure 4). Not infrequently, the tachycardia is well tolerated and does not require specific treatment; trial of antiarrhythmic agents is often attempted but usually to no avail.[23,34-40]

In contrast, when the VT is rapid, persistent, or accompanied by hemodynamic instability, there is a high association (up to 43%) with major medical disorders, such as the LQTS, severe myocarditis (Figure 10), adrenogenital syndrome, large cardiac tumors as well as micro-

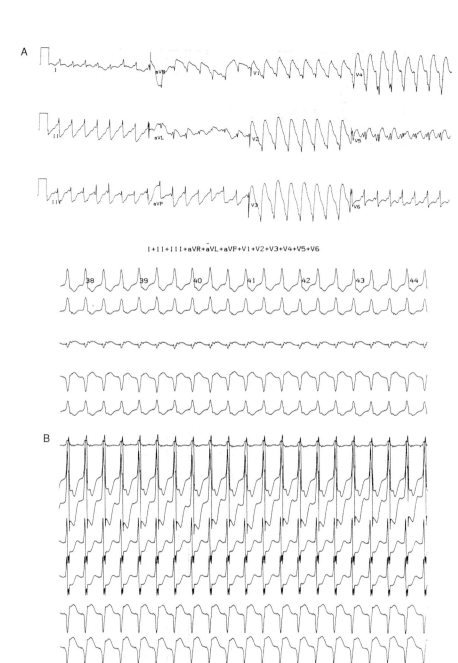

Figure 10. The 12-lead ECG shown in **A** demonstrates sustained wide QRS tachycardia in a 6-month-old boy; histologic findings at autopsy demonstrated acute myocarditis. The 12-lead ECG in **B** is from a critically ill 10-day-old infant; Coxsackie A virus was recovered from nasal and rectal swaps as well as from the cerebrospinal fluid, strongly suggesting viral myocarditis as the cause of the VT, proven by intracardiac recording and pacing. Autopsy was not obtained.

scopic hamartomas[41,42] and electrolyte imbalance, and central nervous system disorders.[40] Treatment is predicated on the underlying condition and the associated hemodynamic state. Infants with the LQTS, myocarditis, or microscopic hamartoma (His-Purkinje cell tumors) may exhibit profound hemodynamic deterioration. Patients with the LQTS often require management with β-blockade, a pacemaker, and possibly an implantable cardioverter-defibrillator (ICD). For the patient with myocarditis, aggressive pharmacologic support with intravenous inotropic agents may be needed as well as intraaortic mechanical pump devices or extracorporeal membrane oxygenator. For patients with cardiac tumors, catheter ablation of the ectopic focus or surgical excision of the tumor may be necessary. Antiarrhythmic agents may be helpful in suppressing the VT but are infrequently sufficient to control the hemodynamically unstable arrhythmia or address the pathological substrate giving rise to the disordered rhythm. Interestingly, it is unusual for VT in the newborn infant to be associated solely with an anatomic malformation.[40]

Idiopathic Ventricular Tachycardia

Idiopathic VT occurs in the absence of identifiable heart disease or predisposing conditions and is reported in all age groups.[43] Recent reviews including patients followed for up to 12 years suggest that idiopathic VT in the young does not necessarily produce symptoms, may disappear spontaneously (particularly in the neonate), and is compatible with a relatively normal life.[1,23,34–39,44–47] On the other hand, a number of reports documented sudden death in eight patients with no structural heart disease.[34,46,48–51] Confusion in the literature regarding the prognosis results from the inclusion of multiple distinct patient populations, such as those with accelerated ventricular rhythm, arrhythmogenic right ventricular (RV) dysplasia, and exercise-related VT, in the same series of idiopathic VT.

Because of the often benign, asymptomatic course of many patients on the one hand and the possibility of medication side effects, proarrhythmic events and failure of antiarrhythmic medications over a long life span on the other, children with VT should undergo evaluation for underlying heart disease. Focus should include the LQTS, myocarditis, cardiomyopathy, cardiac tumor, RV arrhythmogenic dysplasia, or electrolyte imbalance.[1,16] Specific ECG patterns as described below, suppression of the tachycardia with exercise, an asymptomatic state, a relatively low spontaneous tachycardia rate (<150 bpm), and the absence of demonstrable heart disease may allow a conservative approach.[1,35,42–49,52–55] Two specific forms of idiopathic VT with distinctive ECG appearance deserve special attention.

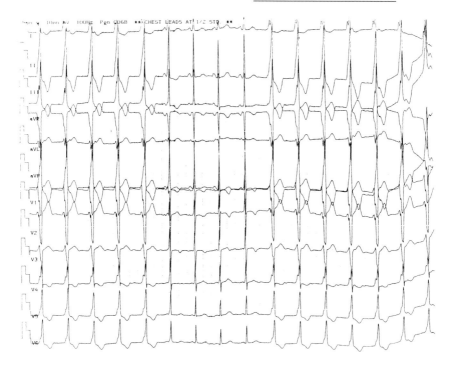

Figure 11. Wide QRS tachycardia in a 5-year-old girl present since birth. Note that the heart rate is similar to the sinus rate and that the QRS morphology is a LBBB pattern with an inferior frontal plane axis, suggesting that the origin of this rhythm was the RVOT.

Right Ventricular Outflow Tract Ventricular Tachycardia

In RV outflow tract (RVOT) VT, the QRS morphology is that of a left bundle-branch block (LBBB) pattern with an inferior frontal plane QRS axis (Figure 11). This form of VT is often catecholamine sensitive, but not uniformly inducible with programmed stimulation.[52,56] Adenosine may successfully terminate this VT, suggesting triggered activity may be the underlying mechanism[57]; β-blocker therapy is often effective, as is radiofrequency (RF) catheter ablation (Figure 12).[58,59] Magnetic resonance imaging (MRI) may detect subtle anatomic abnormalities of the RVOT.[60]

Left Ventricular Outflow Tract Ventricular Tachycardia

In left ventricular (LV) VT, the QRS morphology is right bundle branch with a superior QRS frontal plane axis (Figure 13), suggesting ei-

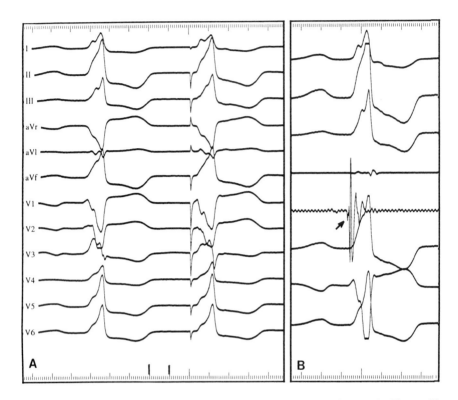

Figure 12. A demonstrates a 12-lead ECG from the same patient as in Figure 11 during pace mapping: the QRS complex on the left is the last QRS complex from the spontaneous clinical VT; the QRS complex on the right is the first paced QRS complex when performing pace mapping from the right posterior aspect of the RVOT. Note the near (11 of 12 ECG leads; V3 is not identical) identity between the spontaneous beat on the left and paced beat on the right. In **B** the top three leads are leads I, II, and III, respectively. The bottom three leads are aVF, V1, and V6, respectively. The middle two leads are intracardiac bipolar (2 mm) leads; the fifth tracing from the top is a bipolar electrogram from a site identical to that of the paced mapping beat in the RVOT shown in **A** and demonstrates a fast action deflection transcribed 25 milliseconds before the surface QRS complex. These tracings together demonstrate that the origin of this patient's tachycardia is the rightward posterior aspect of the RVOT. RF energy delivered at this site abolished the tachycardia. Time interval (between the two dark vertical lines in **A**) is 200 milliseconds.

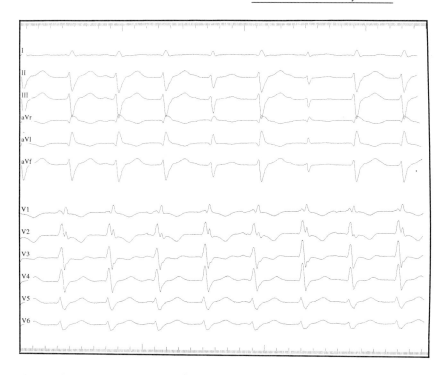

Figure 13. 12-lead ECG from a 7.5-year-old boy with palpitations and wide QRS tachycardia at a CL of 380 milliseconds, characterized by a RBBB configuration and a superior leftward axis. This QRS morphology suggests that the tachycardia arises from the LV, but the precise site cannot be determined from this tracing.

ther an inferior LV or septal origin of the tachycardia, often from the posterior-inferior ventricular His-Purkinje system.[44,45] This form of VT may be induced with programmed atrial as well as ventricular stimulation and is sensitive to verapamil[61–64] but not usually to adenosine.[57] Some authors believe a false tendon in the LV extending from the posteroinferior LV to the septum is responsible for this arrhythmia.[65] RF catheter ablation is highly successful (Figure 14).[53,66,67]

The variable response to EP programmed extrastimulation and to verapamil, adenosine, and isoproterenol underscore the heterogeneity of the mechanisms of these forms of VT. Ventricular reentry, abnormal automaticity, and afterdepolarizations were all implicated.[38,68,69] Pharmacologic treatment, especially with β-blockers or verapamil, depending upon tachycardia characteristics of each individual, may be helpful for these specific types of VT.[38,44,46,50,68] The prognosis for these two forms of tachycardia is generally excellent, and no treatment is required in the absence of symptoms.

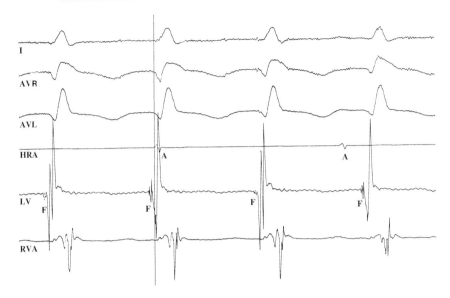

Figure 14. Three ECG and three intracardiac tracings recorded during EP study from the same patient as in Figure 13. Note the ventricular electrogram (LV) recorded very early in ventricular activation and the fast action deflection (F) just preceding the ventricular electrogram. This electrogram (F) was recorded from the posterior fascicle (F) of the left bundle. RF energy delivered at this site abolished the tachycardia. I, AVR, AVL—three ECG leads, HRA—high RA tracing, LV—LV tracing, and RVA—RV apex tracing.

Recent management of young patients with idiopathic VT was greatly influenced by advances in RFA. Successful RFA of the form originating from the RVOT was reported. Identification of early ventricular activation (20–30 milliseconds before the surface QRS) during tachycardia, combined with pace mapping to give an identical ECG reproduction of the tachycardia, are helpful in localizing the focus. Because RVOT myocardial wall is thin, lower energies are used to minimize the risk of perforation in this form.[56,67]

Torsades de Pointes

Torsades de pointes,[70,71] a term introduced in 1966, specifies a ventricular arrhythmia characterized by rapid, wide undulating QRS morphology as if the QRS waveform were spiraling around a single point (Figures 15 and 16). Although the twisting pattern may be seen in ventricular arrhythmias resulting from several different clinical and pathological settings, torsades implies both the spiraling waveform and a preexisting congenital or acquired long QT interval. The nature of the torsades configu-

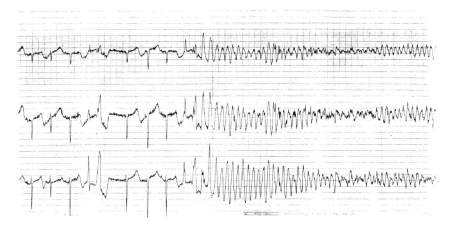

Figure 15. Initiation of torsades de pointes in a 14-year-old girl with the congenital LQTS. Note the T-wave alternans, a characteristic of the LQTS, prior to the onset of torsades.

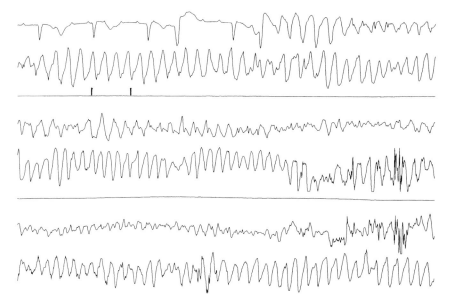

Figure 16. Rhythm strip from 4-year-old boy with congenital complete heart block and a heart rate of 43 bpm. The QT interval has greatly lengthened in response to this bradycardia following the first QRS complex. The second and the third QRS complexes are followed by a relatively normal QT interval for heart rate. The fourth beat is premature and induces pause-dependent accentuation of the T wave and lengthening of the QT interval; the next premature beat, also set up by the pause, induces torsades. This boy was cardioverted with DC current and then treated with temporary transvenous ventricular pacing followed by a permanent transvenous implantable dual chamber pacing system . Time interval (interval between dark vertical lines) equals 1 second.

ration was described as movement of reentrant wavelets in a multilayer cell system around a nonstationary unstable spiral core, resulting from block of potassium repolarizing currents. When there is sufficient inhomogeneity of repolarization, as well as sufficient myocardial mass to support propagation of the wavelet, sustained polymorphic ventricular arrhythmia may develop.[72] This arrhythmia does not support the circulation, and is thus a cause of loss of consciousness and sudden death. In some patients, particularly younger patients with smaller hearts, the torsades may terminate spontaneously. The several different clinical settings that are associated with this ventricular arrhythmia include congenital and acquired forms of the LQTS, responses to antiarrhythmic agents, response to changes in autonomic tone, electrolyte abnormalities, and severe bradycardia.[71,73–76] Recent studies in molecular biology demonstrated, by mutation analysis, several genetic defects for the congenital form of the LQTS associated with subtle differences in QT phenotypes. These studies identified structural abnormalities in one sodium channel and two potassium channels, the latter responsible for conductance of the repolarizing current. It is possible that other channel abnormalities are present in patients who have a normal QT interval at rest but who, in the presence of a number of different stimuli, are subject to torsades.

Congenital Long QT Syndrome

Congenital LQTS (see also Chapter 9) is an inherited disorder comprising a long QT interval on the ECG, recurrent ventricular arrhythmias, particularly torsades de pointes (Figure 15), and sudden death. Patients with the autosomal dominant form, which accounts for over 95% of cases in childhood,[72] have normal hearing, while those patients with the autosomal recessive form have associated congenital neurosensorial deafness. The congenitally long QT interval supplies the EP substrate of delayed repolarization, which underlies the torsades. These patients are particularly sensitive to adrenergic stimulus. Stress associated with an adrenergic surge, particularly emotionally driven, is widely recognized as a herald of torsades in patients with the congenital LQTS.

Recently, positional and candidate cloning studies identified three genes responsible for the congenital LQTS, the putative voltage-gated potassium channel KVLQT1,[77] the HERG potassium channel,[78] and the SCN5A cardiac sodium channel.[79] Linkage studies estimated that ~50% of the LQTS cases are due to defects in the KVLQT1 gene, while HERG and SCN5A defects are the second and third most common causes, respectively.[77] A defect in one of these three genes is responsible for ~90% of the cases of autosomal dominant, LQTS.[80] A fourth LQTS gene was localized to chromosome 4q25–27 in one family[81] and additional families were identified in whom the LQTS is not linked to any of the previously identified loci, suggesting the presence of at least a fifth LQTS gene.[77] A summary of the genes responsible for this syndrome is presented in Table 2.

Determining which gene is affected in a patient with the LQTS may be important in determining the optimal therapy for that patient.[82,83] Preliminary studies revealed that each group of LQTS patients has unique clinical features and may respond very differently to therapeutic interventions.[82–84] Chromosome 7 (LQT2) patients have a decreased number of normal HERG potassium channels per myocardial cell and often have abnormal HERG channels with a diminished capacity to conduct a potassium current.[85] This decreases the rate of outward repolarizing potassium current, thereby prolonging repolarization.[78] In in vitro studies, the potassium current through a homotetramer of four HERG channel proteins is exquisitely sensitive to extracellular potassium concentrations.[85] As extracellular potassium concentration rises, outward potassium current through the HERG channel paradoxically increases as is characteristic of the rapidly activating cardiac delayed rectifier potassium current (I_{Kr}).[85] In seven patients with LQT2 LQTS, an average increase in the serum potassium concentration of 1.4 mEq/L shortened the QT interval an average of 24%, normalized QT dispersion (a measure of spatial heterogeneity of repolarization that is usually increased in patients with LQTS), and improved T-wave abnormalities in six of the seven.[83] Current clinical trials are evaluating the ability of dietary and pharmacotherapeutic increase of the serum potassium concentration to improve the symptoms and decrease the morbidity and mortality of patients with LQT2-type LQTS.[83]

Torsades de pointes in patients with HERG or KVLQT1 defects appears to be adrenergic dependent, occurring during times of stress.[77,78] Previous clinical studies demonstrating the effectiveness of β-blockade in patients with the LQTS[86] likely reflect the benefit of this therapy in patients with HERG and KVLQT1 defects, since they comprise ~80% of the patients with congenital LQTS.[80] The KVLQT1 gene also appears to encode for a voltage-gated potassium channel due to its high homology to the Shaker family of potassium channels.[77] To date, all the mutations of KVLQT1 that cause autosomal dominant LQTS would be predicted to encode for a full-length but potentially defective potassium channel protein.[77,87] This suggests that, in these patients, the defective KVLQT1 proteins may cause prolongation of the QT interval through a dominant negative mechanism.[76] Recently, two Jervell-Lange-Nielsen families (autosomal recessive LQTS) were determined to have a KVLQT1 mutation that would be predicted to encode for a truncated protein, lacking 25 amino acids at the carboxy terminus.[88] This mutation may cause decreased numbers of KVLQT1 potassium channels due to either mutant mRNA or protein instability or may

Table 2

Genes Responsible for the Long QT Syndrome

LQT Locus	Inheritance	Chromosome Location	Responsible Gene	Gene Function	Features	Estimated Percent of Families
LQT1	autosomal dominant	11p15.5	KVLQT1	putative potassium channel	sudden death with excitement	50
LQT2	autosomal dominant	7q35	HERG	potassium channel	exacerbated by hypokalemia	30
LQT3	autosomal dominant	3p21	SCN5A	sodium channel	sudden death with sleep/ bradycardia	10
LQT4	autosomal dominant	4q25–27	Unknown	Unknown	bradycardia U waves	>5
LQT5	autosomal dominant	Unknown	Unknown	Unknown		10
Jervell-Lange-Nielsen	autosomal recessive	Unknown	Unknown	Unknown	patients with sensorineural deafness	rare

* Adapted with permission from Reference 3.

not allow the mutant protein to form the protein-protein interactions required for a functional channel.

Mutations of the cardiac sodium channel (SCN5A) were associated with prolonged sodium inward current during the plateau phase of the action potential due to destabilization of the channel's inactivation gate.[89] While patients with HERG channel defects, and presumably patients with KVLQT1 defects, have diminished outward repolarizing potassium current, patients with SCN5A defects have persistent inward sodium current, likely disrupting the balance between inward and outward currents during the plateau phase and prolonging the action potential.[80] Unlike most LQTS patients, patients with defects in this channel (LQT3-type LQTS) have syncope and sudden death during sleep or rest and appear to be at higher risk of torsades de pointes at slow heart rates.[82] Their QT intervals shorten significantly with exercise and their symptoms may be improved by cardiac pacing.[82] How the negative chronotropic effect of β-blockade affects the symptoms of this specific group of patients was not evaluated. Mexiletene, a sodium channel blocker, shortens the QT interval in patients with LQT3-type LQTS,[82] and its effect on syncope and sudden death in this group of patients is currently being evaluated.

Pause-Dependent Torsades

Pause-dependent torsades is characterized by a pause accentuated U wave following a sudden pause or deceleration of the basic rhythm[71] and may be related to defects in the SCN5A sodium channel or even HERG channel mutations. This form of torsades is usually associated with syncope during stress and may be precipitated by torsades de pointes after a sinus beat following a postextrasystolic pause.[78] Such pause-dependent torsades was observed in patients taking type 1 antiarrhythmic agents at even therapeutic or low serum drug levels (Table 3), patients with hypokalemia or hypomagnesemia, and patients with severe bradycardia such as complete heart block (Figure 16). The typical twisting morphology of pause-dependent torsades, although highly suggestive of torsades, may be associated with other mechanisms of VT, such as those encountered with ischemia or other forms of structural heart disease. Thus the pause-dependent U-wave accentuation is a more specific herald of torsades. This distinction is important as the treatment of pause-dependent torsades is to increase the heart rate by either pacing or the infusion of positive chronotropic agents such as isoproterenol[71]; in contrast, such measures can be deleterious in the congenital form of the LQTS or in VT related to other pathological substrates such as ischemia or abnormal (discontinuous) anisotropic conduction.

_____ Table 3 _____

Antiarrhythmic Agents and Other Medications with Potential Electrophysiological/Prorhythmic Effects

Antiarrhythmic Agents	Cellular Electrophysiological Effect
Class IA—Definite torsades Quinidine Disopyramide Procainamide	Moderately depress conduction, moderately depress repolarization
Class IB—Possible torsades	Depress conduction in abnormal myocardium, no prolongation of repolarization
Class IC—Possible torsades	Strong depression conduction, little repolarization effect
Class II—Only sotalol Sotalol	β-adrenergic antagonists
Class III—Definite torsades Amiodarone Sotalol Bretyllium tosylate	Prolongation of repolarization
Class IV—Only bepridil Bepridil	Depress slow calcium currents
Terfenadine (with)* Erythromycin Claithromycin Ketoconazole Nefazodone Itraconazole Troleandomycin Fluvoxamine Cisapride	Astemizole (with)* Erythromycin Ketoconazole Nefazodone Itraconazole Fluvoxamine

* Medications that alone or in combination have been associated with torsades de pointes.

Catecholamine-Related Polymorphic Ventricular Tachycardia

Catecholamine-related polymorphic VT refers to a rhythm with a spiraling, twisting QRS waveform and a normal corrected QT interval on the resting ECG. Leenhardt and associates[90] reported a group of 21 children (mean age 9.9 years) with emotion or stress-related syncope related to polymorphic VT. These individuals often have polymorphic ventricular premature beats at rest; intense emotional discharge may induce a polymorphic VT that degenerates into ventricular fibrillation. Often there is a family history of sudden death (30%). Lifelong treatment with β-blockers is mandatory as it is highly effective in preventing recurrences. In addition, a pacemaker or an ICD may be necessary.[90] This phenotype may represent a variant of the congenital LQTS and, functionally, an intermediate form between the congenital (adrenergic-dependent) and the acquired (pause-dependent) phenotypes.

Arrhythmogenic Right Ventricular Dysplasia

Arrhythmogenic RV dysplasia, first described in 1977, appears to be a specific pathological entity comprised of RV hypertrophy and either localized or general RV dilatation.[91] Myocardial thinning is present in dilated areas in the apex, infundibulum, and posterobasal region. In the areas of thinning there may be replacement by fibrosis and fat.[92] VT, arising from the abnormal RV and producing a LBBB pattern, is the major clinical manifestation of the disorder. The abnormal RV may be markedly reduced in contractility with a high arrhythmogenic risk for life-threatening VT and fibrillation.[45] Cardiac catheterization or MRI are important in making this diagnosis, as the RV abnormalities are difficult to detect with echocardiogram.[93] Regional abnormalities of sympathetic innervation as detected by scintigraphy are reported to be frequent.[94] The ECG may show an increase in the size of the P wave, incomplete right bundle-branch block (RBBB), and, in 30% of patients, a ventricular postexcitation wave occurring after the QRS complex at the beginning of the ST segment. The most common abnormality is T-wave inversion over the anterior precordium.[91] The VT may be chronic or an incessant form of nonsustained VT, interrupted by isolated sinus beats. The familial occurrence of this disease is particularly high among Italian populations.[95] Pharmacologic management for both inducible and noninducible VT appears to be best achieved with sotalol; amiodarone, an alternative choice, is equivalent to sotalol but carries with it many side effects, especially for long-term use in the young.[96] For those individuals not responding to sotalol, intraoperative epicardial mapping was successful in locating the site of onset of the VT, and successful excision of the arrhythmogenic area was reported.[45]

Cardiac Tumors

Cardiac tumors, including rhabdomyomas associated with tuberous sclerosis and atrial myxomas, which may prolapse into the ventricle, may provide a substrate for ventricular arrhythmias. Diagnosis is made by echocardiogram and angiography; computerized tomograms or MRI may also be useful. Treatment for life-threatening forms may be accomplished with aggressive antiarrhythmic therapy including amiodarone, surgery, or by catheter ablation.[2,41,42,97,98] Microscopic hamartomas were reported in infants with incessant VT, often with a life-threatening course. Identification at surgery with cryoablation can eliminate the tumor and the tachycardia.[41] If the infant has no symptoms, treatment may be deferred. Similar to patients with rhabdomyomas (histologically identical to hamartomas), resolution may occur in some patients.

Obstructive and Nonobstructive Hypertrophic and Dilated Cardiomyopathy

Patients with obstructive and nonobstructive hypertrophic and dilated cardiomyopathy may exhibit VT, even in the newborn period.[99–101] In patients with dilated cardiomyopathy, the incidence of complex ventricular ectopy and nonsustained VT ranges from 60% to 90%.[102] In older patients the dilated form of cardiomyopathy may be associated with a specific form of bundle-branch reentry tachycardia.[103] The wide QRS tachycardia is characteristically due to conduction delay and reentry in the His-Purkinje system demonstrated by LBBB and a long HV interval, in which case RFA of the right bundle may result in cure of the arrhythmia.[103] Although complex ventricular arrhythmia is associated with an increased risk of sudden death in patients with dilated cardiomyopathy, antiarrhythmic therapy was not shown to improve the outcome and, in some cases, actually increases the risk of cardiac arrest, presumably due to proarrhythmic drug effects and electrolyte changes.[102,104] Treatment should be individualized, weighing the severity of ventricular ectopic activity, associated symptoms, and risk-benefit ratio of currently available antiarrhythmic agents, implantable defibrillator, or ablation.

Myocarditis

Myocarditis, even during the neonatal period, may be associated with ventricular ectopic activity including the complex forms of VT (Figure 10). The VT accompanying congestive heart failure may improve with successful treatment of the failure, although aggressive antiarrhythmic therapy may be required during the acute phase. Several reports advocate endomyocardial biopsy for the histological diagnosis of myocarditis in patients with unexplained VT and yield abnormal histology suggesting myocarditis in up to 50%.[105,106] Immunosuppressive treatment with corticosteroids was associated with reduction in VT in a small noncontrolled group of patients.[105] Finally, digoxin toxicity usually manifests as ventricular ectopy, especially with myocarditis or myodystrophic diseases. Careful use of digoxin, or even withholding it in this situation, should be considered.

Exercise-Related Tachycardia

Exercise-related tachycardia is rare in young individuals and is usually associated with heart disease.[107,108] In the child with heart disease, the underlying disorder dictates if and what treatment may be indicated. In the individual with an apparently normal heart and normal cardiac function, treatment should be carefully considered.[108] Symptomatic VT during exercise should be aggressively evaluated and treated, due to the risk of sudden death. In one series of young patients, two of nine patients (22%) with exercise-related VT died suddenly[51]; β-blockers appear to be useful if the probable mechanism is enhanced automaticity as determined by spontaneous onset with isoproterenol infusion as well as non-inducibility by programmed extrastimulation.[109]

Ventricular Tachycardia in Patients Following Congenital Heart Surgery

Since the advent of surgical treatment of patients with congenital heart disease, VT presented potential intermediate or late life-threatening sequelae to surgery, particularly in patients with conotruncal malformations. The most common conotruncal malformation is tetralogy of Fallot; because of the large number of these patients with right ventriculotomy and long-term follow-up, this disorder serves as the prototype for VT following surgery. Patients with tetralogy, especially during the first year of life, except those with the severest forms [pulmonary atresia and ventricular septal defect (VSD)], are now routinely repaired through the tricuspid valve rather than through a ventriculotomy.

In early reports from a number of centers an increased risk of late death was found in postoperative tetralogy patients with conduction defects, particularly those with trifascicular block.[110–112] Other risk factors included poor hemodynamic results and ventricular ectopic activity at rest and during exercise (especially in the presence of elevated RV systolic pressure ≥60 mm Hg).[113–121] In contrast, other investigators have not confirmed this poor outcome following surgery, even after 20 years.[122–128] Age at operation, era of operation, hemodynamic results, cardiomegaly, myocardial performance, conduction disturbances, and ventricular arrhythmias are undoubtedly among the factors that contribute to the risk of VT.[126–132]

A reentry mechanism is probably responsible for most cases of postoperative VT, and the site of origin is usually in the infundibulum, around the septal patch, and at the ventriculotomy incision.[119–121,133,134] Endocardial excision of the site of onset of the tachycardia resulted in cessation of the tachycardia in these patients[135]; in addition, RF current was applied to sites of slow conduction with successful disruption of the reentry circuit and elimination of the tachycardia.[136–138]

Medical treatment of asymptomatic nonsustained ventricular ectopic activity in the clinical setting of late postoperative tetralogy of Fallot is no longer routinely advised. Asymptomatic low-grade ventricular activity is not treated but monitored by periodic Holter monitoring. A 0.21% yearly mortality rate of patients following repair of tetralogy of Fallot in patients with frequent (>1000/24 hours) or complex ventricular premature beats is the computed incidence among patients repaired 1–2 decades ago, during the era of right ventriculotomy.[139] Sustained (>30 beats, hemodynamic symptoms, or cardiovascular collapse) monomorphic VT that is inducible during EP study requires an aggressive approach with either surgical or catheter delivered ablation.[120,122,133,135–138] Antiarrhythmic therapy with amiodarone or combined drug treatment is an option when ablative therapy is not available or unsuccessful[139–141]; rarely, an implantable defibrillator may be required.

Ventricular Fibrillation

Ventricular fibrillation is a terminal lethal arrhythmia and is characterized by a very rapid ventricular rate with irregular polymorphic complexes. Maintenance of ventricular fibrillation requires not only EP changes but also a critical mass; this may explain the rarity of ventricular fibrillation in the newborn infant. When ventricular fibrillation occurs in the older child, underlying causes that can alter these EP properties (hypoxemia, halothane anesthesia, changes in potassium) should be explored.

Idiopathic Ventricular Fibrillation

Idiopathic ventricular fibrillation is estimated to account for 1% of out-of-hospital sudden deaths.[142] This arrhythmia occurs in a relatively young population with a mean age of 33–36 years; ~25% of patients are under age 20 years.[143,144] A history of syncope is present in 25% of patients. Polymorphic VT or fibrillation is inducible with programmed stimulation in only 40% to 55% of patients.[143,144] A specific subset of patients with RBBB and persistent ST segment elevation in leads V_1 to V_3 was described.[145] These patients are at high risk for recurrent cardiac arrest and may require an implantable defibrillator.[146]

Management

Management of young patients with VT is highly dependent upon age, type of tachycardia, associated symptoms, and the state of the myocardium. The focus of evaluation is to clarify each of the preceding variables. The duration of tachycardia, nonsustained versus sustained, is important, as is clarification of any associated symptoms. The presence of predisposing factors should be ascertained, such as other medications, electrolyte imbalance, central lines, or infection; treatment of the underlying cause usually results in arrhythmia resolution. The presence of structural heart disease is critical, as symptoms in this population associated with an arrhythmia will be pursued aggressively. In the absence of structural heart disease, more subtle abnormalities of the myocardium need to be considered as ventricular arrhythmia may be the initial manifestation of cardiomyopathy.

Besides a careful history and physical examination, an ECG and continuous 24-hour Holter recording are obtained; patients with abnormal findings or more than rare premature ventricular contractions (PVCs) usually undergo an echocardiogram. Certain conditions, such as RV dysplasia, may warrant MRI or angiography to make the diagnosis. Exercise testing is performed to evaluate activity-related symptoms and the response of an arrhythmia to exercise (suppression or exacerbation) and to assess drug efficacy in certain situations (β-blocker therapy for long QT or RVOTVT). Signal-averaged ECGs to detect delayed activation of small portions of the myocardium may prove useful in identifying patients at high risk for sudden death.[142,147-149]

Indications for intracardiac EP testing for patients with ventricular arrhythmias were summarized.[150] The asymptomatic patient with PVCs or complex ventricular arrhythmia does not require intracardiac study. The patient with structural heart disease and complex ventricular arrhythmia is considered a class II indication for study (divided opinion regarding the usefulness of EP testing). Patients with structural heart disease and unexplained syncope are considered a class I indication (general agreement that EP testing will provide useful information); patients without heart disease but with unexplained syncope are considered class II indications. Any patient surviving a cardiac arrest (not associated with infarction) should undergo EP testing, as should patients with sustained VT (not associated with LQTS) who require guidance for drug therapy. Patients with LQTS do not require intracardiac EP testing.

Treatment Strategy for Ventricular Tachycardia

A treatment strategy for VT is summarized in Table 4. The pharmacology, pharmacokinetics, doses, metabolism, side effects, toxicity, and proarrhythmic effects of the various antiarrhythmic agents are outlined in Chapter 10. In certain situations one may have to settle for reduction in severity of ventricular ectopic activity rather than its total abolition. The acute therapy for VT is described in Chapter 11, and the use of an ICD is discussed in Chapter 14.

The results of the Cardiac Arrhythmia Suppression Trial (CAST) study[151,152] underscore the complexity of antiarrhythmic therapy. The increased mortality in middle-aged men on flecainide or encainide with ventricular ectopic activity following myocardial infarction markedly influenced the use of all class I (Vaughan-Williams classification) antiarrhythmic agents, especially in asymptomatic individuals.[153] Although the EP effects of these medications on single-cell preparations are critical to the understanding of their action, other factors such as autonomic tone, the multi-

Table 4 Continued

Type VT	Etiology/ Mechanism	Age	Symptoms Related to Tachycardia/ Heart Failure	Ventricular Function	Associated Structural Heart Disease	Treatment	Comments
VT	Mitral valve prolapse	Older children	+	Normal	—	β-blockers	Very rare finding in childhood years
Torsades de pointes	Congenital long QT syndrome	All	++++	Normal	None	β-blockers for patients with potassium channel defects; mexilitene for patients with sodium channel defects	Pacemaker and/or ICD may be necessary; potassium supplements
Torsades de pointes	Pause dependent atrioventricular block—severe bradycardia Drug toxicity Na and K channel blockers Low Ca, K, Mg	All	+++	Normal	All forms heart disease	Emergency: pacing/or isoproterenol infusion to increase heart rate	Prorhythmic effect usually occurs within 4–7 d but may appear years after successful use
Torsades de pointes	Normal QT No medications Idiopathic	All	+++	Normal	Normal	β-blockers, ICD	Polymorphic ventricular tachycardia; possible long QT variant

AVR, accelerated ventricular rhythm; ICD, implantable cardioverter-defibrillator; IHSS, idiopathic hypertrophic subaortic stenosis; IV, intravenous; LBBB, left bundle branch block; LV, left ventricle; RFA, radiofrequency ablation; RVOT, right ventricular outflow tract; VT, ventricular tachycardia.

layer cellular milieu, and the effects on the channels, receptors, and pumps of the cell wall of the myocyte clearly play an important role in both the therapeutic and toxic effects.[20,21,154,155]

Sports Participation

Recommendations regarding involvement in recreational or organized competitive sports in young patients with VT are available[156]; these guidelines are based on limited data and represent the thoughtful views of "experts." The goal of maximizing freedom of exercise choice without incurring increased risk of an exercise-related VT is the challenge for the physician advising these young potentially active patients. One recent classification of sports segregates exercise into two general types: dynamic and static.[157] Each sports activity is classified by the level of intensity of both static and dynamic exercise required to perform the sport during competition (Table 5). By way of example, sports such as golf or bowling are low static and low dynamic, labeled type IA by this system. Low-static and high-dynamic sports include cross-country skiing, running, and soccer, ie., type IC. The intensity of the sport increases as the grade increases along both the static and dynamic axis (Table 5).

The Task Force report [156] recommends that individuals, and especially athletes, with nonsustained or sustained VT on an ECG, exercise test, or a 24-hour ECG recording during exercise avoid all sports for 6 months. This injunction applies whether the individual is treated or untreated. If there are no clinical recurrences and VT is not induced by exercise or exercise testing and/or EP study (if this was the mode of initial induction) and the individual has no structural heart disease, full sports activity and competition can be resumed. In the individual with structural heart disease and VT, moderate- and high-intensity activity (greater than type IA) is proscribed, regardless of whether the VT is suppressed. The implantation of ICD does not override these recommendations. An exception to these recommendations is the asymptomatic individual or athlete with brief ($\leq$8–10 consecutive ventricular beats, usually <150 bpm) episodes of nonsustained monomorphic VT and no structural heart disease. If exercise testing (preferably during the exercise with ambulatory ECG monitoring) suppresses or does not worsen the VT, participation in all sports is permissible. Individuals with accelerated ventricular rhythm may participate in all sports.

Table 6 outlines suggested recommendations for sports activity in individuals with VT. Recommendations for recreational sports encompass these same guidelines; however, due to the reduced emotional intensity of this level of activity, recommendations and restrictions can be tailored to the specific functional and cardiac pathophysiological state of the individual.

_____ **Table 5** _____

Classification of Sports*

	A: Low Dynamic	B: Moderate Dynamic	C: High Dynamic
I: Low static	Bowling Golf	Baseball Softball Table tennis Tennis (doubles) Volleyball	Badminton Cross-country skiing Field hockey Racquetball/squash Long-distance running Soccer Tennis (singles)
II: Moderate static	Archery Auto racing Diving Equestrian Motorcycling	Fencing Field events (jumping) Figure skating Football (American) Rodeo Rugby Running (sprint) Surfing	Basketball Ice hockey Football (Australian) Lacrosse Swimming Team handball Running (middle distance)
III: High static	Sledding Field events (throwing) Gymnastics Sailing Rock climbing Waterskiing Weightlifting	Body building Downhill skiing Wrestling	Boxing Canoeing Cycling Decathlon Rowing Speed skating

* Adapted with permission from Reference 157.

_____ **Table 6** _____

Guidelines for Sports Activity Competitive and Recreational

Type VT	Recommendations
AVR	All sports activity
VT—RVOT	All sports activity if <150 bpm and asymptomatic
VT—LV	All sports activity if <150 bpm and asymptomatic
VT—myocarditis	≤Type IA
VT—tumor	≤Type IA
VT—cardiomyopathy	≤Type IA
VT—mitral valve prolapse	All sports activity if <150 bpm and asymptomatic
Torsades de pointes	≤Type IA

AVR—Accelerated ventricular rhythm; VT—Ventricular tachycardia; VT-LV—Ventricular tachycardia-left ventricle; VT-RVOT—Ventricular tachycardia-right ventricular outflow tract.

In summary, chronic therapy must be individualized to the severity of the ventricular ectopic activity, the association of underlying heart disease, the presence of symptoms, and the assessment of the risk-benefit ratio. Careful observation and long-term follow-up will help clarify the natural history of ventricular arrhythmias in childhood.

References

1. Yabek SM. Ventricular arrhythmias in children with an apparently normal heart. *J Pediatr* 1991;119:1–11.
2. Zeigler VL, Gillette PC, Crawford FA Jr, et al. New approaches to treatment of incessant ventricular tachycardia in the very young. *J Am Coll Cardiol* 1990;16:681–685.
3. Russell MW. The long QT syndromes. *Prog Pediatr Cardiol* 1996;6:43–51.
4. Wit AL, Rosen MR. Cellular electrophysiology of cardiac arrhythmias. I. Arrhythmias caused by abnormal impulse generation. *Mod Concepts Cardiovasc Dis* 1981;50:1–6.
5. Wit AL, Rosen MR. Cellular electrophysiology of cardiac arrhythmias. II. Arrhythmias caused by abnormal impulse generation. *Mod Concepts Cardiovasc Dis* 1981;50:7–12.
6. Wellens HJJ, Schuilenburg RM, Durrer D. Electrical stimulation of the heart in patients with ventricular tachycardia. *Circulation* 1972;46:216–226.
7. Wellens HJJ, Durer DR, Lie KI. Observations on mechanisms of ventricular tachycardia in man. *Circulation* 1976;54:237–244.
8. El-sherif N, Scherlag BJ, Lazzara R, et al. Re-entrant ventricular arrhythmias in the late myocardial infarction period. 1. Conduction characteristics in the infarction zone. *Circulation* 1977;55:686–702.
9. El-sherif N, Hope RR, Scherlag BJ, et al. Re-entrant ventricular arrhythmias in the late infarction period. 2. Patterns of initiation and termination of re-entry. *Circulation* 1977;55:702–719.
10. Josephson ME, Horowitz LN, Farshidi A, et al. Recurrent sustained ventricular tachycardia. 1. Mechanisms. *Circulation* 1978;57:431–440.
11. Josephson ME, Horowitz LN, Farshidi A, et al. Recurrent sustained ventricular tachycardia 2. Endocardial mapping. *Circulation* 1978;57:440–447.
12. Rosen MR, Reder RF. Does triggered activity have a role in the genesis of cardiac arrhythmias? *Ann Intern Med* 1981;94:794–801.
13. Rosen MR, Fisch C, Hoffman BF, et al. Can accelerated atrioventricular junctional escape rhythms be explained by delayed afterdepolarizations? *Am J Cardiol* 1980;45:1272–1282.
14. Benson DW Jr, Smith WM, Dunnigan A, et al. Mechanisms of regular, wide QRS tachycardia in infants and children. *Am J Cardiol* 1982;49:1778–1788.
15. Gaum WE, Biancaniello T, Kaplan S. Accelerated ventricular rhythm in childhood. *Am J Cardiol* 1979;43:162–164.
16. Van Hare GF, Stanger P. Ventricular tachycardia and accelerated ventricular rhythm presenting in the first month of life. *Am J Cardiol* 1991;67:42–45.
17. MacLellan-Tobert SG, Porter CJ. Accelerated idioventricular rhythm: a benign arrhythmia in childhood. *Pediatrics* 1995;96:122–125.
18. Calkins H, Kalbfleisch SJ, el-Atassi R, et al. Relation between efficacy of radiofrequency catheter ablation and site of origin of idiopathic ventricular tachycardia. *Am J Cardiol* 1993;71:827–833.

19. Stevenson WG, Sager PT, Friedman PL. Entrainment techniques for mapping atrial and ventricular tachycardias. *J Cardiovasc Electrophysiol* 1995;6:201–216.
20. Seliem MA, Benson DW Jr, Strasburger JF, et al. Complex ventricular ectopic activity in patients less than 20 years of age with or without syncope, and the role of ventricular extrastimulus testing. *Am J Cardiol* 1991;68:745–750.
21. Katritsis D, Camm AJ. Antiarrhythmic drug classifications and the clinician: a gambit in the land of chaos. *Clin Cardiol* 1994;17:142–148.
22. The Task Force of the Working Group on Arrhythmias of the European Society of Cardiology: Review. The "Sicilian Gambit." A new approach to the classification of antiarrhythmic drugs based on their actions on arrhythmogenic mechanisms. *Eur Heart J* 1991;12:1112–1131.
23. Tsuji A, Nagashima M, Hasegawa S, et al. Long-term follow-up of idiopathic ventricular arrhythmias in otherwise normal children. *Jpn Circ J* 1995;59:654–662.
24. Morganroth J, Michelson EL, Horowitz LN, et al. Limitations of routine long-term electrocardiographic monitoring to assess ventricular ectopic frequency. *Circulation* 1978;58:408–414.
25. Young BK, Katz M, Klein SA. Intrapartum fetal cardiac arrhythmias. *Obstet Gynecol* 1979;54:427–432.
26. Southall DP, Richards J, Hardwick RA, et al. Prospective study of fetal heart rate and rhythm patterns. *Arch Dis Child* 1980;55:506–511.
27. Southall DP, Richards J, Mitchell P, et al. Study of cardiac rhythm in healthy newborn infants. *Br Heart J* 1980;43:14–20.
28. Jones RW, Sharp C, Rabb LR, et al. 1028 neonatal electrocardiograms. *Arch Dis Child* 1979;54:427–431.
29. Montague TJ, Taylor PG, Stockton R, et al. The spectrum of cardiac rate and rhythm in normal newborns. *Pediatr Cardiol* 1982;2:33–38.
30. Morgan BC, Deane PG, Guntheroth WG. Long-term continuous electrocardiographic recording in pediatric patients. *Pediatrics* 1965;36:792–797.
31. Brodsky M, Wu D, Denes P, et al. Arrhythmias documented by 24 hour continuous electrocardiographic monitoring in 50 male medical students without apparent heart disease. *Am J Cardiol* 1977;39:390–395.
32. Palatini P, Maraglino G, Sperti G, et al. Prevalence and possible mechanisms of ventricular arrhythmias in athletes. *Am Heart J* 1985;110:560–567.
33. Gaum WE, Schwartz DC, Kaplan S. Ventricular tachycardia in infancy: evidence for a reentrant mechanism. *Circulation* 1980;62:401–406.
34. Bergdahl DM, Stevenson JG, Kawabori I, et al. Prognosis in primary ventricular tachycardia in the pediatric patient. *Circulation* 1980;62:897–901.
35. Rocchini AP, Chun PO, Dick M. Ventricular tachycardia in children. *Am J Cardiol* 1981;47:1091–1097.
36. Hernandez A, Strauss A, Kleiger RE, et al. Idiopathic paroxysmal ventricular tachycardia in infants and children. *J Pediatr* 1973;86:182–188.
37. Noh CI, Gillette PC, Case CL, et al. Clinical and electrophysiological characteristics of ventricular tachycardia in children with normal hearts. *Am Heart J* 1990;120:1326–1333.
38. Rahilly GT, Prystowsky EN, Zipes DP, et al. Clinical and electrophysiologic findings in patients with repetitive monomorphic ventricular tachycardia and otherwise normal electrocardiogram. *Am J Cardiol* 1982;50:459–468.
39. Attina DA, Mori F, Falorni PL, et al. Long-term follow-up in children without heart disease with ventricular premature beats. *Eur Heart J* 1987;8:21–23.
40. Stevens DC, Schreiner RL, Hurwitz RA, et al. Fetal and neonatal ventricular arrhythmia. *Pediatrics* 1979;63:771–777.

41. Garson A Jr, Smith RT Jr, Moak JP, et al. Incessant ventricular tachycardia in infants: myocardial hamartomas and surgical cure. *J Am Coll Cardiol* 1987;10:619–626.
42. Garson A, Gillette PC, Titus J, et al. Surgical treatment of ventricular tachycardia in infants. *N Engl J Med* 1984;310:1443–1445.
43. Slama R, Leclercq JF, Coumel P. Paroxysmal ventricular tachycardia in patients with apparently normal hearts. In: Zipes DP, Jalife J, eds. *Cardiac Electrophysiology and Arrhythmias*. New York: Grune & Stratton; 1985:545–552.
44. Vetter VL, Josephson ME, Horowitz LN. Idiopathic recurrent sustained ventricular tachycardia in children and adolescents. *Am J Cardiol* 1981;47:315–322.
45. Fontaine G, Guiraudon G, Frank R, et al. Surgical management of ventricular tachycardia unrelated to myocardial ischemia or infarction. *Am J Cardiol* 1982;49:397–410.
46. Steffens TG, Pierce PL, Zegerius RJ. Multiple ventricular premature beats in five adolescents. *Eur J Cardiol* 1978;8:177–184.
47. Fulton DR, Chung KJ, Tabakin BS, et al. Ventricular tachycardia in children without heart disease. *Am J Cardiol* 1985;55:1328–1331.
48. Rowland TW, Schweiger MJ. Repetitive paroxysmal tachycardia and sudden death in a child. *Am J Cardiol* 1984;53:1729.
49. Pfammatter JP, Paul T, Kallfelz HC. Recurrent ventricular tachycardia in asymptomatic young children with an apparently normal heart. *Eur J Pediatr* 1995;154:513–517.
50. Radford DJ, Izukawa T, Rowe RD. Evaluation of children with ventricular arrhythmias. *Arch Dis Child* 1977;52:345–353.
51. Deal BJ, Miller SM, Scagliotti D, et al. Ventricular tachycardia in a young population without overt heart disease. *Circulation* 1986;73:1111–1118.
52. Ritchie AH, Kerr CR, Qi A, et al. Nonsustained ventricular tachycardia arising from the right ventricular outflow tract. *Am J Cardiol* 1989;64:594–598.
53. Gaita F, Giustetto C, Leclercq JF, et al. Idiopathic verapamil-responsive left ventricular tachycardia: clinical characteristics and long-term follow-up of 33 patients. *Eur Heart J* 1994;15:1252–1260.
54. Alpert MA, Mukerji V, Bikkina M, et al. Pathogenesis, recognition, and management of common cardiac arrhythmias. I. Ventricular premature beats and tachyarrhythmias. *South Med J* 1995;88:1–21.
55. Gursoy S, Brugada R, Brugada J, et al. Which ventricular tachycardia is dangerous? *Clin Cardiol* 1992;15:43–44.
56. O'Connor BK, Case CL, Sokoloski MC, et al. Radiofrequency catheter ablation of right ventricular outflow tachycardia in children and adolescents. *J Am Coll Cardiol* 1996;27:869–874.
57. Wilber DJ, Baerman J, Olshansky B, et al. Adenosine-sensitive ventricular tachycardia. Clinical characteristics and response to catheter ablation. *Circulation* 1993;87:126–134.
58. Morady F, Kadish AH, DiCarlo L, et al. Long-term results of catheter ablation of idiopathic right ventricular tachycardia. *Circulation* 1990;82:2093–2099.
59. Klein LS, Shih H-T, Hackett FK, et al. Radiofrequency catheter ablation of ventricular tachycardia in patients without structural heart disease. *Circulation* 1992;85:1666–1674.
60. Carlson MD, White RD, Trohman RG, et al. Right ventricular outflow tract ventricular tachycardia: detection of previously unrecognized anatomic abnormalities using cine magnetic resonance imaging. *J Am Coll Cardiol* 1994;24:720–727.
61. Lin F-C, Finley CD, Rahimtoola SH, et al. Idiopathic paroxysmal ventricular tachycardia with a QRS pattern of right bundle branch block and left axis

deviation: a unique clinical entity with specific properties. *Am J Cardiol* 1983;52:95–100.

62. German LD, Packer DL, Bardy GH, et al. Ventricular tachycardia induced by atrial stimulation in patients without symptomatic cardiac disease. *Am J Cardiol* 1983;52:1202–1207.

63. Klein GJ, Millman PJ, Yee R. Recurrent ventricular tachycardia responsive to verapamil. *Pacing Clin Electrophysiol* 1984;7:938–948.

64. Ohe T, Shimomura K, Aihara N, et al. Idiopathic sustained left ventricular tachycardia: clinical and electrophysiologic characteristics. *Circulation* 1988;77:560–568.

65. Thakur RK, Klein GJ, Sivaram CA, et al. Anatomic substrate for idiopathic left ventricular tachycardia. *Circulation* 1996;93:497–501.

66. Wen M-S, Yeh S-J, Wang C-C, et al. Radiofrequency ablation therapy in idiopathic left ventricular tachycardia with no obvious structural heart disease. *Circulation* 1994;89:1690–1696.

67. Coggins DL, Lee RJ, Sweeney J, et al. Radiofrequency catheter ablation as a cure for idiopathic tachycardia of both left and right ventricular origin. *J Am Coll Cardiol* 1994;23:1333–1341.

68. Ohe T, Aihara N, Kamakura S, et al. Long-term outcome of verapamil-sensitive sustained left ventricular tachycardia in patients without structural heart disease. *J Am Coll Cardiol* 1995;25:54–58.

69. Sung RJ, Keung EC, Nguyen NX, et al. Effects of beta-adrenergic blockade on verapamil-responsive and verapamil-irresponsive sustained ventricular tachycardias. *J Clin Invest* 1988;81:688–699.

70. Dessertenne F. La tachycardie ventriculaire a deux foyers opposes variables. *Arch Mal Coeur Vaiss* 1966;59:263–272.

71. Jackman WM, Friday KJ, Anderson JL, et al. The long QT syndromes: a critical review, new clinical observations and a unifying hypothesis. *Prog Cardiovasc Dis* 1988;31:115–172.

72. Starmer CF, Romashko DN, Reddy RS, et al. Proarrhythmic response to potassium channel blockade. Numerical studies of polymorphic tachyarrhythmias. *Circulation* 1995;92:595–605.

73. Garson A Jr, Dick M, Fournier A, et al. The long QT syndrome in children. An international study of 287 patients. *Circulation* 1993;87:1866–1872.

74. Vincent GM, Timothy KW, Leppert M, et al. The spectrum of symptoms and QT intervals in carriers of the gene for the long-QT syndrome. *N Engl J Med* 1992;327:846–852.

75. Schwartz PJ, Moss AJ, Vincent GM, et al. Diagnostic criteria for the long QT syndrome. An update. *Circulation* 1993;88:782–784.

76. Moss AJ, Schwartz PJ, Crampton RS, et al. The long QT syndrome. Prospective longitudinal study of 328 families. *Circulation* 1991;84:1136–1144.

77. Wang Q, Curran ME, Splawski I, et al. Positional cloning of a novel potassium channel gene: *KVLQT1* mutations cause cardiac arrhythmias. *Nat Genet* 1996;12:17–23.

78. Curran ME, Splawski I, Timothy KW, et al. A molecular basis for cardiac arrhythmia: *HERG* mutations cause long QT syndrome. *Cell* 1995;80:795–803.

79. Wang Q, Shen J, Splawski I, et al. *SCN5A* mutations associated with an inherited cardiac arrhythmia, long QT syndrome. *Cell* 1995;80:805–811.

80. Roden DM, Lazzara R, Rosen M, et al. Multiple mechanisms in the long-QT syndrome. Current knowledge, gaps, and future directions. The SADS Foundation Task Force on LQTS. *Circulation* 1996;94:1996–2012.

81. Schott JJ, Charpentier F, Peltier S, et al. Mapping of a gene for long QT syndrome to chromosome 4q25–27. *Am J Hum Genet* 1995;57:1114–1122.

82. Schwartz PJ, Priori SG, Locati EH, et al. Long QT syndrome patients with mutations of the *SCN5A* and *HERG* genes have differential responses to Na$^+$ channel blockade and to increases in heart rate. Implications for gene-specific therapy. *Circulation* 1995;92:3381–3386.

83. Compton SJ, Lux RL, Ramsey MR, et al. Genetically defined therapy of inherited long-QT syndrome. Correction of abnormal repolarization by potassium. *Circulation* 1996;94:1018–1022.

84. Moss AJ, Zareba W, Benhorin J, et al. ECG T-wave patterns in genetically distinct forms of the hereditary long QT syndrome. *Circulation* 1995;92:2929–2934.

85. Sanguinetti MC, Jiang C, Curran ME, et al. A mechanistic link between an inherited and an acquired cardiac arrhythmia: *HERG* encodes the IKr potassium channel. *Cell* 1995;81:299–307.

86. Schwartz PJ, Bonazzi O, Locati E, et al. Pathogenesis and therapy of the idiopathic long QT syndrome. *Ann NY Acad Sci* 1992;644:112–114.

87. Russell MW, Dick M II, Collins FS, et al. KVLQT1 mutations in three families with familial or sporadic long QT syndrome. *Hum Mol Genet* 1996;5:1319–1324.

88. Neyroud N, Tesson F, Denjoy I, et al. A novel mutation in the potassium channel gene KVLQT1 causes the Jervell and Lange-Nielsen cardioauditory syndrome. *Nat Genet* 1997;15:186–189.

89. Bennett PB, Yazawa K, Makita N, et al. Molecular mechanism for an inherited cardiac arrhythmia. *Nature* 1995;376:683–685.

90. Leenhardt A, Lucet V, Denjoy I, et al. Catecholaminergic polymorphic ventricular tachycardia in children. A 7-year follow-up of 21 patients. *Circulation* 1995;91:1512–1519.

91. Marcus FI, Fontaine GH, Guiraudon G, et al. Right ventricular dysplasia: a report of 24 adult cases. *Circulation* 1982;65:384–398.

92. Lobo FV, Heggtveit HA, Butany J, et al. Right ventricular dysplasia: morphological findings in 13 cases. *Can J Cardiol* 1992;8:261–268.

93. Pietras RJ, Lam W, Bauernfeind R, et al. Chronic recurrent right ventricular tachycardia in patients without ischemic heart disease: clinical, hemodynamic, and angiographic findings. *Am Heart J* 1983;105:357–366.

94. Wichter T, Hindricks G, Lerch H, et al. Regional myocardial sympathetic dysinnervation in arrhythmogenic right ventricular cardiomyopathy. An analysis using ^{123}I-meta-iodobenzylguanidine scintigraphy. *Circulation* 1994;89:667–683.

95. Wichter T, Borggrefe M, Haverkamp W, et al. Efficacy of antiarrhythmic drugs in patients with arrhythmogenic right ventricular disease. Results in patients with inducible and noninducible ventricular tachycardia. *Circulation* 1992;86:29–37.

96. Nava A, Thiene G, Canciani B, et al. Familial occurrence of right ventricular dysplasia: a study involving nine families. *J Am Coll Cardiol* 1988;12:1222–1228.

97. Caldwell PD, Ricketts HJ, Dillard DH, et al. Ventricular tachycardia in a child: an indication for angiography? *Am Heart J* 1974;88:777–781.

98. Kohli V, Mangru V, Pearse LA, et al. Radiofrequency ablation of ventricular tachycardia in an infant with cardiac tumors. *Am Heart J* 1996;132:198–200.

99. Savage DD, Seides SF, Maron BJ, et al. Prevalence of arrhythmias during 24-hour electrocardiographic monitoring and exercise testing in patients with obstructive and nonobstructive hypertrophic cardiomyopathy. *Circulation* 1979;59:866–875.

100. Ingham RE, Mason JW, Rossen RM, et al. Electrophysiologic findings in patients with idiopathic hypertrophic subaortic stenosis. *Am J Cardiol* 1978;41:811–816.

101. Finley JP, Radford DJ, Freedom RM. Torsade de pointes ventricular tachycardia in a newborn infant. *Br Heart J* 1978;40:421–424.

102. DeMaria R, Gavazzi A, Caroli A, et al. Ventricular arrhythmias in dilated cardiomyopathy as an independent prognostic hallmark. Italian Multicenter Cardiomyopathy Study (SPIC) Group. *Am J Cardiol* 1992;69:1451–1457.

103. Blanck Z, Akhtar M. Ventricular tachycardia due to sustained bundle branch block reentry: diagnostic and therapeutic considerations. *Clin Cardiol* 1993; 16:619–622.

104. Dargie HJ, Cleland JGF, Leckie BJ, et al. Relation of arrhythmias and electrolyte abnormalities to survival in patients with severe chronic heart failure. *Circulation* 1987:75(suppl IV):98–107.

105. Ino T, Okubo M, Akimoto K, et al. Corticosteroid therapy for ventricular tachycardia in children with silent lymphocytic myocarditis. *J Pediatr* 1995;126:304–308.

106. Wiles HB, Gillette PC, Harley RA, et al. Cardiomyopathy and myocarditis in children with ventricular ectopic rhythm. *J Am Coll Cardiol* 1992;20:359–362.

107. Bricker JT, Traweek MS, Smith RT, et al. Exercise-related ventricular tachycardia in children. *Am Heart J* 1986;112:186–188.

108. Coumel P, Leenhardt A, Haddad G. Exercise ECG: prognostic implications of exercise induced arrhythmias. *Pacing Clin Electrophysiol* 1994;17:417–427.

109. DiCarlo LA Jr, Susser F, Winston SA. The role of beta-blockade for ventricular tachycardia induced with isoproterenol: a prospective analysis. *Am Heart J* 1990;120:1347–1355.

110. Quattlebaum TG, Varghese J, Neill CA, et al. Sudden death among postoperative patients with tetralogy of Fallot: a follow-up study of 243 patients for an average of twelve years. *Circulation* 1976;54:289–293.

111. Krongrad E. Prognosis for patients with congenital heart disease and postoperative intraventricular conduction defects. *Circulation* 1978; 57:867–870.

112. Hougen TJ, Dick M II, Freed MD, et al. His bundle electrogram after intracardiac repair of tetralogy of Fallot. *Am J Cardiol* 1978;41:552–558.

113. James JW, Kaplan S, Chou T. Unexpected cardiac arrest in patients after surgical correction of tetralogy of Fallot. *Circulation* 1975;52:691–695.

114. Garson A Jr, Gillette PC, Gutgesell HP, et al. Stress-induced ventricular arrhythmia after repair of tetralogy of Fallot. *Am J Cardiol* 1980;46:1006–1012.

115. James FW, Kaplan S, Schwartz DC, et al. Response to exercise in patients after total surgical correction of tetralogy of Fallot. *Circulation* 1976;54:671–679.

116. Kavey RW, Blackman MS, Sondheimer HM. Incidence and severity of chronic ventricular dysrhythmias after repair of tetralogy of Fallot. *Am Heart J* 1982;103:342–350.

117. Rosing DR, Borer JS, Kent KM, et al. Long-term hemodynamic and electrocardiographic assessment following operative repair of tetralogy of Fallot. *Circulation* 1978;58(suppl I):209–217.

118. Garson A Jr, Nihill MR, McNamara DG, et al. Status of the adult and adolescent after repair of tetralogy of Fallot. *Circulation* 1979;59:1232–1240.

119. Horowitz LN, Vetter VL, Harken AH, et al. Electrophysiologic characteristics of sustained ventricular tachycardia occurring after repair of tetralogy of Fallot. *Am J Cardiol* 1980;46:446–452.

120. Garson A, Porter C, Gillette PC. Ventricular tachycardia induction during electrophysiologic study after repair of tetralogy of Fallot. *Circulation* 1981;64(suppl IV): 227.

121. Kugler JD, Pinsky WW, Cheatham JP, et al. Sustained ventricular tachycardia after repair of tetralogy of Fallot: new electrophysiologic findings. *Am J Cardiol* 1983;51:1137–1143.

122. Wessel HU, Bastanier CK, Paul MH, et al. Prognostic significance of arrhythmia in tetralogy of Fallot after intracardiac repair. *Am J Cardiol* 1980;46:843–848.

123. Fuster V, McGoon DC, Kennedy MA, et al. Long-term evaluation (12 to 22 years) of open heart surgery for tetralogy of Fallot. *Am J Cardiol* 1980;46:635–642.

124. Katz NM, Blackstone EH, Kirklin JW, et al. Late survival and symptoms after repair of tetralogy of Fallot. *Circulation* 1982;65:403–410.

125. Downar E, Harris L, Kimber S, et al. Ventricular tachycardia after surgical repair of tetralogy of Fallot: results of intraoperative mapping studies. *J Am Coll Cardiol* 1992;20:648–655.

126. Walsh EP, Rockenmacher S, Keane CJF, et al. Late results in patients with tetralogy of Fallot repaired during infancy. *Circulation* 1988;77:1062–1067.

127. Vaksmann G, Fournier A, Davignon A, et al. Frequency and prognosis of arrhythmia after operative "correction" of tetralogy of Fallot. *Am J Cardiol* 1990;66:346–349.

128. Chandar JS, Wolff GS, Garson A Jr, et al. Ventricular arrhythmias in postoperative tetralogy of Fallot. *Am J Cardiol* 1990;65:655–661.

129. Murphy JG, Gersh BJ, Mair DD, et al. Long-term outcome in patients undergoing surgical repair of tetralogy of Fallot. *N Engl J Med* 1993;329:593–599.

130. Cullen S, Celermajer DS, Franklin RCG, et al. Prognostic significance of ventricular arrhythmia after repair of tetralogy of Fallot: a 12-year prospective study. *J Am Coll Cardiol* 1994;23:1151–1155.

131. Joffe H, Georgakopoulos D, Celermajer DS, et al. Late ventricular arrhythmia is rare after early repair of tetralogy of Fallot. *J Am Coll Cardiol* 1994;23:1146–1150.

132. Deal BJ, Scagliotti D, Miller SM, et al. Electrophysiologic drug testing in symptomatic ventricular arrhythmias after repair of tetralogy of Fallot. *Am J Cardiol* 1987;59:1380–1385.

133. Swerdlow CD, Oyer PE, Pitlick PT. Septal origin of sustained ventricular tachycardia in a patient with right ventricular outflow tract obstruction after correction of tetralogy of Fallot. *Pacing Clin Electrophysiol* 1986;9:584–588.

134. Boersma L, Brugada J, Kirchhof C, et al. Mapping of reset of anatomic and functional entry in anisotropic rabbit ventricular myocardium. *Circulation* 1994;89:852–862.

135. Misaki T, Tsubota M, Watanabe G, et al. Surgical treatment of ventricular tachycardia after surgical repair of tetralogy of Fallot. Relation between intraoperative mapping and histological findings. *Circulation* 1994;90:264–271.

136. Burton ME, Leon AR. Radiofrequency catheter ablation of right ventricular outflow tract tachycardia late after complete repair of tetralogy of Fallot using the pace mapping technique. *Pacing Clin Electrophysiol* 1993;16:2319–2325.

137. Biblo LA, Carlson MD. Transcatheter radiofrequency ablation of ventricular tachycardia following surgical correction of tetralogy of Fallot. *Pacing Clin Electrophysiol* 1994;17:1556–1560.

138. Chinushi M, Aizawa Y, Kitazawa H, et al. Successful radiofrequency catheter ablation for macroreentrant ventricular tachycardias in a patient with tetralogy of Fallot after corrective surgery. *Pacing Clin Electrophysiol* 18:1713–1716, 1995.

139. Garson A Jr. Ventricular arrhythmias after repair of congenital heart disease: who needs treatment? *Cardiol Young* 1991;1:177–181.

140. Fenrich AL Jr, Perry JC, Freidman RA. Flecainide and amiodarone: combined therapy for refractory tachyarrhythmias in infancy. *J Am Coll Cardiol* 1995; 25:1195–1198.

141. Perry JC, Knilans TK, Marlow D, et al. Intravenous amiodarone for life-threatening tachyarrhythmias in children and young adults. *J Am Coll Cardiol* 1993;22:95–98.
142. Vaksman G, el Kohen M, Lacroix D, et al. Influence of clinical and hemodynamic characteristics on signal-average electrocardiogram in postoperative tetralogy of Fallot. *Am J Cardiol* 1993;71:317–321.
143. Viskin S, Belhassen B. Idiopathic ventricular fibrillation. *Am Heart J* 1990; 120:661–671.
144. Wever EFD, Hauer RNW, Oomen A, et al. Unfavorable outcome in patients with primary electrical disease who survived an episode of ventricular fibrillation. *Circulation* 1993;88:1021–1029.
145. Brugada P, Brugada J. Right bundle branch block, persistent ST segment elevation and sudden cardiac death: a distinct clinical and electrocardiographic syndrome. A multicenter report. *J Am Coll Cardiol* 1992;20:1391–1396.
146. Meissner MD, Lehmann MH, Steinman RT, et al. Ventricular fibrillation in patients without significant structural heart disease: a multicenter experience with implantable cardioverter-defibrillator therapy. *J Am Coll Cardiol* 1993; 21:1406–1412.
147. Stelling JA, Danford DA, Kugler JD, et al. Late potentials and inducible ventricular tachycardia in surgically repaired congenital heart disease. *Circulation* 1990;82:1690–1696.
148. Janousek J, Paul T, Bartakova H. Role of late potentials in identifying patients at risk for ventricular tachycardia after surgical correction of congenital heart disease. *Am J Cardiol* 1995;75:146–150.
149. Daliento L, Caneve F, Turrini P, et al. Clinical significance of high-frequency, low-amplitude electrocardiographic signals and QT dispersion in patients operated on for tetralogy of Fallot. *Am J Cardiol* 1995;76:408–411.
150. Lemery R, Brugada P, Janssen J, et al. Nonischemic sustained ventricular tachycardia: clinical outcome in 12 patients with arrhythmogenic right ventricular dysplasia. *J Am Coll Cardiol* 1989;14:96–105.
151. The Cardiac Arrhythmia Suppression Trial (CAST) Investigators: Preliminary report: effect of encainide and flecainide on mortality in a randomized trial of arrhythmia suppression after myocardial infarction. *N Engl J Med* 1989; 321:406–412.
152. Echt DS, Liebson PR, Mitchell LB, et al. Mortality and morbidity in patients receiving encainide, flecainide, or placebo. The Cardiac Arrhythmia Suppression Trial. *N Engl J Med* 1991;324:781–788.
153. Vaughan Williams EM. Significance of classifying antiarrhythmic actions since the Cardiac Arrhythmia Suppression Trial. *J Clin Pharmacol* 1991;31:123–135.
154. Reiffel JA, Estes NAM III, Waldo AL, et al. A consensus report on antiarrhythmic drug use. *Clin Cardiol* 1994;17:103–116.
155. Janse MJ. What a clinician needs to know about the mechanisms of action of antiarrhythmic drugs. *Clin Cardiol* 1991;14:65–67.
156. Zipes DP, Garson A Jr. 26th Bethesda Conference: Recommendations for determining eligibilty for competition in athletes with cardiovascular abnormalities. Task Force 6: Arrhythmias. *J Am Coll Cardiol* 1994;24:892–899.
157. Mitchell JH, Haskell WL, Raven PB. Classification of sports. *J Am Coll Cardiol* 1994;24:864–866.

Chapter 8

Syncope—Diagnosis and Management

Grace S. Wolff, MD
Ming L. Young, MD
and Dolores F. Tamer, MD

Syncope is the loss of consciousness and postural tone followed by complete recovery within a few minutes. It is a common occurrence in adults and children and is only rarely life threatening. In patients referred for "syncope," the most common cause is neurocardiac. The incidence of neurocardiac syncope ranges between 23% and 93% of patients referred for evaluation of this problem.[1-3] In some series cardiac causes account for as much as 28% and neurological or psychological causes for 11% and 18%, respectively.[2,3]

This chapter is divided into four sections: (1) the various causes of syncope, (2) the evaluation of the patient with syncope with an extensive discussion of tilt-table testing, (3) mechanisms, and (4) current management options.

Causes

Neurocardiac Syndrome

Neurocardiac syncope has also been referred to as vasovagal syncope or the common "faint." Neurocardiac syncope is the final response to a complex interplay of physiological factors involving, but not limited to, the

From Deal B, Wolff G, Gelband H, (eds.). *Current Concepts in Diagnosis and Management of Arrhythmias in Infants and Children.* Armonk, NY: Futura Publishing Co., Inc.; © 1998.

autonomic and cardiovascular systems. The responses were divided into three categories: (1) cardioinhibitory, when there is predominant bradycardia or asystole, (2) vasodepressor, when there is predominant hypotension, and (3) mixed, when there are components of both. In those patients tested with orthostatic maneuvers, the incidence of these responses varies from 4% to 20% for cardioinhibitory[4–8] and 13% to 30% for vasodepressor; the majority are mixed.

Precipitating Events

There are many triggers of neurocardiac syncope, but prolonged standing is probably the most common. Hair grooming is frequently associated with syncope. Lewis and Frank[9] reported 15 children between the ages of 5 and 13 years who had "seizures" related to hair grooming; most of the patients were standing at the time of the grooming. The authors suggested that the pain from scalp stimulation initiated the syncope or seizure. Similarly, "hair-burning syncope" was described by White and Toor,[10] and seizurelike activity occurred during hair grooming with a hot curling iron.

Syncope provoked by pain or fear is a well-known trigger in both adults and children. Syncope during venipuncture is a common setting. Pavlin and associates[11] performed a prospective study on 141 patients in an ambulatory surgical center. During venous cannulation, 11% of these patients had presyncope or syncope, increasing to 17% in the younger patient. If there was a previous history of syncope or presyncope the incidence was 50% for this younger population and females were affected more commonly than males.

Breathholding spells are a form of neurocardiac syncope presenting in early childhood. The typical presentation is syncope during a crying spell, associated with color change due to breathholding. As early as 1957 Gastaut[12] suggested that the syncope was related to cardiorespiratory reflexes. He described comparable findings in children with breathholding spells and adults with syncope. In a significant percentage of both groups, ocular pressure caused cardiac arrest. Electroencephalographic (EEG) monitoring did not show seizure activity during tonic and opisthotonic posturing. Instead, slow waves predominated. Classic cardioinhibitory and vasodepressor syncope were described. Similarly, Lombroso and Lerman[13] reported findings in 92 children who were tested with ocular pressure (a maneuver now proscribed). Three groups were defined, and the largest consisted of children with the traditional stimulus for breathholding, ie, vigorous crying, apnea, and cyanosis. In this group asystole was less common than in the second group of pallid breathholders who demonstrated severe pallor and syncope or seizure after a minimal stimulus. The third group possessed features of both. In the majority of patients these spells started in the first few weeks of life and only a few after 2 years of age. The breathholding spells stopped in the majority by 4–5 years of age. However, in 17% of the patients syncopal attacks occurred again later in life. This connection between early breathholding spells and later syncopal episodes was stressed by Lombroso and Lerman[13] and Lerman-Sagie and colleagues.[14] DiMario and coworkers[15,16] identified dysregulation of the autonomic system in both pallid and cyanotic breathholders. Emery[17] reported two cases of breathholding that were associated with prolonged seizures (40–45 minutes) which required intravenous anticonvulsant therapy. Therefore, rarely, breathholding spells may precipitate "status epilepticus."

Other triggers of neurocardiac syncope include cough syncope and asthma.[14,18] Haslam and Freigang[18] reported 12 children with cough syncope. The episodes were more common during sleep and during periods of bronchospasm. In nearly half of the children convulsive movements were associated with the syncopal episode. Therapy was geared toward aggressive control of bronchospasm.

Malignant neuroendocrine syncope may occur in asthmatics who are dependent upon β-agonists. Grubb and associates[19] reported a case of a young man who collapsed after using an aerosol with β-agonist. Subsequently, with isoproterenol stimulation during tilt study, there was a positive response manifested by decrease in blood pressure and pulse. We saw two asthmatic patients who required resuscitation, both of whom had bradycardia. Exaggerated neurocardiac response may be one mechanism for sudden death in these patients, although ventricular arrhythmia may also be significant.

Although exercise-related syncope should alert one to the possibility of an underlying malignant cause, it is not uncommon for neurocardiac syncope to occur following strenuous exercise. Grubb and colleagues[20] reported a study of 24 young athletes with neurocardiac syncope. All had extensive evaluation to eliminate the possibility of cardiac or neurological disorder. Tilt studies were useful in identifying the diagnosis in these patients. A careful history is necessary to determine whether syncope occurred during peak exertion or immediately following a strenuous effort. The abrupt withdrawal of sympathetic tone immediately following exertion is thought to be important in triggering syncope. Rarely neurocardiac syncope may occur during or at peak exercise, but this clinical situation should raise suspicion of an underlying malignant cause.

Cardiac Syncope

While neurocardiac syncope is the most common form and is usually benign, other causes may lead to sudden death. Cardiac disease accounts for 30% to 80% of sudden deaths in the pediatric population and 50% to

85% in young adults.[21-29] In these patients, history of prior syncope is a fairly common finding, particularly exercise-related syncope.[21,29] Thus, syncope in a patient with underlying heart disease should be considered an ominous event until proven otherwise.

Structural heart diseases more frequently associated with sudden death are cardiomyopathy and postoperative congenital heart disease. Other causes include myocarditis, aortic stenosis, anomalous coronary artery, pulmonary artery hypertension, and right ventricular (RV) dysplasia, the latter more common in Italian populations.[26]

Cardiac arrhythmias more frequently associated with sudden death are ventricular tachycardia (VT)/fibrillation, congenital long QT syndrome (LQTS), and Wolff-Parkinson-White (WPW) syndrome.[23,24,27]

Cardiomyopathy

In patients with dilated cardiomyopathy, the occurrence of syncope is a poor prognostic indicator. In general, a 5-year survival rate of 0–50% has been described for dilated cardiomyopathy[30,31] with a significant positive impact on survival when cardioverter defibrillator therapy is used.[25] For hypertrophic cardiomyopathy the yearly attrition has been reported as high as 5.9%[32] The mechanism of syncope in hypertrophic cardiomyopathy may be due to inadequate cardiac output related to obstruction, atrial arrhythmias, or ventricular arrhythmias, perhaps triggered by subendocardial ischemia.

Postoperative Congenital Heart Disease

Those who have undergone surgery for repair of congenital heart defects are vulnerable to sudden death, usually due to arrhythmia. In children who had the Mustard procedure for transposition of the great vessels, the incidence of late sudden death ranges from 2.4% to 6.4%.[33,34] Predictors of sudden death included the presence of active arrhythmias, atrial tachycardia, and atrial flutter (AF). Garson and coworkers[35] reported a 17% mortality for patients with flutter (the majority had surgery for congenital heart disease). Death occurred at a mean of 2.4 years after the onset of flutter. Although the follow-up period is shorter for patients who had the Fontan procedure for single ventricle or hypoplastic RV, the incidence of cardiac arrhythmias is high. In some series,[36-38] the development of AF in the early period after surgery was associated with a particularly high mortality.

Patients who have had repair of tetralogy of Fallot or double outlet RV[39,40] are at risk for ventricular arrhythmias and occasionally atrial tachycardia. After repair of tetralogy the risk is probably low but after repair of double outlet RV, the presence of VT is associated with a mortality of 35%; when atrial fibrillation or flutter are also associated, the mortality is 59%.[40]

Primary Arrhythmias

While atrial and ventricular arrhythmias in the setting of congenital cardiac defects are particularly foreboding, these arrhythmias may also cause syncope and sudden death in overtly healthy young populations. Deal and associates[41] identified VT as a cause of syncope and sudden death in such children. Frequently there are underlying microscopic ventricular abnormalities. In these patients the presence of the arrhythmia may be the initial presentation of cardiomyopathy, which is difficult to detect by noninvasive evaluation.

The congenital LQTS is one of the more frequent causes of syncope or sudden death in children.[42] The incidence of sudden death is higher in patients with a very long QTc (0.6 milliseconds) and in those noncompliant with medication. Infancy is a particularly high-risk period for these patients, especially in the presence of bradycardia and/or "seizures."

Finally,WPW syndrome is associated with sudden death. The mechanism of cardiac arrest in these patients is thought to be rapid conduction of atrial tachycardia (atrial fibrillation) over the accessory connection to the ventricles, provoking ventricular fibrillation. Although such patients frequently have a history of supraventricular tachycardia (SVT), cardiac arrest may be the first arrhythmia, particularly in young patients. In a multicenter study of children with cardiac arrest and WPW syndrome, arrest was the initial documented arrhythmia in 48%.[43] Radiofrequency (RF) catheter ablation is effective and safe for treatment of these arrhythmias in children and adults. The statistics from the pediatric ablation registry,[44] established in 1991 for tracking these patients, support a gratifying success rate of 90%.

Neurological Syncope

Neurological disorders account for 7% to 11% of patients who present with syncope. Sometimes it is difficult to distinguish a primary neurological disorder from simple neurocardiac syncope. This was demonstrated in a study by Linzer and colleagues,[45] who reported 12 patients who were initially diagnosed as having epilepsy. They cautioned that, when the EEG is normal or near normal, one should search for other causes, notably the LQTS. In that report, five patients had neurocardiac syncope but the others had cardiac arrhythmias. Some of the patients had been treated for a seizure disorder for as long as 20 years. The authors found that the most important diagnostic tests for identifying the correct diagnosis in these patients were Holter study, event recording, and head-up tilt (HUT) table studies. Another interesting entity that may be misdiagnosed as a "seizure disorder" is the video game-related seizure. Graf and coworkers[46] reported the occurrence of seizures in 10 patients and reviewed 25 cases from the literature. The authors concluded that the seizurelike events were triggered by visual stimuli, particularly when they were "repetitive, high-intensity, multicolored or white flashes, rapid changes of scene, swift displacement of images, appearance of line patterns and rolling or flickering TV patterns."

Neurocutaneous and neuromuscular disorders are associated with syncope and seizure and may be due to primary central nervous system (CNS) disease or to arrhythmias related to cardiac involvement as is seen in Kearns-Sayre syndrome.[47] This syndrome is associated with progressive conduction disease and may present with acute atrioventricular (AV) block.

Lintermans[48] reported on the utility of cardiac echocardiography in the management of patients with neurological disorders with associated cardiac components such as tuberous sclerosis with rhabdomyomas and Friedreich ataxia with hypertrophic cardiomyopathy. Kohli and associates[49] reported the occurrence of malignant VT as the cause of syncope in a 3-month-old infant with tuberous sclerosis. RF ablative therapy at the site of an intracardiac tumor eliminated the tachycardia focus and the syncope in this patient.

Temporal lobe epilepsy may be heralded by syncope.[50] Constantin and colleagues[51] and Zeiler and Zeitlhofer[52] reported the occurrence of bradycardia and syncope in complex partial seizures.

Syncope may accompany basilar migraine. It may augur the occurrence of the headache and other associations such as vertigo, paresthesia, and dysarthria.[53] Though clinical seizures are rarely associated with migraine, EEG abnormalities are common.[54]

Psychological Syncope

Psychological disorders are not uncommonly associated with syncope. According to some authors the incidence may be as high as 40% with panic, depressive, and conversion reactions predominating.[55,56] Koenig and coworkers[56] found that bedside hyperventilation testing was helpful in distinguishing those patients with a psychogenic cause. The high incidence of psychiatric disorders in these series contrasts with others and may reflect selection bias in populations and modes of investigation. HUT studies were not performed.

Endocrine Syncope

Endocrinopathies are rare causes of syncope or seizures. The signs of the primary disorder are usually evident. Hypothalamic and pituitary tumors may produce symptoms because of mass effect or because of hormonal secretion. Fifteen percent of all CNS tumors in children originate from the hypothalamus.[57] Diabetes insipidus and inappropriate secretion of antidiuretic hormone should be considered.[58]

Parathyroid and thyroid disorders[59–61] and abnormalities of glucose metabolism[62–64] may be associated with syncope. Miller and associates[61] reported the occurrence of third-degree heart block and syncope in a patient with Graves disease. Normal conduction was restored with control of the hyperthyroid state. Syncope may be a signal of underlying adrenal insufficiency and multiple endocrine neoplasia.[65,66] Differentiating an endocrinological etiology for syncope is usually accomplished by careful history, physical examination, and blood electrolyte determination.

Evaluation of Syncope

As is clearly evident, there are multiple potential causes of syncope or seizure and various precipitants or historical events. In evaluating the patient with syncope the object is to exclude malignant causes. The clues to differentiating benign from malignant causes reside primarily in the history, physical examination, and a limited number of investigational studies.

History

A careful history is the single most useful tool for identifying the likely cause of syncope. Suspicion should be raised when there is a family history of sudden death, heart disease (acquired or congenital), genetic diseases associated with sudden death (such as LQTS), arrhythmias, pacemakers, or neurologic or endocrine disease. Moreover, further exploration should be prompted by the personal history of congenital or acquired heart disease; cardiac surgery; palpitations; drug therapy for asthma, allergies and colds; psychotropic drug use; or unusual diets. The history surrounding the syncopal attack usually provides essential information to aid in differential diagnosis. Specific areas of interest would be the activity or circumstances at the time of the episode, eg, level of activity, dietary intake, sleep, illness or fever prior to the episode, resuscitation, palpitations, or occurrence of seizure activity. Syncope with standing, painful stimulation, or fear support the diagnosis of ''benign syncope,'' particularly when associated with feelings of warmth, nausea, sweatiness, or headache. An awareness of palpitations or rapid heart rate prior to syncope is not common in neurocardiac syncope and raises the possibility of an arrhythmia. Syncope on awakening to an alarm or during swimming or running should raise the possibility of LQTS. Syncopal occurrence during exercise may implicate anomalies of the coronary arteries or cardiomyopathy.

The physical examination should focus on cardiovascular, neurological, psychological and endocrine systems. An electrocardiogram (ECG) should be obtained and reviewed for bradycardia, PR interval, QT interval, abnormal Q waves and ST changes, atrial or ventricular ectopy, or preexcitation.

Based upon these results, in most instances a clear picture of the underlying etiology should emerge. For example, a neurocardiac cause is most likely in a teenager who had a syncopal episode during choir practice or in a 1-year-old with a temper tantrum. On the other hand, a cardiac cause is likely in the teenager who faints while engaged in playing football.

A basic evaluation should be done for patients with clear neurocardiac syncope, epilepsy, and migraine. This should include history and physical examination and ECG. A tilt study or EEG may be indicated depending upon history and physical findings. A tilt study may be necessary if the diagnosis of neurocardiac syncope is unclear or there is a seizure component with the syncope. A moderate evaluation should be done for the other groups discussed. Moderate evaluation includes the basic and all or some of the following: electrolytes, cardioscan/event recorder, echocardiogram and exercise study. A full evaluation includes the moderate evaluation plus catheterization, angiography, and electrophysiological (EP) study, and should be considered in patients with unexplained exertional syncope. Patients with cardiomyopathy and congenital and surgically repaired heart disease frequently require EP investigation. All syncopal patients with WPW should have an EP study and probably ablative therapy if SVT is identified as the cause of symptoms.

Tilt Testing

Populations and Methodology

There are extensive reports of HUT studies in both adults and children. This study is based on the ability to reproduce symptoms of neurocardiac syncope by simply having patients stand for a variable period while monitoring heart rate and blood pressure. Several series[4,7,67–69] suggested a higher incidence of neurocardiac syncope among females, which may represent selection bias in the population studies. Other investigations found an equal distribution among males and females[20] when the study population was comprised of athletes. In the studies cited there were variations in methodology including a supine period ranging between 5 and 19 minutes, and the upright period ranged between 10 and 49 minutes. Some workers did not include isoproterenol stimulation but most investigators utilized this type of provocation if the baseline tilt study was negative.

Sheldon[70] also compared a single stage tilt with 5 μg per minute of isoproterenol to the protocol utilizing incremental doses of the drug. He found a 79% concordance. Ovadia and Thoele[71] analyzed esmolol withdrawal as a unique method for provocation. Although sensitivity and specificity could not be identified, the authors concluded that the esmolol withdrawal study was at least equivalent to isoproterenol, safer, and less likely to produce false-positive results.

Of a number of studies[4,6,7,20,49,67,68,70,71] the incidence of a positive result ranged between 44% and 80%, the lower incidence[7] in a population in which baseline tilting was the only provocation.

Reproducibility

In studies in both adults and children, reproducibility of findings ranges between 67% and 87%.[8,72,73]

Sensitivity and Specificity

In a study in young adults[74] and two studies in children,[7,75] sensitivity and specificity determinations of tilt testing were made. In the studies in children, the sensitivity ranged between 45% to 57% and specificity between 83% to 100%. In the study of young adults[74] there was poor sensitivity and poor specificity, the former being 75% and the latter 35% to 55%. The rate of false-positive studies was high. The authors suggested that isoproterenol stimulation results in the falsely high positive rate in the controls. If the control population was exposed only to HUT without isoproterenol, the positive rate was 17%. Therefore, it appears more valid to study patients with a prolonged tilt without isoproterenol stimulation.

Although tilt testing may be helpful to clarify the diagnosis of neurocardiac syncope, its reliability and accuracy in pediatric patients is less than optimal. Clearly, clinical history and assessment are the most essential elements for this diagnosis.

Mechanisms

The mechanisms involved in neurocardiac syncope are probably similar to those involved in acute hypovolemia. Schadt and Ludbrook[76] conducted an extensive literature review on responses to acute hypovolemia. They described two separate physiological phases. The first phase is a sympathoexcitatory phase, which occurs before the blood loss exceeds 30%. The afferent limb for this phase is decreased traffic from the mechanoreceptors at the base of the ventricles with efferent feedback characterized by tachycardia and increased systemic vascular resistance due to decreased vagal activity and increased sympathetic activity. The second phase (when blood loss is more extreme) is sympathoinhibitory. The mechanoreceptors are stimulated by stretch of the myocardial fibers generated by an ''empty'' ventricle; the efferent feedback results in withdrawal of sympathetic tone and increase in vagal tone. There is general vasodilatation except in the skin. There is decreased release of norepinephrine from postganglionic sympathetic fibers and compensatory increases in epinephrine from the adrenal glands. Renin-angiotensin increases as does vasopressin. A similar mechanism may be involved in neurocardiac syncope.

In an effort to identify mechanisms for positive responses to HUT, various parameters were measured. Balaji and coworkers[4] analyzed catecholamine levels during the supine and standing positions. He found that patients who were tilt positive had elevated epinephrine levels in the supine position compared to the tilt-negative patients. There were no significant differences between the groups in reference to norepinephrine or standing epinephrine values. There was also a significant difference in the blood pressure response to isoproterenol. In the tilt-positive group the blood pressure was lower. There was no difference in the heart rate response to isoproterenol between the groups. Response to phenylephrine was the same in both groups.

These findings contrast with the study of Perry and Garson,[77] who found significantly lower values of norepinephrine in the study group in both the supine and standing positions but no differences in epinephrine. Heart rate response to isoproterenol was greater in the tilt-positive group.

Sra et al[78] noted increased levels of epinephrine in both the supine and standing positions in the tilt positive group versus the control group. It is noteworthy that these were true controls and not patients with a history of syncope. These investigators also found a significant surge in epinephrine levels just prior to hypotension and syncope. There was no change in norepinephrine levels. Because of the discordance between the norepinephrine and epinephrine levels, the investigators suggested that this reflected a predominance of adrenomedullary activity and inhibition of neuronal sympathetic activity.

Mehta and associates[79] studied endothelin levels in syncopal children who were tilt positive and tilt negative compared to a control group. There was a significantly elevated level of endothelin in both former groups compared to controls. This was evident when measurements were taken with the patients in the supine position. This suggested that there is an alteration in basal vascular tone with compensatory increase in the endothelium-derived vasoconstrictor. This situation may be similar to that reported by Stewart and colleagues[80] in patients with congestive heart failure. They have high basal levels of endothelin and fail to show an increase in endothelin levels with tilt.

Several authors studied vascular responses to lower body negative pressure. Sneddon et al[81] found increased forearm vascular resistance when tilt-positive patients were exposed to minor negative pressure in the supine position. When forearm vascular measurements were made during upright tilt, there was a significantly smaller increase in resistance than in the tilt-negative group.[82] These two studies support both augmented cardiopulmonary and impaired vasoconstrictor responses as contributing to neurocardiac syncope.

Studies of heart rate variability were similar in tilt-positive patients versus tilt-negative and control patients.[83] This was true for both the low-frequency and high-frequency power spectra reflecting sympathetic and parasympathetic inputs, respectively. These resting studies were confirmed by Pruvot,[84] who also demonstrated an increase in parasympathetic and sympathetic activity *during* the tilt.

Plasma renin activity was measured by Uchiyama and coworkers[85] in a group of syncopal children. There were no differences in the baseline activity. In those patients who had a positive (syncopal) response to upright position, the renin activity was higher than in those with a negative response or in the normal group.

Wallbridge and associates[86] studied syncopal patients (adults) and identified increased levels of β-endorphins in the tilt-positive (before symptoms) versus the tilt-negative groups. The pretilt levels were similar. Similar findings were reported by Perna and colleagues,[87] who studied syncopal patients at rest and during syncope. There was a significant increase in β-endorphins during syncope similar to that seen in septic shock. The basal levels were similar to controls.

In summarizing the findings of these various studies, there are some general patterns that emerge despite some conflicting results. Fairly firm is the conclusion that there is basal motor dysregulation and augmented responses of cardiopulmonary receptors. Receptor site dysregulation is suggested by the elevated levels of epinephrine and endothelin in the unstressed state.

Management

For any treatment strategy for neurocardiac syncope, consideration must be given to the self-limiting nature of the problem, with gradual improvement over time. In addition, with long-term follow-up, a clear advantage to any treatment regimen is not established. A decision to treat should be based on the frequency and severity of episodes and the ability of the patient to recognize predisposing factors and avoid them (standing for prolonged periods in the heat) or to respond rapidly to prodromal symptoms (sit promptly with the onset of dizziness). Dietary modifications may be very helpful, as many adolescents will skip breakfast and lunch and experience syncope in the early afternoon. With these considerations, no further therapy may be necessary.

In children the primary therapy for neurocardiac syncope is an increase in fluid and salt intake. In the study of Mangru and coworkers[5] normal saline infusion was given following a positive tilt study. The study was negative in 84% of patients after the saline. On clinical follow-up the majority were asymptomatic or improved on sodium chloride therapy and/ or fludrocortisone.

A traditional therapy for neurocardiac syncope was β-blockade. The efficacy for various β-blockers ranges from 60% to 96%.[4,68,88–90] Sra and colleagues[91] demonstrated that intravenous esmolol during HUT predicted the response to oral metoprolol. O'Marcaigh and coworkers[92] showed a closer concordance between intravenous and oral metoprolol than that found in Muller's[90] study population.

In an important study in adults, Brignole and cowokers[93] demonstrated that there was no difference in response to treatment with atenolol and placebo with an 80% efficacy in the former and 73% in the latter. This is similar to the results of a study by Morillo and associates[94] in presyncopal and syncopal adults. There was a 68% to 90% efficacy with no treatment compared to various treatment regimens including fludrocortisone, β-blockers, α-agonists, and disopyramide. Morillo et al[95] also found that there was no difference in response to treatment with disopyramide and no treatment. On the other hand, Kelly and associates[96] demonstrated a 93% efficacy in patients treated with high dose disopyramide. Other agents utilized in children and adults include α-agonists[97] and methyl xanthines[98] with an efficacy of 94% and 82% respectively. Sertraline[99] was effective in 50% of children who were intolerant or unresponsive to other medications.

Pacemaker therapy was utilized in some patients who have severe cardioinhibitory syncope, sometimes called malignant syncope, with asystole for ≥5 seconds. A pacemaker is often ineffective since the cardioinhibitory response may be overcome by the pacemaker but a vasodepressor component may persist.[100] Therefore, combined therapies were utilized with pacemakers, including β-blockers and disopyramide.[65,101–103] Deal et al[104] reported that medical therapy without pacemakers was successful in 18 pediatric patients who had asystole (median duration 10 seconds) during tilt testing. From that study and the study of Dhala and associates,[105] the outcome is similarly favorable for syncopal patients with and without asystole.

An apparent conclusion from these studies is that nearly anything is effective for the treatment of neurocardiac syncope. Therefore, the most prudent approach would be to first utilize education and behavior control and increase fluid and salt intake; finally, fludrocortisone, β-blockers or α-agonists may be helpful. If fludrocortisone is used, one must be aware of the possibility of electrolyte disturbance and even myocardial changes.[106] Brignole and colleagues[93] suggest that the high incidence rate for spontaneous remission of syncope in untreated patients may be due to recognition of prodromal symptoms with consequent self-imposed maneuvers to avoid syncope or the psychological effect of the study and assurance of favorable outcome. Sheldon and coworkers,[107] on the basis of a study of 338 patients, formulated graphs for prediction of recurrent syncope. Stratification for risk may give direction to those who deserve more intensive intervention. In that study, the tilt test and clinical encounter served as the sole intervention producing a significant reduction in the frequency of syncope following the study. Because of the tendency to "grow out" of the propensity to faint, it is even more judicious to avoid drug therapy in children if possible.

References

1. Strieper MJ, Auld DO, Hulse JE, et al. Evaluation of recurrent pediatric syncope: Role of tilt table testing. *Pediatrics* 1994;93:660–662.
2. Ozme S, Alehan D, Yalaz K, et al. Causes of syncope in children: a prospective study. *Int J Cardiol* 1993;40:111–114.
3. Gordon TA, Moodie DS, Passalacqua M, et al. A retrospective analysis of the cost-effective workup of syncope in children. *Cleve Clin J Med* 1987;54:391–394.
4. Balaji S, Oslizlok PC, Allen MC, et al. Neurocardiogenic syncope in children with a normal heart. *J Am Coll Cardiol* 1994;23:779–785.
5. Mangru N, Young ML, Mas MS, et al. Usefulness of tilt table test with saline infusion in management of children with neurocardiac syncope. *Am Heart J.* 1996;131:953–959.
6. Pongiglione G, Fish FA, Strasburger JF, et al. Heart rate and blood pressure response to upright tilt in young patients with unexplained syncope. *J Am Coll Cardiol* 1990;16:165–170.
7. Ross BA, Hughes S, Anderson E, et al. Abnormal responses to orthostatic testing in children and adolescent with recurrent unexplained syncope. *Am Heart J* 1991;122:748–754.
8. Fish FA, Strasburger JF, Benson DW Jr. Reproducibility of a symptomatic response to upright tilt in young patients with unexplained syncope. *Am J Cardiol* 1992;70:605–609.
9. Lewis DW, Frank LM. Hair-grooming syncope seizures. *Pediatrics* 1993;91:836–838.
10. White LE, Toor SS. Hair burning syncope. *Pediatrics* 1993;92:638–649.
11. Pavlin DJ, Links S, Rapp SE, et al. Vaso-vagal reactions in an ambulatory surgery center. *Anesth Analg* 1993;76:931–935.
12. Gastaut H. Electro-encephalographic study of syncope. *Lancet* 1957;275(part II):1018–1025.
13. Lombroso CT, Lerman P. Breathholding spells (cyanotic and pallid infantile syncope). *Pediatrics* 1967;39:563–581.
14. Lerman-Sagie T, Lerman P, Mukamel M, et al. A prospective evaluation of pediatric patients with syncope. *Clin Pediatr* 1994;33:67–70.
15. DiMario FJ Jr, Chee CM, Berman PH. Pallid breath-holding spells. Evaluation of the autonomic nervous system. *Clin Pediatr* 1990;29:17–24.
16. DiMario FJ Jr, Burleson JA. Autonomic nervous system function in severe breath-holding spells. *Pediatr Neurol* 1993;9:268–274.
17. Emery ES. Status epilepticus secondary to breath-holding and pallid syncopal spells. *Neurology* 1990:12:45–47.
18. Haslam RH, Freigang B. Cough syncope mimicking epilepsy in asthmatic children. *Can J Neurol Sci* 1985;12:45–47.

19. Grubb BP, Wolfe DA, Nelson LA, et al. Malignant vasovagally mediated hypotension and bradycardia: a possible cause of sudden death in young patients with asthma. *Pediatrics* 1992;90:983–986.
20. Grubb BP, Temesy-Armos PN, Samoil D, et al. Tilt table testing in the evaluation and management of athletes with recurrent exercise-induced syncope. *Med Sci Sports Exerc* 1993;25:24–28.
21. Driscoll DJ, Edwards WD. Sudden unexpected death in children and adolescents. *J Am Coll Cardiol* 1985;5:118B–121B.
22. Shen WK, Edwards WD, Hammill SC, et al. Sudden unexpected nontraumatic death in 54 young adults: a 30-year population-based study. *Am J Cardiol* 1995;76:148–152.
23. Klitzner TS. Sudden cardiac death in children. *Circulation* 1990;82:629–632.
24. Silka MJ, Kron J, Walance CG, et al. Assessment and follow-up of pediatric survivors of sudden cardiac death. *Circulation* 1990;82:341–349.
25. Silka MJ, Kron J, Dunnigan A, et al. Sudden cardiac death and the use of implantable cardioverter-defibrillators in pediatric patients. *Circulation* 1993;87:800–807.
26. Daliento L, Turrini P, Nava A, et al. Arrhythmogenic right ventricular cardiomyopathy in young versus adult patients: similarities and differences. *J Am Coll Cardiol* 1995;25:655–664.
27. Liberthson RR. Sudden death from cardiac causes in children and young adults. *N Engl J Med* 1996;334:1039–1044.
28. Steinberger J, Lucas RV Jr, Edwards JE, et al. Causes of sudden unexpected cardiac death in the first two decades of life. *Am J Cardiol* 1996;77:992–995.
29. Maron BJ, Shirani J, Poliac LC, et al. Sudden death in young competitive athletes: clinical, demographic, and pathological profiles. *JAMA* 1996;276:199–204.
30. Taliercio CP, Seward JB, Driscoll DJ, et al. Idiopathic dilated cardiomyopathy in the young: clinical profile and natural history. *J Am Coll Cardiol* 1985;6:1126–1131.
31. Griffin ML, Hernandez A, Martin TC, et al. Dilated cardiomyopathy in infants and children. *J Am Coll Cardiol* 1988;11:139–144.
32. McKenna W, Deanfield J, Faruqui A, et al. Prognosis in hypertrophic cardiomyopathy: role of age and clinical, electrocardiographic and hemodynamic features. *Am J Cardiol* 1981;47:532–538.
33. Flinn CJ, Wolff GS, Dick M II, et al. Cardiac rhythm after the Mustard procedure for complete transposition of the great arteries. *N Engl J Med* 1984;310:1635–1638.
34. Gelatt M, Hamilton RM, McCrindle BW, et al. Arrhythmia and mortality after the Mustard procedure: a 30-year single-center experience. *J Am Coll Cardiol* 1997; 29:194–201.
35. Garson A, Bink-Boelkens M, Hesslein PS, et al. Atrial flutter in the young: a collaborative study of 380 cases. *J Am Coll Cardiol* 1985;6:871–878.
36. Balaji S, Gewillig M, Bull C, et al. Arrhythmias after the Fontan procedure. Comparison of total cavopulmonary connection and atriopulmonary connection. *Circulation* 1991;84(suppl III):162–167.
37. Gewillig M, Wyse RK, de Leval MR, et al. Early and late arrhythmias after the Fontan operation: predisposing factors and clinical consequences. *Br Heart J* 1992;67:72–79.
38. Peters NS, Somerville J: Arrhythmias after the Fontan procedure. *Br Heart J* 1992;68:199–204.
39. Chandar JS, Wolff GS, Garson A Jr, et al. Ventricular arrhythmias in postoperative tetralogy of Fallot. *Am J Cardiol* 1990;65:655–661.

40. Shen W-K, Holmes DR Jr, Porter CJ, et al. Sudden death after repair of double-outlet right ventricle. *Circulation* 1990;81:128–136.
41. Deal BJ, Miller SM, Scagliotti D, et al. Ventricular tachycardia in a young population without overt heart disease. *Circulation* 1986;73:1111–1118.
42. Garson A Jr, Dick M II, Fournier A, et al. The long QT syndrome in children. An international study of 287 patients. *Circulation* 1993;87:1866–1872.
43. Deal BJ, Dick M, Beerman L, et al. Cardiac arrest in young patients with Wolff-Parkinson White Syndrome. *Pacing Clin Electrophysiol* 1995;18:815.
44. Kugler JD, Danford DA, Deal BJ, et al. Radiofrequency catheter ablation for tachyarrhythmias in children and adolescents. The Pediatric Electrophysiology Society. *N Engl J Med* 1994;330:1481–1487.
45. Linzer M, Grubb BP, Ho S, et al. Cardiovascular causes of loss of consciousness in patients with presumed epilepsy: a cause of the increased sudden death rate in people with epilepsy? *Am J Med* 1994;96:146–154.
46. Graf WD, Chatrian G-E, Glass ST, et al. Video game-related seizures: a report on 10 patients and a review of the literature. *Pediatrics* 1994;93:551–556.
47. Clark DS, Myerburg RJ, Morales AR, et al. Heart block in Kearns–Sayre Syndrome. *Chest* 1982;68:727.
48. Lintermans JP. Echocardiography in neurological disorders. *Eur J Pediatr* 1987;146:15–20.
49. Kohli V, Mangru N, Pearse LA, et al. Radiofrequency ablation of ventricular tachycardia in an infant with cardiac tumors. *Am Heart J* 1996;132:198–200.
50. Mikati M, Holmes GL. Temporal lobe epilepsy. In: Wyllie E, ed. *The Treatment of Epilepsy: Principals and Practices.* Philadelphia: Lea & Febiger; 1993:513.
51. Constantin L, Martins JB, Fincham RW, et al. Bradycardia and syncope as manifestations of partial epilepsy. *J Am Coll Cardiol* 1990;15:900–905.
52. Zeiler K, Zeitlhofer J. Syncopal consciousness disorders and drop attacks from the neurologic viewpoint. *Wien Klin Wochenschr* 1988;100:93–99.
53. Pellock JM. The differential diagnosis of epilepsy: non-epileptic paroxysmal disorders. In: Wyllie E, ed. *The Treatment of Epilepsy: Principles and Practices.* Philadelphia: Lea & Febiger; 1993:703.
54. Prensky AL, Sommer D. Diagnosis and treatment of migraine in children. *Neurology* 1979;29:506–510.
55. Linzer M, Varia I, Pontinen M, et al. Medically unexplained syncope: relationship to psychiatric illness. *Am J Med* 1992;92(suppl IA):18–25.
56. Koenig D, Linzer M, Pontinen M, et al. Syncope in young adults: evidence for a combined medical and psychiatric approach. *J Intern Med* 1992;232:169–176.
57. Christy NP, Warren MP. Other clinical syndromes of the hypothalamus and anterior pituitary, including tumor mass effects. In: DeGroot LJ, ed. *Endocrinology.* Philadelphia: WB Saunders Co; 1989:419–453.
58. Baylis PH. Vasopressin and its neurophysin. In: DeGroot LJ, ed. *Endocrinology.* Philadelphia: WB Saunders Co; 1989:213–229.
59. Parfitt AM. Surgical, idiopathic and other varieties of parathyroid hormone-deficient hypoparathyroidism. In: DeGroot LJ, ed. *Endocrinology.* Philadelphia: WB Saunders Co; 1989:1049–1064.
60. Utiger RD. Hypothyroidism. In: DeGroot LJ, ed. *Endocrinology.* Philadelphia: WB Saunders Co; 1989:702–721.
61. Miller RH, Corcoran FH, Baker WP. Second and third degree atrioventricular block with Graves' disease: a case report and review of the literature. *Pacing Clin Electrophysiol* 1980;3:702–711.
62. Service FJ. Hypoglycemia. In: DeGroot LJ, ed. *Endocrinology.* Philadelphia: WB Saunders Co; 1989:1524–1548.

63. Foster DW, McGarry D. Acute complications of diabetes: ketoacidosis, hyperosmolar coma, lactic acidosis. In: DeGroot LJ, ed. *Endocrinology.* Philadelphia: WB Saunders Co; 1989:1439–1453.

64. Burman WJ, McDermott MT, Bornemann M. Familial hyperinsulinism presenting in adults. *Arch Intern Med* 1992;152:2125–2127.

65. Bethune JE. The diagnosis and treatment of adrenal insufficiency. In: DeGroot LJ, ed. *Endocrinology.* Philadelphia: WB Saunders Co; 1989:1647–1659.

66. Zahner J, Borchard F, Schmitz U, et al. Thymus carcinoid in multiple endocrine neoplasms type I. *Dtsch Med Wochenschr* 1994;119:135–140.

67. Thilenius OG, Quiñones JA, Husayni TS, et al. Tilt test for diagnosis of unexplained syncope in pediatric patients. *Pediatrics* 1991;87:334–338.

68. Thilenius OG, Ryd KJ, Husayni J. Variations in expression and treatment of transient neurocardiogenic instability. *Am J Cardiol* 1992;69:1193–1195.

69. Grubb BP, Temesy-Armos P, Moore J, et al. Head-upright tilt-table testing in evaluation and management of the malignant vasovagal syndrome. *Am J Cardiol* 1992;69:904–908.

70. Sheldon R. Evaluation of a single-stage isoproterenol-tilt table test in patients with syncope. *J Am Coll Cardiol* 1993;22:114–118.

71. Ovadia M, Thoele D. Esmolol tilt testing with esmolol withdrawal for the evaluation of syncope in the young. *Circulation* 1994;89:228–235.

72. Chen XC, Chen MY, Remole S, et al. Reproducibility of head-up tilt-table testing for eliciting susceptibility to neurally mediated syncope in patients without structural heart disease. *Am J Cardiol* 1992;69:755–760.

73. De Buitleir M, Grogan EW Jr, Picone MF, et al. Immediate reproducibility of the tilt-table test in adults with unexplained syncope. *Am J Cardiol* 1993;71:304–307.

74. Kapoor WN, Brant N. Evaluation of syncope by upright tilt testing with isoproterenol. A nonspecific test. *Ann Intern Med* 1992;116:358–363.

75. Fouad FM, Sitthisook S, Vanerio G, et al. Sensitivity and specificity of the tilt table test in young patients with unexplained syncope. *Pacing Clin Electrophysiol* 1993;16:394–400.

76. Schadt JC, Ludbrook J. Hemodynamic and neurohumoral responses to acute hypovolemia in conscious mammals. *Am J Physiol* 1991;260:H305–H318.

77. Perry JC, Garson A Jr. The child with recurrent syncope: autonomic function testing and beta-adrenergic hypersensitivity. *J Am Coll Cardiol* 1991;17:1168–1171.

78. Sra JS, Murthy V, Natale A, et al. Circulatory and catecholamine changes during head-up tilt testing in neurocardiogenic (vasovagal) syncope. *Am J Cardiol* 1994;73:33–37.

79. Mehta M, Wolff G, Young M-L, et al. Usefulness of endothelin-1 as a predictor of response to head-up tilt-table testing in children with syncope. *Am J Cardiol* 1995;76:86–88.

80. Stewart DJ, Cernacek P, Costello KB, et al. Elevated endothelin-1 in heart failure and loss of normal response to postural change. *Circulation* 1992;85:510–517.

81. Sneddon JF, Counihan PJ, Bashir Y, et al. Assessment of autonomic function in patients with neurally mediated syncope: augmented cardiopulmonary baroreceptor responses to graded orthostatic stress. *J Am Coll Cardiol* 1993;21:1193–1198.

82. Sneddon JF, Counihan PJ, Bashir Y, et al. Impaired immediate vasoconstrictor responses in patients with recurrent neurally mediated syncope. *Am J Cardiol* 1993;71:72–76.

83. Sneddon JF, Bashir Y, Murgatroyd FD, et al. Do patients with neurally mediated syncope have augmented vagal tone? *Am J Cardiol* 1993;72:1314–1315.
84. Pruvot E. Autonomic dysfunction in vasovagal syncope occurs during head-up tilt test: results of heart rate variability analysis. *Am J Cardiol* 1994;74:209.
85. Uchiyama M, Otsuka T, Sakai K. Response of plasma renin activity to postural change in vasovagal syncope in children, with observations on syncope. *Horm Res* 1986;23:147–150.
86. Wallbridge DR, MacIntyre HE, Gray CE, et al. Increase in plasma beta endorphins precedes vasodepressor syncope. *Br Heart J* 1994;71:446–448.
87. Perna GP, Ficola U, Salvatori MP, et al. Increase of plasma beta endorphins in vasodepressor syncope. *Am J Cardiol* 1990;65:929–930.
88. Grubb BP, Temesy-Armos P, Moore J, et al. The use of head-upright tilt table testing in the evaluation and management of syncope in children and adolescents. *Pacing Clin Electrophysiol* 1992;15:742–748.
89. Scott WA, Pongiglime G, Bromberg BI, et al. Comparison of treatments for neurally mediated syncope. *Circulation* 1994;90:523.
90. Müller G, Deal BJ, Strasburger JF, et al. Usefulness of metoprolol for unexplained syncope and positive response to tilt testing in young persons. *Am J Cardiol* 1993;71:592–595.
91. Sra JS, Murthy VS, Jazayeri MR, et al. Use of intravenous esmolol to predict efficacy of oral beta-adrenergic blocker therapy in patients with neurocardiogenic syncope. *J Am Coll Cardiol* 1992;19:402–408.
92. O'Marcaigh AS, MacLellan-Tobert SG, Porter CJ. Tilt-table testing and oral metoprolol therapy in young patients with unexplained syncope. *Pediatrics* 1994;93:278–283.
93. Brignole M, Menozzi C, Gianfranchi L, et al. A controlled trial of acute and long-term medical therapy in tilt-induced neurally mediated syncope. *Am J Cardiol* 1992;70:339–342.
94. Morillo CA, Zandri S, Klein GJ, et al. Neurally mediated syncope: long-term follow-up of patients with and without pharmacological therapy. *Circulation* 1994;90:1–54.
95. Morillo CA, Leitch JW, Yee R, et al. A placebo-controlled trial of intravenous and oral disopyramide for prevention of neurally mediated syncope induced by head-up tilt. *J Am Coll Cardiol* 1993;22:1843–1848.
96. Kelly PA, Mann DE, Adler SW, et al. Low dose disopyramide often fails to prevent neurogenic syncope during head-up tilt testing. *Pacing Clin Electrophysiol* 1994;17:573–576.
97. Strieper MJ, Campbell RM. Efficacy of alpha-adrenergic agonist therapy for prevention of pediatric neurocardiogenic syncope. *J Am Coll Cardiol* 1993;22:594–597.
98. Nelson SD, Stanley M, Love CJ, et al. The autonomic and hemodynamic effects of oral theophylline in patients with vasodepressor syncope. *Arch Intern Med* 1991;151:2425–2429.
99. Grubb BP, Samoil D, Kosinski D, et al. Use of sertraline hydrochloride in the treatment of refractory neurocardiogenic syncope in children and adolescents. *J Am Coll Cardiol* 1994;24:490–494.
100. Sra JS, Jazayeri MR, Avitall B, et al. Comparison of cardiac pacing with drug therapy in the treatment of neurocardiogenic (vasovagal) syncope with bradycardia or asystole. *N Engl J Med* 1993;328:1085–1090.
101. Oslizlok P, Allen M, Griffin M, et al. Clinical features and management of young patients with cardioinhibitory response during orthostatic testing. *Am J Cardiol* 1992;69:1363–1365.

102. Perry JC, Friedman RA, Moak JP, et al. Bradycardia and syncope in children not controlled by pacing: beta-adrenergic hypersensitivity. *Pacing Clin Electrophysiol* 1991;14:391–394.
103. Fitzpatrick A, Theodorakis G, Ahmed R, et al. Dual chamber pacing aborts vasovagal syncope induced by head-up 60 degrees tilt. *Pacing Clin Electrophysiol* 1991;14:13–19.
104. Deal BJ, Strieper M, Scagliotti D, et al. The medical therapy of cardioinhibitory syncope in pediatric patients. *Pacing Clin Electrophysiol.* 1997;20:1759–1761.
105. Dhala A, Natale A, Sra J, et al. Relevance of asystole during head-up tilt testing. *Am J Cardiol* 1995;75:251–254.
106. Weber KT, Sun Y, Campbell SE, et al. Chronic mineralocorticoid excess and cardiovascular remodeling. *Steroids* 1995;60:125–132.
107. Sheldon R, Rose S, Flanagan P, et al. Risk factors for syncope recurrence after a positive tilt-table test in patients with syncope. *Circulation* 1996;93:973–981.

Long QT Syndrome

Michael P. Carboni, MD
and Arthur Garson Jr, MD, MPH

Background

In 1957, Jervell and Lange-Neilsen first described a family with congenital nerve deafness, prolongation of the QT interval, and a high incidence of syncope and sudden death transmitted in an autosomal recessive pattern.[1] A similar syndrome was then reported by Romano and associates in 1963 and by Ward in 1964, except hearing was normal and the hereditary pattern was more consistent with autosomal dominant transmission.[2-5]

Evidence continues to accumulate that a syndrome exists in which patients demonstrate cardiac electrical instability and, because of this instability, have a propensity for life-threatening arrhythmias [characteristically torsades de pointes (Figure 1) and ventricular fibrillation] and sudden death. Most, but not all, of these patients have a long QT interval (Figure 2); few have abnormal hearing and about half have hereditary transmission (autosomal dominant most commonly).[4,6] In fact, not all people with a prolonged QT interval have the syndrome and, therefore, are not at risk for sudden death; conversely, rare patients with a normal QT interval may have the syndrome. Therefore, the QT interval is only a marker. The most graphic demonstration of this is that, when patients with a prolonged QT interval take propranolol, the QT interval may not shorten, but they may be protected from sudden death.

Approximately 21% of symptomatic adult patients with the long QT syndrome (LQTS) who go untreated die within a year of their first syncopal

From Deal B, Wolff G, Gelband H, (eds.). *Current Concepts in Diagnosis and Management of Arrhythmias in Infants and Children.* Armonk, NY: Futura Publishing Co., Inc.; © 1998.

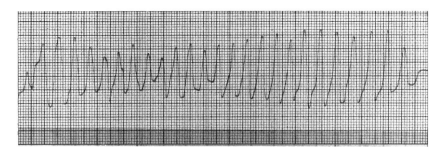

Figure 1. Example of torsades de pointes seen in a child with LQTS.

episode or cardiac event. Mortality in untreated patients approaches 60% within 10 years.[7] With proper therapy, 10-year mortality can be reduced to 3% to 4%.[7] For these reasons, it is of the utmost importance to attempt to diagnose which individuals have the syndrome and, therefore, are likely to have sudden death.

In children, diagnosis of LQTS can be difficult. These patients are frequently misdiagnosed as having benign syncope or seizures.[8–10] Prolongation of the QT interval may be subtle and the computer interpretation on a 12-lead electrocardiogram (ECG) may be inaccurate. Therefore, we recommend routine measurement of the QT interval by hand, especially when considering the diagnosis of LQTS.

In this chapter we will review the ECG findings in LQTS, the results of recent genetic studies in identifying markers for LQTS, followed by a discussion of the clinical evaluation and treatment of these patients.

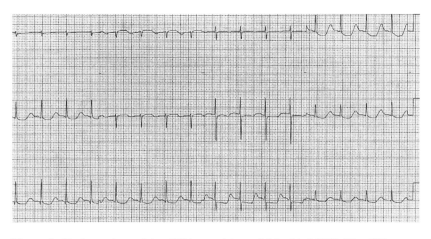

Figure 2. Prolongation of the QT interval in a child with LQTS. The QTc measured 0.63 seconds.

Electrocardiographic Findings

QT Interval

Measurement of the QT interval in children can be problematic. The QT interval is not the same in all leads. By consensus, lead II is used. In children, it is generally not normal to have a significant U wave in lead II; therefore, significant U waves in lead II should be included in the measurement. Sometimes, lead II has a nearly isoelectric T wave and other leads should be examined; lead V_5 is probably next best. The QT interval must be corrected for heart rate. Traditionally, we use Bazett's formula proposed in 1918: corrected QT (QTc) = measured QT interval divided by the square root of the RR interval.[11] The original work was done in awake adults using only lead II. The normal QTc was <0.44 seconds. Since that time, numerous problems with this method of correction were found. First, the normal QTc depends on the state of sympathetic or parasympathetic tone. For example, QTc increases with sleep and may be prolonged shortly after waking.[12,13] These variations may be seen during Holter recordings and are one reason not to diagnose LQTS by Holter monitor alone. Also, measurement of the same complexes on Holter recordings versus standard surface ECG may differ by 0.04 seconds (eg, 0.42 to 0.46 seconds) in either direction.[14]

Additionally, infants and children have considerable sinus arrhythmia. Over several beats, the QT interval generally stays the same while the RR interval may change drastically, thus changing the QTc. We recently conducted a study measuring the QT interval and its correction in 143 subjects; 63 of these had known symptomatic LQTS and 80 were normal controls.[15] The standard QT correction following the shortest RR interval was <0.47 seconds in 96.2% of controls but in only 1.6% of LQTS patients. Alternatively, the QTc following the shortest RR interval was >0.46 seconds in 3.8% of controls but in 98.4% of those with the LQTS. Also, variation of the QT interval during sinus arrhythmia assessed in lead II was found to be >0.03 seconds in none of the control patients but in 33% of LQTS patients. Therefore, in the presence of sinus arrhythmia, LQTS should be considered in a patient whose QT interval varies by >0.03 seconds or whose longest QTc following the shortest RR interval is >0.46 seconds.

Even in the absence of sinus arrhythmia, in many infants the QTc may be slightly longer than 0.44 seconds. In the study by Leistner et al, the upper limit of the normal QTc interval at 1 month of age is 0.453 seconds; at 2 months, 0.468 seconds; at 3 months, 0.470 seconds; and at 4 months, 0.468 seconds.[16] These are somewhat longer than those reported by Schwartz, where the QTc did not exceed 0.44 seconds throughout infancy.[4] Since the data are conflicting, it is wise to be suspicious of a QTc >0.44

seconds in any infant or child, but this finding should not be used in isolation.

T-Wave Morphology and QT Dispersion

Special attention should be paid to the morphology of the T waves. Large, notched T waves ("humps") (Figure 3) or T-wave alternans (successive T waves alternating in polarity from upright to inverted every other beat) are suspicious for LQTS, even in the absence of a prolonged QTc.[17-23] These T-wave abnormalities are markers for regional heterogeneity of repolarization and may indicate individuals at risk for cardiac events. In patients with LQTS, T-wave morphology may be phenotypically different, depending on the genetic mutation.[23] For example, patients with mutations of the *HERG* gene on chromosome 7 (LQT2) have low-amplitude, delayed T waves. In comparison, individuals with a mutation in the *SCN5A* sodium channel gene on chromosome 3 (LQT3) appear to have T waves of normal duration and amplitude, but are significantly late in onset. Genetic mutations on chromosome 11 (LQT1) lead to broad-based, prolonged T waves. Overlap exists in the phenotypic expression of T waves among the groups, making it difficult to accurately predict the genotypic pattern of individuals with LQTS.

In addition to T-wave morphology, QT dispersion was described as a potential indicator of patients with LQTS and individuals at risk.[19] A greater dispersion of the QT interval suggests heterogenous repolarization of the myocardium, allowing a properly timed premature ventricular beat to trigger reentrant ventricular tachycardia (VT; ie, torsades de pointes). Some authors have proposed that the efficacy of β-blocker therapy may also be followed by QT dispersion, which may normalize with adequate treat-

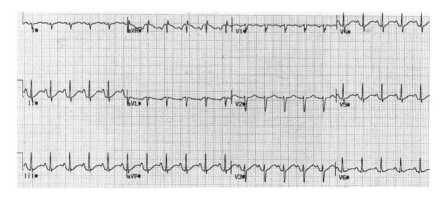

Figure 3. Notched T waves ("humps") seen in a 3-year-old patient with LQTS. Note subtle notching near peak of the T waves in almost all leads.

ment.[19] Catecholamines were shown to enhance T-wave abnormalities and increase QT dispersion in patients with LQTS.[24-28] Notched T waves, T-wave alternans, and QT dispersion are all indicative of patients with high probability of having LQTS. Each define high-risk patients in association with a significantly prolonged QTc, but not independently.[17-19,22,23]

Genetic Analysis and Molecular Mechanisms

Genetic linkage analysis confirmed the inherited basis of patients with LQTS.[29] The genetic analysis of LQTS evolved rapidly, leading to the current understanding that LQTS is a sarcolemmal ion-channel disorder, predominantly affecting sodium and potassium channels. The difference in affected ion channel may translate into distinct clinical entities, with varying responses to medication. In 1991, Keating et al detected a DNA marker on the short arm of chromosome 11 (11p15) near the Harvey *ras*-1 locus linked to a cohort of families with LQTS.[30] Further investigation of other families led to the discovery of additional linkage to chromosomes 7 (7q35–36), 3 (3p21–24), and, most recently, chromosome 4 (4q25–27).[31,32] Despite these findings, not all families with LQTS showed linkage to any known locus, supporting the existence of additional heterogeneity.[31,33-37]

Proteins encoded by genes on these chromosomes appear to modulate ion channels involved in the cardiac action potential. Gene mutations change protein structure and channel function, altering normal cardiac repolarization and therefore increasing the risk for ventricular arrhythmias in patients with LQTS. These findings lend support for a cellular basis for this syndrome with sympathetic neural influences playing a secondary role.[38]

Further analysis of LQTS patients with linkage to chromosome 11 (LQT1) demonstrated that the gene responsible lies outside the *ras* locus.[34,39,40] This gene, KVLQT1, encodes a protein structurally similar to a voltage-gated potassium channel.[39] Mutations in this gene may promote inhibition of channel closure, prolonging repolarization and predisposing these patients to significant ventricular arrhythmias.

LQT2: *HERG*

In 1994, Jiang and coworkers demonstrated linkage of a cohort of families with LQTS to chromosome 7 (LQT2).[31] Subsequently, this locus, 7q35–36, was demonstrated to be the *H*uman *E*ther-a-go-go-*R*elated *G*ene (*HERG*).[41] This gene encodes for a potassium channel with characteristics resembling the rapid component of the delayed rectifier, I_{Kr}.[42-44] Mutations of this gene likely result in the abnormal expression of inward potassium current, resulting in repolarization and ventricular arrhythmias. Torsades de pointes in patients with *HERG* defects appear to be adrenergic related,

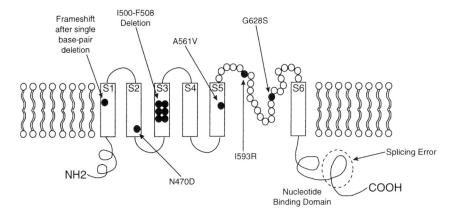

Figure 4. *HERG* ion channel domain with six transmembrane segments and a pore region. Each potassium channel is made of four domains (tetramer). Represented are the locations of mutations of *HERG* that were described so far.

occurring during periods of stress or excitation.[39,41] Antiarrhythmic medications that result in block of I_{Kr} (eg, quinidine) were associated with torsades de pointes; measures to increase the serum potassium levels in these patients may decrease the incidence of torsades.

Multiple mutations in *HERG* were reported in various families and are illustrated in Figure 4.[41,45] Those described include intragenic deletions, missense mutations, and a splice-donor mutation. Despite the description of *HERG* mutations, the exact molecular mechanism responsible for LQTS was not entirely elucidated. Also, how each individual mutation affects *HERG* function is not yet entirely known.

Dysfunction of I_{Kr} in LQT2 patients results in decreased outward potassium current, preventing termination of the plateau phase of the action potential. Mutations result in loss of *HERG* function through reduction in potassium channel numbers, alteration in channel structure and, therefore, channel function, or alteration in permeability and selectivity of the channel.[45]

LQT3: *SCN5A*

Jiang and colleagues[31] also reported linkage in an additional group of LQTS family members to chromosome 3 (LQT3). This locus, 3p21–24, was later demonstrated to be the human cardiac sodium channel gene, *SCN5A*.[46] Further investigation of LQT3 families allowed the identification of a nine nucleotide deletion in the linker between domains III and IV (Figure 5) of the sodium channel.[38] The mutant gene was designated ΔKPQ after the three amino acids deleted: lysine (K), proline (P), and

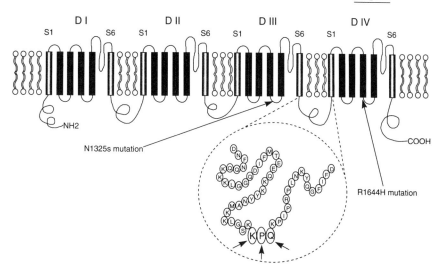

Figure 5. Representation of the human cardiac sodium channel composed of four domains (DI–DIV) with six transmembrane segments. Linker portion is between domains III and IV. The mutations of the *SCN5A* gene are demonstrated. Small arrows in the inset point to the three amino acid deletion designated ΔKPQ. In addition, two missense mutations are indicated by larger arrows.

glutamine (Q). Two additional mutations in *SCN5A*-linked families were also described (Figure 5).[47]

The linker portion of the sodium channel was shown to play an important role in normal channel inactivation. Alteration in its function results in continued inward sodium currents during the plateau phase, prolonging the action potential and allowing for significant ventricular arrhythmias. Studies demonstrated that the sustained inward sodium current is due to intermittent reopenings of multiple sodium channels during the action potential.[48,49]

Unlike many long QT patients, patients with LQT3 tend to have syncope and sudden death during sleep or rest and appear to be at higher risk during periods of slow heart rates.[50] Potentially, optimal therapy for these patients may be cardiac pacing and treatment with a sodium channel blocking medication (mexiletine).

Arrhythmogenesis

Studies using monophasic action potentials demonstrated direct evidence of early afterdepolarizations (EADs) in congenital and acquired LQTS.[24–26,51,52] Additionally, catecholamines play a significant role in enhancing EADs.[24–27] Excessive prolongation of action potential duration could result in reactivation of L-type calcium channels leading to afterde-polarizations. Early EADs or triggered activity is a likely mechanism for the initiation of torsades de pointes.

In addition, dispersion of the QT interval was implicated in the mechanism of ventricular arrhythmias.[17-19] Heterogeneity in repolarization of the myocardium predisposes individuals to torsades de pointes and could account for a reentry mechanism in the perpetuation of torsades de pointes. Catecholamines were also shown to enhance these repolarization abnormalities.[24-28]

Investigations of the molecular mechanisms for LQT2 and LQT3 prompted studies using various drugs to control the ion channels and reduce the risk of ventricular arrhythmias. Schwartz and associates[50] used the sodium channel-blocking drug mexiletine to assess the response of LQTS patients with mutations of the *SCN5A* (LQT3) and *HERG* (LQT2) genes. Mexiletine did shorten the QT interval in LQT3 patients as would be expected and did little in LQT2 patients and controls. In addition, while increases in heart rate modestly decreased the QT interval in LQT2 patients and controls, LQT3 patients experienced an accentuated reduction in the QT interval. These findings may account for the clinical findings that LQT3 patients seem to have significant cardiac events at rest or asleep, whereas LQT2 patients experience events during exercise or stress.

Sato and colleagues[53] report on the use of a potassium channel opener, nicorandil, in a patient with LQTS who experienced multiple syncopal episodes during exercise (most likely LQT2). They demonstrated a significant reduction in EADs during electrophysiological (EP) study and, with prolonged therapy, documented normalization of T-wave morphology and elimination of syncopal episodes. Shimizu and coworkers[27] demonstrated suppression of epinephrine-induced EADs and ventricular arrhythmias, as well as improvement in repolarization variables, with the combined use of verapamil and propranolol.

Analysis of patients with various mutations proposed differences in phenotypic expression of LQTS and variable risks for arrhythmias and sudden death. Gene carriers were shown to have relatively longer QTc intervals and present with symptoms more often than noncarriers.[12] A QTc of >0.47 seconds had a 100% positive predictive value in gene carriers. Only 6% of gene carriers had QTc intervals of <0.44 seconds. However, within the group of gene carriers, QTc duration could not predict who was at risk for syncope or sudden death.

Clinical Diagnosis of Long QT Syndrome

The clinical presentation of patients and their families is varied.[54-56] Children may present with syncope related to exercise, noise, or anger; seizures; or sudden death. Patients are sometimes misdiagnosed as having benign syncope or a seizure disorder.[8–10,57] The QTc may be significantly prolonged, borderline, or normal.[55,56]

Genetic Heterogeneity

Since the demonstration of genetic linkage, variations in the clinical presentation of LQTS patients was described based on the genetic mutation. For example, individuals with LQT2 (mutation in the *HERG* potassium channel) appear to have significantly greater proportion of cardiac events occurring during stress or exercise.[52] LQT3 patients experience more cardiac events during rest or sleep, when the heart rate is slower. As described earlier, the various genotypes may have differences in repolarization abnormality markers (ie, T waves and QT intervals). The findings will play an important role in determining gene-specific therapies and risks for significant cardiac events.

Criteria

Because of the broad range of presentations also seen in adults with LQTS, Schwartz[4] proposed certain major and minor criteria for the diagnosis of the syndrome (modified for diagnosis in children). Recently, these criteria were revised for all ages to better reflect newly reported information regarding ECG characteristics, clinical history, and family history of LQTS patients.[58] Individual criteria are assigned point values that reflect their relative importance in the diagnosis of LQTS (Table 1). The total point score (range 0–9) was arbitrarily divided into three probability categories for adults: one point or less, low probability of having LQTS; two to three points, intermediate probability; and four or more points, high probability. The greater number of points are assigned for a QTc of 0.48 seconds or greater. Fewer points are given for QTc intervals between 0.44 and 0.47 seconds. This is to reflect gender and age differences in the QTc interval as well as overlap of this interval in LQTS gene carriers and noncarriers.[33,59,60] Other criteria include a heart rate less than the second percentile for age and large, bizarre, notched T waves. Vincent found that, in children with LQTS, the heart rate is less than normal up to 3 years of age and then normalizes.[61]

The role of Holter monitoring in the diagnosis of LQTS was not established. As discussed earlier, QTc measurements on Holter recordings may vary significantly in either direction when compared to measurements from standard ECGs.[14] For this reason, the interpretation of QT intervals on Holter recording is problematic. We, therefore, do not recommend measurement of the QTc interval on a Holter recording to establish the diagnosis of LQTS. Abnormalities such as profound bradycardia, significant ventricular arrhythmias, and T-wave disturbances may be helpful in con-

_____ **Table 1** _____

1993 Long QT Syndrome Criteria*

	Points
ECG Findings[†]	
Q Tc[‡]	
>0.47 s	3
0.46–0.47 s	2
0.45 s (males)	1
Torsades de pointes	2
T-wave alternans	1
Notched T waves (three leads)	1
Low heart rate for age[§]	0.5
Clinical History	
Syncope	
With stress	2
Without stress	1
Congenital deafness	0.5
Family History[‖]	
Definite LQTS[¶]	1
Unexplained sudden death in immediate family members age <30 y of age	0.5

[†] In the absence of secondary causes for ECG features.

[‡] Calculated by Bazett's formula.

[§] Resting heart rate below the second percentile for age.

[‖] Can not include the same family member in A and B.

[¶] Defined as an LQTS score of four or greater.

* Adapted with permission from Reference 58.

firming the diagnosis of LQTS.[55,56,62–64] These tests are also helpful in assessing treatment effectiveness. One must take care in assessing bradycardia and pauses on Holter recordings in patients with LQTS receiving therapy with β-blockers. It may be difficult to determine what may be a response to the β-blocker and what may be a sign of the LQTS.

Exercise testing may also be helpful with the diagnosis of LQTS. It is stated that, in patients with the LQTS, the QT interval does not shorten appropriately with exercise and these patients fail to achieve a normal maximum heart rate.[5,63,65,66] In our experience, it is difficult to measure the QT interval during peak exercise, and the characteristic response in children is variously reported.[67] According to Schwartz,[7] the QTc measurement 1 minute after exercise may provide a sensitive indicator for patients with the prolonged QT interval syndrome. Yu and colleagues[68] published values for the QTc interval in exercise in normal adults. The baseline measurement was 0.420 seconds. During exercise, the QTc ranged from 0.440–0.443 seconds. One minute after exercise, the QTc returned to baseline, at 0.422 seconds. In the 2nd minute after exercise, it was 0.408 seconds and then gradually returned back to 0.420 seconds by the 10th minute after exercise. Presumably, if the QTc 1 minute after exercise is >0.440 seconds, this is suggestive of the syndrome. Coumel and coworkers[6] suggested that patients with exercise-related VT had a variant of LQTS. This is a helpful finding if positive; however, Von Bernuth and associates[69] reported on exercise testing in 23 children and young adults with idiopathic LQTS and found exercise-related VT in only one of these patients; five of them later died suddenly. Therefore, the absence of exercise-related VT in patients with the long QT interval syndrome is not helpful.[28]

Infusions of epinephrine and isoproterenol were shown to be somewhat useful in the diagnosis of individuals with LQTS.[24,28,63,65,66] Catecholamines enhance repolarization abnormalities as well as EAD, and occasionally precipitate torsades de pointes.

Invasive EP studies in children with the LQTS are poor at predicting those at risk for sudden death. In a multicenter study, 74% of 60 patients who underwent programmed stimulation had no ventricular arrhythmia.[56]

Studies specifically in children with LQTS were recently reported. We examined 287 patients with either idiopathic prolonged QT interval (QTc of >0.44 seconds) or a family history of LQTS and unexplained syncope, seizure, or cardiac arrest.[56] The age at diagnosis ranged from in utero (fetal bradycardia) to 21 years (mean of 7 years). The initial presentation was a cardiac arrest in 9%, syncope in 26%, seizures in 10%, and presyncope or palpitations in 6%. The majority of these children (85%) had symptoms related to exercise. Thirty-nine percent of patients were asymptomatic. On the ECG, 27% of all patients had a QTc of ≥0.55 seconds and 13% had a QTc of ≥0.60 seconds. Of those with a QTc >0.55 seconds, 59% were symptomatic at presentation. They were also younger and had more bradycardia and ventricular arrhythmias on routine ECG than those with a shorter QTc. Seventeen of 287 patients were found to have a normal QTc interval (≤0.44 seconds): 11 had a positive family history and 6 had cardiac arrest, syncope, or seizure. Three patients with a normal QTc interval at presentation were found to have a QTc of ≥0.46 seconds at follow-up, all of whom developed symptoms or sudden death. During the 5 years of follow-up, sudden death occurred in 8% of the patients (about two thirds were asymptomatic prior to sudden death). Eighty-two percent of all patients received treatment which included β-blockers (78%), phenytoin (5%), mexiletine (3%), left stellectomy (2%), or implantation of a pacemaker (15%) or defibrillator (1%). Of the patients experiencing sudden death, 40% were receiving propranolol, 10% another β-blocker, and 20%

received a pacemaker. Seventeen percent of those with sudden death received no treatment (one patient presented with only a positive family history for LQTS).

There are several implications of this study. First, reports of children with the LQTS differ compared to those in adults. The initial symptom in a child with LQTS may be cardiac arrest (9% in this study) as compared to predominately syncope in adults.[70] This may be due to the fact that survivors into adulthood have a less severe form of the syndrome.[71] Arguments could be made that children who meet criteria for the diagnosis of LQTS should be treated even if asymptomatic, given that their first symptom may be a cardiac arrest. In this study, 12% of asymptomatic patients later developed symptoms and 4% experienced sudden death. On the other hand, the patient with a normal QTc who is asymptomatic and has a positive family history of LQTS is at low risk of sudden death. Therefore, one could consider observing this patient until symptoms develop or the QT interval becomes prolonged. No patient in this study who presented with a normal QTc developed symptoms or experienced sudden death without prolongation of the QT interval at follow-up.

Second, children with a QTc of >0.55 seconds are at high risk for sudden death. No relation was noted between the presence of continued symptoms or ventricular arrhythmias and the occurrence of sudden death in this group, making it difficult to predict which children with extremely long QT intervals will experience sudden death. Because their risk is extremely high, implantation of a defibrillator should be considered earlier in these patients than in those with shorter QTc intervals.

Third, the criteria that define "effective" treatment may need to be reassessed. Five percent of children felt to be treated "effectively" experienced sudden death in this study. Fewer patients with sudden death had Holter recordings and treadmill tests at follow-up than the survivors. This perhaps implies that these tests may contribute important information in treatment effectiveness.

Special Situations in Long QT Syndrome

Neonates

Neonates exhibit prolongation of the QT interval, which may be transient or may be an early indicator of the LQTS. Villain and colleagues[72] described 15 neonates with idiopathic prolongation of the QTc interval on routine ECG after 4 days of life (0.46 seconds to >0.70 seconds).[72] Patients were evaluated because of cardiac arrest, apnea, seizures, or arrhythmias. Eight infants experienced first- and second-degree atrioventricular (AV) block (all with a QTc of >0.60 seconds), and six of these infants were also found to have monomorphic VT or torsades de pointes. Of the 15 neonates, 4 died in the 1st month of life. All of these infants had a markedly prolonged QTc (>0.65 seconds) with signs of repolarization abnormalities and a combination of AV block and ventricular arrhythmia. Of the surviving infants, five were asymptomatic with a QTc which normalized by 1 year of age, all with an initial QTc of <0.50 seconds. The remaining six infants had a QTc >0.50 seconds and continued with β-blocker therapy at follow-up with no significant arrhythmias. One infant also required a permanent pacemaker. It is difficult to know whether these represent transient sympathetic imbalance or electrical instability that may occur in the 1st year of life and then disappear. It is also difficult to know how to manage the patient with previous symptoms and a prolonged QT interval who completely normalizes by 1 year of age. In two of the patients with continued normal QT interval and without recurrent symptoms, β-blockade was discontinued and there was no lengthening of the QT interval and no reappearance of symptoms or arrhythmias. These findings support previous reports by Schwartz and coworkers[73] and Di Segni and associates.[74]

High-Grade Atrioventricular Block

There is an association of a prolonged QT interval with high-grade (usually complete) AV block.[75] In our study of 287 patients with LQTS, 5% presented with AV block (most often 2:1) prior to treatment.[56] Esscher[76] reviewed 273 cases with congenital complete AV block and found that 59 (22%) had a prolonged QT interval when corrected for heart rate. It could be said that this was simply an artifact of the correction due to extreme bradycardia, except that 50 of these 59 patients had syncopal episodes. It is not known whether the syncope was due to tachyarrhythmias or bradycardia. We had one patient, who was previously thought to be completely normal, present with a syncopal episode at the age of 4 years. His ECG revealed complete AV block with a ventricular escape rate of 45 beats per minute and a QTc of 0.53 seconds. He arrived in the emergency room unconscious, but by history he had a heart rate over 200 beats per minute. Therefore, it is possible that the syncope was due to VT rather than paroxysmal AV block. Solti and colleagues[77] described a similar experience with congenital heart block in association with QT interval prolongation. Syncopal episodes were more frequent in this group than in the controls of congenital heart block alone. These attacks were more often associated with VT than AV block. In all children with congenital complete AV block, the QT interval should be measured carefully. Batisse and coworkers[78] reported on five infants in the 1st year of life with congenital complete AV block and a prolonged QT interval. One of these infants died suddenly, and, in another, the QT interval shortened by 1 year of age and AV conduction returned to normal. Nicolic and associates[79] reported on an infant with the same combination of problems in whom a long period of asystole was recorded; the patient underwent a permanent pacemaker implantation without complications. In Villain's series of patients,[73] four of the eight infants with AV block died and one required a permanent pacemaker. Therefore, it seems that in infants and children with the combination of prolonged QT interval and complete AV block, the prognosis may be poor either from extreme bradycardia or VT. These children should probably be treated relatively aggressively with the combination of a permanent pacemaker and β-blockade.

The cause of this combination remains speculative. If the primary problem were the prolonged QT interval with long action potential durations, the His bundle or both bundle branches could have extremely long action potentials leading to functional block. This is supported in the report by Takamizawa and colleagues,[80] in which an infant with a prolonged QT interval and 2:1 AV block was given mexiletine. The QT interval shortened and 1:1 conduction returned. Van Hare and coworkers[81] report a study of two patients with prolonged QT interval and second-degree AV block in which they conclude that the block "is functional in nature and results from interrelationships between ventricular rate, action potential duration, and His-Purkinje system refractoriness." Others[82–85] have also documented sinus node dysfunction in similar groups of patients.

Treatment of Long QT Syndrome

Children with the long QT interval syndrome can present with a cardiac arrest or sudden death without preceding symptoms. In general, resuscitation from cardiac arrest in children is much less successful than in adults. One possible reason for this is that the adult ventricle is more likely to fibrillate than the ventricle in a child and, therefore, it would seem reasonable that the degree of insult needed to fibrillate the ventricle of a child could be greater than in an adult. Another reason that children with LQTS might be different from adults is selection bias: the adult has survived childhood. Therefore, while it is stated that sudden death practically never occurs in adults without preceding symptoms, we saw that this is not true in children, in whom the first symptom may be sudden death. We recommend that in children meeting the criteria for LQTS, treatment should be instituted whether the child is symptomatic or not.

A careful and extensive clinical history of the patient and the patient's family is essential. A prior history of syncope, near-fainting spells, or seizures should be investigated in detail. Syncope with exertion, particularly swimming, raises a red flag for LQTS. In patients with recurrent syncope, an attempt should be made to determine whether episodes are tachycardia (stress, exertion) or bradycardia (during sleep, on awakening) related or associated with loud noises. Associated medication use or unusual diets should be examined. A family history of sudden death at an early age, recurrent syncope, hearing loss, or a diagnosis of "epilepsy" needs to be examined.

We would begin treatment with a β-blocking agent. Weintraub[55] and Garson[56] found propranolol and other β-blockers (atenolol, nadolol, metoprolol) equally effective in treating LQTS children with no differences in sudden death or requirement for additional agents. This is in contrast to a study by Trippel and Gillette,[86] which showed that atenolol was effective in only four of ten patients with LQTS. Two of the remaining six patients experienced sudden death and the other four required additional medication or surgical sympathectomy for continued symptoms. In the patient in whom compliance is a concern, use of a long-acting β-blocker should be nonetheless considered. When initiating β-blocker therapy, it is important to document an adequate response to the dose used. This is best accomplished by demonstration of a blunted heart rate response to exercise by treadmill testing and Holter monitoring. Baseline testing should be performed prior to the initiation of drug therapy since there may be bradycardia before treatment. Some authors[19] proposed that the efficacy of β-blocker therapy may also be followed by QT dispersion, which may normalize with adequate treatment, although this was disputed by Linker and coworkers.[18]

In the presence of continued symptoms despite adequate β-blockade, the next step may be somewhat controversial. Further medical options include the addition of other antiarrhythmics such as phenytoin or mexiletine and, potentially, calcium channel or α-blockers.[27,48,87,88]

Left stellate ganglionectomy was proposed by Locati and associates[89] to "eliminate the hyperactive left stellate output." There was variation in the success of this operation.[90–93] Most patients continue to take β-blockers even after surgery. Schwartz and colleagues[94] reported on 85 patients worldwide with LQTS who have received left stellate ganglionectomy for persistent syncope despite prior therapy. They describe a significant reduction in the number of patients experiencing life-threatening arrhythmias, symptoms, and cardiac events. In children, the operation was not performed sufficiently frequently to make a conclusion as to its success.

The use of a permanent pacemaker may be necessitated by profound bradycardia produced with β-blockade. A pacemaker may also be useful in preventing the pause after a bigeminal cycle. It is thought that the compensatory pause following the premature beat is part of the pathophysiology of the rapid tachyarrhythmia that follows. Therefore, if a pacemaker is implanted and the long pause is prevented following a premature beat, this may eliminate or reduce episodes of torsades de pointes.[95,96] This was supported by reports that pacemaker therapy prevented torsades de pointes or bradycardia and reduced symptoms but did not provide complete protection.[97,98]

Finally, the use of implantable cardioverter-defibrillators in children was recently reported.[99-103] This device has the same appearance as an implantable pacemaker, although current models of the defibrillator are larger. Epicardial implantation of the electrodes is likely necessary in most children, although endocardial placement was described.[104] The device senses ventricular fibrillation and, after confirming the diagnosis by a number of algorithms, delivers shocks of up to 30 J. Some newer devices combine pacemaker function with cardioverter-defibrillator capabilities. This may be the desired therapy for patients with LQTS who persist with syncope on β-blocker therapy or who experience cardiac arrest.[105] Questions arise regarding its use in the patient with LQTS and one time aborted cardiac arrest. Continued investigation in this population of children is needed.

Selection of one or more of these therapeutic options is patient and institution dependent. Children with LQTS should avoid competitive athletics.[106] In addition, medications that prolong the QT interval or are associated with torsades de pointes continue to be described.[107-109] In fact, *HERG* was reported as a target for the antihistamine, terfenadine.[44,110] These medications should be avoided in any individual felt to have LQTS regardless of the QT interval.

Currently, genetic screening should be undertaken in families with LQTS when more than one generation is affected to identify the affected gene and members at risk and potentially to influence treatment strategies. Individuals with normal QT intervals and no syncope may transmit a defective gene, resulting in symptomatic LQTS in their offspring.[111] At this time, genetic testing is not available for "sporadic" cases; this will likely change in the near future.

Summary

Risk of significant cardiac events in patients with LQTS is continuously being assessed. The strongest independent predictor for experiencing cardiac events appears to be the QTc interval.[55-57,70] Those with a QTc >0.50 seconds have a significantly greater risk for cardiac events than those with normal or borderline QTc intervals. Also, significant sinus tachycardia or bradycardia are indicators for patients at risk. Therefore, optimization of heart rate with β-blocker or pacemaker therapy would be beneficial. In addition to clinical presentation, other variables that should raise attention are abnormal T waves, female gender, and family history. Zareba and co-workers[112] studied the risk of cardiac events in family members of patients with LQTS. Similar variables indicated family members at risk, especially first-degree female relatives, or those with QTc >0.50 seconds. Sinus tachycardia was less indicative of significant risk, but important in combination with other variables. Clearly, further analysis of patients and their families is needed to define those at risk and determine therapeutic strategies most effective.

Acquired Long QT Interval Syndromes

There are four general categories of conditions that can cause an acquired LQTS.

1. Electrolytes: hypocalcemia, hypomagnesemia, liquid protein diets, and malnutrition resulting from anorexia nervosa.[113] Hypocalcemia appears to be the most common cause of acquired long QT interval syndrome.
2. Drugs (Table 2): phenothiazines, tricyclic antidepressants, vasodilators (lidoflazine), organophosphates, macrolide antibiotics (eg, erythromycin), sulfamethoxazole, antifungals (eg, ketoconazole, fluconazole), terfenadine (antihistamine),[44,107,108,110] cisapride,[109] inhalation anesthetics,[114] procainamide, and disopyramide, with

_____ **Table 2** _____

Drugs Associated with Prolonged Q-T Interval and Torsades de Pointes

Antiarrhythmic Agents
    Class Ia: Quinidine, disopyramide, procainamide
    Class Ib: Lidocaine, mexiletine
    Class Ic: Flecainide, propafenone
    Class III: Amiodarone, sotalol

Antibiotics
    Macrolides (erythromycin, clarithromycin, azithromycin)
    Trimethoprim/sulfamethoxazole
    Pentamidine (intravenous)

Antidepressants
    Tricyclics (amitriptyline, nortriptyline, imipramine, desipramine, doxepin)

Antifungals
    Ketoconazole, fluconazole, itraconazole

Antihistamines
    Terfenedine, astemizole

Antipsychotics

Gastrointestinal Agents
    Cisapride

Diuretics
    Indapamide
    Secondary hypokalemia

quinidine being the most common to cause drug-induced long QT interval syndrome. It is difficult to predict which patient will develop the "idiosyncratic" reaction of torsades de pointes due to quinidine treatment. This reaction generally occurs early in the course of treatment as the serum concentration is increasing, generally with subtherapeutic plasma concentrations, and may be exacerbated by hypokalemia.[115] In a patient taking any such drug (especially quinidine), if the QTc prolongs by greater than 33% or if the absolute QT interval is greater than 600 milliseconds, patients are more likely to have torsades de pointes.[113,116,117] While amiodarone prolongs the QT interval in almost all patients, it is rare for this drug to produce torsades de pointes, although it does occur.[118]

Erythromycin was shown to prolong ventricular repolarization to a large extent by block of I_{Kr}.[119,120] As with other medications which block potassium channel function, patients receiving erythromycin are at risk for QT prolongation and ventricular arrhythmias, especially when receiving erythromycin in combination with other potassium channel-blocking medications.[121] Terfenadine was shown to also block I_{Kr} channels, resulting in QT prolongation and increased risk for torsades de pointes.[44,110,122] The parent compound appears to have the greatest effect on potassium channels; therefore, use of terfenadine with medications that decrease its hepatic metabolism increase its potential arrhythmic effects.[122,123] Ketoconazole is an antifungal medication that inhibits hepatic clearance of drugs and frequently is used in combination with erythromycin and terfenadine.[124] Combined use of terfenadine with erythromycin or ketoconazole or use of erythromycin with ketoconazole is associated with increased risk of QTc prolongation and ventricular arrhythmias.[125] Caution should be exhibited when using these drugs in combination. Any individual with even suspected congenital LQTS should not receive any medications listed in Table 2.

3. Central nervous system (CNS) trauma and injury (especially subarachnoid hemorrhage) lengthen the QT interval. These were associated with cardiac subendocardial lesions that could prolong the QT interval; alternatively, this may be a reflection of sympathetic imbalance based on the CNS.

4. Primary myocardial problems such as myocarditis, ischemia, hypertrophic and dilated cardiomyopathies,[126] and mitral valve prolapse may also cause the QT interval to prolong.

Conclusion

Increased awareness of the LQTS and its myriad presentations improved the diagnostic capability and treatment options for these patients, resulting in improved survival. Recent rapid advances in genetic markers and our understanding of the cellular mechanisms will likely translate into gene/mechanism-specific therapy, and improve the ability to screen family members at potential risk.

References

1. Jervell A, Lange-Nielsen F. Congenital deaf-mutism, functional heart disease with prolongation of the QT and sudden death. *Am Heart J* 1957;54:59–68.
2. Romano C, Gemme G, Pongiglione R. Aritmie cardiache rare delle¢eta pediatrica. *Clin Pediatr* 1963;45:565.
3. Ward O. A new familial cardiac syndrome in children. *J Ir Med Assoc* 1964;54:103.
4. Schwartz PJ. The sudden infant death syndrome. In: *Reviews in Perinatal Medicine*, Vol 4. New York: Raven Press; 1981.
5. Schwartz PJ, Periti M, Malliani A. The long QT syndrome. *Am Heart J* 1975;89:378–390.
6. Coumel P, Leclercq J, Lucet V. Possible mechanisms of the arrhythmias in the long QT syndrome. *Eur Heart J* 1985;6(suppl D):115–129.
7. Schwartz PJ. Idiopathic long QT syndrome: progress and questions. *Am Heart J* 1985;109:399–411.
8. Horn CA, Beekman RH, Dick M II, et al. The congenital long QT syndrome. An unusual cause of childhood seizures. *Am J Dis Child* 1986;140:659–661.
9. Pacia SV, Devinsky O, Luciano DJ, et al. The prolonged QT syndrome presenting as epilepsy: a report of two cases and literature review. *Neurology* 1994;44:1408–1410.
10. Singh B, al Shahwan SA, Habbab MA, et al. Idiopathic long QT syndrome: asking the right question. *Lancet* 1993;341:741–742.
11. Bazett HC. An analysis of the time relations of electrocardiograms. *Heart* 1918;7:353–370.
12. Browne KF, Prystowsky EN, Zipes DP. Diurnal variation of QT interval in man. *Circulation* 1982;66:II-128.
13. Molnar J, Zhang F, Weiss J, et al. Diurnal pattern of QTc interval: how long is prolonged? Possible relation to circadian triggers of cardiovascular events. *J Am Coll Cardiol* 1996;27:76–83.
14. Christiansen JL, Guccione P, Garson A Jr. Difference in QT interval measurement on ambulatory ECG compared with standard ECG. *Pacing Clin Electrophysiol* 1996;19:1296–1303.
15. Garson A Jr. How to measure the QT interval—what is normal? *Am J Cardiol* 1993;72:14B–16B.
16. Leistner HL, Haddad GG, Lai TL, et al. Heart rate pattern during sleep in an infant with congenital prolongation of the QT interval (Romano-Ward syndrome). *Chest* 1983;84:191–194.
17. Benhorin J, Merri M, Alberti M, et al. Long QT syndrome. New electrocardiographic characteristics. *Circulation* 1990;82:521–527.
18. Linker NJ, Colonna P, Kekwick CA, et al. Assessment of QT dispersion in symptomatic patients with congenital long QT syndromes. *Am J Cardiol* 1992;69:634–638.
19. Priori SG, Napolitano C, Diehl L, et al. Dispersion of the QT interval. A marker of therapeutic efficacy in the idiopathic long QT syndrome. *Circulation* 1994;89:1681–1689.

20. Malfatto G, Beria G, Sala S, et al. Quantitative analysis of T wave abnormalities and their prognostic implications in the idiopathic long QT syndrome. *J Am Coll Cardiol* 1994;23:296–301.

21. Moss AJ, Zareba W, Benhorin J, et al. ECG T-wave patterns in genetically distinct forms of the hereditary long QT syndrome. *Circulation* 1995;92:2929–2934.

22. Zareba W, Moss AJ, le Cessie S, et al. T wave alternans in idiopathic long QT syndrome. *J Am Coll Cardiol* 1994;23:1541–1546.

23. Lehmann MH, Suzuki F, Fromm BS, et al. T wave "humps" as a potential electrocardiographic marker of the long QT syndrome. *J Am Coll Cardiol* 1994;24:746–754.

24. Shimizu W, Ohe T, Kurita T, et al. Early afterdepolarizations induced by isoproterenol in patients with congenital long QT syndrome. *Circulation* 1991;84:1915–1923.

25. Shimizu W, Ohe T, Kurita T, et al. Epinephrine-induced ventricular premature complexes due to early afterdepolarizations and effects of verapamil and propranolol in a patient with congenital long QT syndrome. *J Cardiovasc Electrophysiol* 1994;5:438–444.

26. Zhou JT, Zheng LR, Liu WY, et al. Early afterdepolarizations in the familial long QTU syndrome. *J Cardiovasc Electrophysiol* 1992;3:431–436.

27. Shimizu W, Ohe T, Kurita T, et al. Effects of verapamil and propranolol on early afterdepolarizations and ventricular arrhythmias induced by epinephrine in congenital long QT syndrome. *J Am Coll Cardiol* 1995;26:1299–1309.

28. Schechter E, Anderson J, Prabhu S, et al. Epinephrine infusion in the congenital long-QT syndrome. *J Am Coll Cardiol* 1986;7:155A.

29. Keating MT. Genetic approaches to cardiovascular disease. Supravalvular aortic stenosis, Williams syndrome, and long-QT syndrome. *Circulation* 1995;92:142–147.

30. Keating M, Atkinson D, Dunn C, et al. Linkage of a cardiac arrhythmia, the long QT syndrome, and the Harvey ras-1 gene. *Science* 1991;252:704–706.

31. Jiang C, Atkinson D, Towbin JA, et al. Two long QT syndrome loci map to chromosomes 3 and 7 with evidence for further heterogeneity. *Nat Genet* 1994;8:141–147.

32. Schott JJ, Charpentier F, Peltier S, et al. Mapping of a gene for long QT syndrome to chromosome 4q25–27. *Am J Hum Genet* 1995;57:1114–1122.

33. Vincent GM, Timothy KW, Leppert M, et al. The spectrum of symptoms and QT intervals in carriers of the gene for the long-QT syndrome. *N Engl J Med* 1992;327:846–852.

34. Curran M, Atkinson D, Timothy K, et al. Locus heterogeneity of autosomal dominant long QT syndrome. *J Clin Invest* 1993;92:799–803.

35. Benhorin J, Kalman YM, Medina A, et al. Evidence of genetic heterogeneity in the long QT syndrome. *Science* 1993;260:1960–1962.

36. Towbin JA, Li H, Taggart RT, et al. Evidence of genetic heterogeneity in Romano-Ward long QT syndrome. Analysis of 23 families. *Circulation* 1994;90:2635–2644.

37. Vincent GM. Heterogeneity in the inherited long QT syndrome. *J Cardiovasc Electrophysiol* 1995;6:137–146.

38. Wang Q, Shen J, Splawski I, et al. SCN5A mutations associated with an inherited cardiac arrhythmia, long QT syndrome. *Cell* 1995;80:805–811.

39. Wang Q, Curran ME, Splawski I, et al. Positional cloning of a novel potassium channel gene: KVLQT1 mutations cause cardiac arrhythmias. *Nat Genet* 1996;12:17–23.

40. Kainulainen K, Swan H, Miettinen H, et al. Linkage of the long QT syndrome to the short arm of chromosome 11: use of five highly polymorphic markers towards more detailed localization of the mutant gene. *Hum Genet* 1995;96:395–400.
41. Curran ME, Splawski I, Timothy KW, et al. A molecular basis for cardiac arrhythmia: HERG mutations cause long QT syndrome. *Cell* 1995;80:795–803.
42. Sanguinetti MC, Jiang C, Curran ME, et al. A mechanistic link between an inherited and an acquired cardiac arrhythmia: HERG encodes the IKr potassium channel. *Cell* 1995;81:299–307.
43. Trudeau MC, Warmke JW, Ganetzky B, et al. HERG, a human inward rectifier in the voltage-gated potassium channel family. *Science* 1995;269:92–95.
44. Roy M, Dumaine R, Brown AM. HERG, a primary human ventricular target of the nonsedating antihistamine terfenadine. *Circulation* 1996;94:817–823.
45. Benson DW, MacRae CA, Vesely MR, et al. Missense mutation in the pore region of HERG causes familial long QT syndrome. *Circulation* 1996;93:1791–1795.
46. George AL Jr, Varkony TA, Drabkin HA, et al. Assignment of the human heart tetrodotoxin-resistant voltage-gated Na$^+$ channel alpha-subunit gene (SCN5A) to band 3p21. *Cytogenet Cell Genet* 1995;68:67–70.
47. Wang Q, Shen J, Li Z, et al. Cardiac sodium channel mutations in patients with long QT syndrome, an inherited cardiac arrhythmia. *Hum Mol Genet* 1995;4:1603–1607.
48. Bennett PB, Yazawa K, Makita N, et al. Molecular mechanism for an inherited cardiac arrhythmia. *Nature* 1995;376:683–685.
49. Dumaine R, Wang Q, Keating MT, et al. Multiple mechanisms of Na+ channel-linked long QT syndrome. *Circ Res* 1996;78:916–924.
50. Schwartz PJ, Priori SG, Locati EH, et al. Long QT syndrome patients with mutations of the SCN5A and HERG genes have differential responses to Na+ channel blockade and to increases in heart rate. Implications for gene-specific therapy. *Circulation* 1995;92:3381–3386.
51. Bonatti V, Rolli A, Botti G. Recording of monophasic action potentials of the right ventricle in long QT syndromes complicated by severe ventricular arrhythmias. *Eur Heart J* 1983;4:168–179.
52. Jackman WM, Szabo B, Friday KJ, et al. Ventricular tachyarrhythmias related to early afterdepolarizations and triggered firing: relationship of QT interval prolongation and potential therapeutic role for calcium channel blocking agents. *J Cardiovasc Electrophysiol* 1990;1:170–195.
53. Sato T, Hata Y, Yamamoto M, et al. Early afterdepolarizations abolished by potassium channel opener in a patient with idiopathic long QT syndrome. *J Cardiovasc Electrophysiol* 1995;6:279–282.
54. Moss AJ, Schwartz PJ, Crampton RS, et al. The long QT Syndrome. Prospective longitudinal study of 328 patients. *Circulation* 1991;84:1136–1144.
55. Weintraub RG, Gow RM, Wilkinson JL. The congenital long QT syndromes in childhood. *J Am Coll Cardiol* 1990;16:674–680.
56. Garson A Jr, Dick M II, Fournier A, et al. The long QT syndrome in children. An international study of 287 patients. *Circulation* 1993;87:1866–1872.
57. Pfammatter JP, Donati F, Durig P, et al. Cardiac arrhythmias mimicking primary neurological disorders: a difficult diagnostic situation. *Acta Paediatr* 1995;84:569–572.
58. Schwartz PJ, Moss AJ, Vincent GM, et al. Diagnostic criteria for the long QT syndrome. An update. *Circulation* 1993;88:782–784.
59. Moss AJ. Measurement of the QT interval and the risk associated with QTc interval prolongation: a review. *Am J Cardiol* 1993;72:23B–25B.

60. Rautaharju PM, Zhou SH, Wong S, et al. Sex differences in the evolution of the electrocardiographic QT interval with age. *Can J Cardiol* 1992;8:690–695.
61. Vincent GM. The heart rate of Romano-Ward syndrome patients. *Am Heart J* 1986;112:61–64.
62. Eggeling T, Osterhues HH, Hoeher M, et al. Value of Holter monitoring in patients with the long QT syndrome. *Cardiology* 1992;81:107–114.
63. Eggeling T, Hoeher M, Osterhues HH, et al. Significance of noninvasive diagnostic techniques in patients with long QT syndrome. *Am J Cardiol* 1992;70:1421–1426.
64. Makarov LM, Belokon NA, Laan MI, et al. Holter monitoring in the long QT syndrome of children and adolescents. *Cor Vasa* 1990;32:474–483.
65. Vincent GM, Jaiswal D, Timothy KW. Effects of exercise on heart rate, QT, QTc and QT/QS2 in the Romano-Ward inherited long QT syndrome. *Am J Cardiol* 1991;68:498–503.
66. Shimizu W, Ohe T, Kurita T, et al. Differential response of QTU interval to exercise, isoproterenol, and atrial pacing in patients with congenital long QT syndrome. *Pacing Clin Electrophysiol* 1991;14:1966–1970.
67. Vetter VL, Berul C, Sweeten TL. Response of corrected QT interval to exercise, pacing, and isoproterenol. *Cardiol Young* 1993;3(suppl 1):63.
68. Yu PN, Bruce RA, Lovejoy FW Jr, et al. Observations on the change of ventricular systole (QT interval) during exercise. *J Clin Invest* 1950;29:279–289.
69. Von Bernuth G, Bernsau U, Gutheil H, et al. Tachyarrhythmic syncopes in children with structurally normal hearts with and without QT prolongation in the electrocardiogram. *Eur J Pediatr* 1982;138:206–210.
70. Moss AJ, Schwartz PJ, Crampton RS, et al. The long QT syndrome: a prospective international study. *Circulation* 1985;71:17–21.
71. Schwartz PJ, Locati E, Priori SG, et al. The long QT syndrome. In: Zipes DP, Jalife J, eds. *Cardiac Electrophysiology: From Cell to Bedside*. Philadelphia: WB Saunders Co; 1990;589–605.
72. Villain E, Levy M, Kachaner J, et al. Prolonged QT interval in neonates: benign, transient, or prolonged risk of sudden death. *Am Heart J* 1992;124:194–197.
73. Schwartz PJ, Montemerlo M, Facchini M, et al. The QT interval throughout the first 6 months of life: a prospective study. *Circulation* 1982;66:496–501.
74. Di Segni E, David D, Katzenstein M, et al. Permanent overdrive pacing for the suppression of recurrent ventricular tachycardia in a newborn with long QT syndrome. *J Electrocardiol* 1980;13:189–192.
75. Trippel DL, Parsons MK, Gillette PC. Infants with long-QT syndrome and 2:1 atrioventricular block. *Am Heart J* 1995;130:1130–1134.
76. Esscher EB. Congenital complete heart block in adolescence and adult life. A follow-up study. *Eur Heart J* 1981;2:281–288.
77. Solti F, Szatmary L, Vecsey T, et al. Congenital complete heart block associated with QT prolongation. *Eur Heart J* 1992;13:1080–1083.
78. Batisse A, Belloy C, Fermont L, et al. Prolonged QT interval with functional A-V block in neonates and young infants. *Arch Pediatr* 1981;38:657–662.
79. Nikolic G, Arnold J, Coles DM. Torsade de pointes and asystole in a child with complete heart block and prolonged QT interval. *Aust Paediatr J* 1983;19:187–191.
80. Takamizawa K, Takao A, Ohta F. Mexiletine for successful treatment of the long QT syndrome. In: *Proceedings of the Second World Congress of Pediatric Cardiology*. New York: Springer-Verlag; 1985.

81. Van Hare GF, Franz MR, Roge C, et al. Persistent functional atrioventricular block in two patients with prolonged QT intervals: elucidation of the mechanism of block. *Pacing Clin Electrophysiol* 1990;13:608–618.
82. Case CL, Gillette PC. Conduction system disease in a child with long QT syndrome. *Am Heart J* 1990;120:984–986.
83. Kugler JD. Sinus nodal dysfunction in young patients with long QT syndrome. *Am Heart J* 1991;121:1132–1136.
84. Scott WA, Dick M II. Two:one atrioventricular block in infants with congenital long QT syndrome. *Am J Cardiol* 1987;60:1409–1410.
85. Matsuoka S, Akita H, Takahashi Y, et al. Assessment of sinus node function in patients with congenital long QT syndrome. *Jpn Circ J* 1991;55:487–489.
86. Trippel DL, Gillette PC. Atenolol in children with ventricular arrhythmias. *Am Heart J* 1990;119:1312–1316.
87. Friesen RM, Duncan P, Tweed WA, et al. Appraisal of pediatric cardiopulmonary resuscitation. *Can Med Assoc J* 1982;126:1055–1058.
88. Bricker JT, Garson A Jr, Gillette PC. A family history of seizures associated with sudden cardiac deaths. *Am J Dis Child* 1984;138:866–868.
89. Locati E, Schwartz PJ, Moss AJ, et al. Long-term survival after left cervicothoracic sympathectomy in high risk long QT syndrome patients with refractory ventricular arrhythmias. *J Am Coll Cardiol* 1986;7:235A.
90. Packer DL, Coltorti F, Smith MS, et al. Sudden death after left stellectomy in the long QT syndrome. *Am J Cardiol* 1984;54:1365–1366.
91. Till JA, Shinebourne EA, Pepper J, et al. Complete denervation of the heart in a child with congenital long QT and deafness. *Am J Cardiol* 1988;62:1319–1321.
92. Bockeria LA, Mikhailin SI. The results of surgery for tachyarrhythmias in children. *Pacing Clin Electrophysiol* 1990;13:1990–1995.
93. Ouriel K, Moss AJ. Long QT syndrome: an indication for cervicothoracic sympathectomy. *Cardiovasc Surg* 1995;3:475–478.
94. Schwartz PJ, Locati EH, Moss AJ, et al. Left cardiac sympathetic denervation in the therapy of congenital long QT syndrome. A worldwide report. *Circulation* 1991;84:503–511.
95. Kay G, Plumb VJ, Arciniegas JG, et al. Torsade de pointes: the long-short initiating sequence and other clinical features: observations in 32 patients. *J Am Coll Cardiol* 1983;2:806–817.
96. Viskin S, Alla SR, Barron HV, et al. Mode of onset of torsade de pointes in congenital long QT syndrome. *J Am Coll Cardiol* 1996;28:1262–1268.
97. Eldar M, Griffin JC, Abbott JA, et al. Permanent cardiac pacing in patients with the long QT syndrome. *J Am Coll Cardiol* 1987;10:600–607.
98. Moss AJ, Liu JE, Gottlieb S, et al. Efficacy of permanent pacing in the management of high-risk patients with long QT syndrome. *Circulation* 1991;84:1524–1529.
99. Kron J, Oliver RP, Norsted S, et al. The automatic implantable cardioverter-defibrillator in young patients. *J Am Coll Cardiol* 1990;16:896–902.
100. Breithardt G, Wichter T, Haverkamp W, et al. Implantable cardioverter defibrillator therapy in patients with arrhythmogenic right ventricular cardiomyopathy, long QT syndrome, or no structural heart disease. *Am Heart J* 1994;127:1151–1158.
101. Silka MJ, Kron J, Dunnigan A, et al. Sudden cardiac death and the use of implantable cardioverter-defibrillators in pediatric patients. The Pediatric Electrophysiology Society. *Circulation* 1993;87:800–807.
102. Kaminer SJ, Pickoff AS, Dunnigan A, et al. Cardiomyopathy and the use of implanted cardio-defibrillators in children. *Pacing Clin Electrophysiol* 1990;13:593–597.

103. Saxon LA, Shannon K, Wetzel GT, et al. Familial long QT syndrome: electrical storm and implantable cardioverter device therapy. *Am Heart J* 1996;131:1037–1039.
104. Kron J, Silka MJ, Ohm OJ, et al. Preliminary experience with nonthoracotomy implantable cardioverter defibrillators in young patients. The Medtronic Transvene Investigators. *Pacing Clin Electrophysiol* 1994;17:26–30.
105. Sokoloski MC, O'Conner BK, Taylor SJ, et al. Pacemaker cardioverter defibrillators in young patients. *J Am Coll Cardiol* 1995;25:53A.
106. Twenty-sixth Bethesda Conference. Recommendations for determining eligibility for competition in athletes with cardiovascular abnormalities. *J Am Coll Cardiol* 1994;24:845–899.
107. Morganroth J, Brown AM, Critz S, et al. Variability of the QTc interval: impact on defining drug effect and low-frequency cardiac event. *Am J Cardiol* 1993;72:26B–31B.
108. Koh KK, Rim MS, Yoon J, et al. Torsade de pointes induced by terfenadine in a patient with long QT syndrome. *J Electrocardiol* 1994;27:343–346.
109. Bran S, Murray WA, Hirsch IB, et al. Long QT syndrome during high-dose cisapride. *Arch Intern Med* 1995;55:765–768.
110. Crumb WJ Jr, Wible B, Arnold DJ, et al. Blockade of multiple human cardiac potassium currents by the antihistamine terfenadine: possible mechanism for terfenidine-associated cardiotoxicity. *Mol Pharmacol* 1995;47:181–190.
111. Russell MW, Dick M II, Collins FS, et al. KVLQT1 mutations in three families with familial or sporadic long QT syndrome. *Hum Mol Genet* 1996;5:1319–1324.
112. Zareba W, Moss AJ, le Cessie S, et al. Risk of cardiac events in family members of patients with long QT syndrome. *J Am Coll Cardiol* 1995;26:1685–1691.
113. Clark M, Lazzara R, Jackman W. Torsade de pointes: serum drug levels and electrocardiographic warning signs. *Circulation* 1982;66(suppl II):71.
114. Schmeling WT, Warltier DC, McDonald DJ, et al. Prolongation of the QT interval by enflurane, isoflurane, and halothane in humans. *Anesth Analg* 1991;72:137–144.
115. Webb CL, Dick M II, Rocchini AP, et al. Quinidine syncope in children. *J Am Coll Cardiol* 1987;9:1031–1037.
116. Barton CW, Dick M II, Rosenthal A. Quinidine syncope in children. *J Am Coll Cardiol* 1985;5:429–433.
117. Itoh S, Munemura S, Satoh H. A study of the inheritance pattern of Romano-Ward syndrome: prolonged QT interval, syncope, and sudden death. *Clin Pediatr* 1982;21:20–24.
118. Kugler, JD. Control of torsade de pointes by tocainide in children with congenital and acquired prolonged QT interval. In: *Proceedings of the Second World Congress of Pediatric Cardiology*. New York: Springer-Verlag; 1985.
119. Rubart M, Pressler ML, Pride HP, et al. Electrophysiological mechanisms in a canine model of erythromycin-associated long QT syndrome. *Circulation* 1993;88:1832–1844.
120. Oberg KC, Bauman JL. QT interval prolongation and torsade de pointes due to erythromycin lactobionate. *Pharmacotherapy* 1995;15:687–692.
121. Gitler B, Berger LS, Buffa SD. Torsade de pointes induced by erythromycin. *Chest* 1994;105:368–372.
122. Woosley RL, Chen Y, Freiman JP, et al. Mechanism of the cardiotoxic actions of terfenadine. *JAMA* 1993;269:1532–1536.
123. Honig PK, Woosley RL, Zamani K, et al. Changes in the pharmacokinetics and electrocardiographic pharmacodynamics of terfenadine with concomitant administration of erythromycin. *Clin Pharmacol Ther* 1992;52:231–238.

124. Monahan BP, Ferguson CL, Killeavy ES, et al. Torsades de pointes occurring in association with terfenadine. *JAMA* 1990;264:2788–2790.
125. Hanrahan JP, Choo PW, Carlson W, et al. Terfenadine-associated ventricular arrhythmias and QTc interval prolongation. A retrospective cohort comparison with other antihistamines among members of a health maintenance organization. *Ann Epidemiol* 1995;5:201–209.
126. Martin AB, Garson A Jr, Perry JC. Prolonged QT interval in hypertrophic and dilated cardiomyopathy in children. *Am Heart J* 1994;127:64–70.

Pharmacologic Therapy
of Arrhythmias

James C. Perry, MD

The use of available pediatric antiarrhythmic agents changed considerably due to the widespread use of catheter ablative techniques. The efficacy and safety of these curative procedures brought about a reexamination of the need for aggressive antiarrhythmic drug therapies.

Degree of Medical Control Versus
Ablation Success

Options for antiarrhythmic therapy are now based on the relative balance of efficacy rates, safety issues, and natural history data for arrhythmias in children compared to ablative therapy. Medical efficacy rates for arrhythmia "control" vary considerably. Patients with rare episodes of supraventricular tachycardia (SVT) may require little or no therapy whereas potentially life-threatening atrial and ventricular tachyarrhythmias (VTs) demand far more aggressive medical control. Complete medical control of many SVTs may be achieved in 50% to 60% of patients[1] over a given year, but this observation is confounded by the natural history aspects of arrhythmias. Medical control may be deemed adequate if there are rare recurrences, shorter episodes, or fewer symptoms. For resistant arrhythmias, medical therapy can become quite complex. This is especially true for the patient in whom ablative therapy is not an option, when ablation is attempted but proved unsuccessful, or when other antiarrhythmic interven-

From Deal B, Wolff G, Gelband H, (eds.). *Current Concepts in Diagnosis and Management of Arrhythmias in Infants and Children*. Armonk, NY: Futura Publishing Co., Inc.; © 1998.

tional devices (eg, defibrillators, pacemakers) are utilized in conjunction with drug therapy.

For catheter ablation, success rates depend on the mechanism of tachycardia and the underlying cardiac anatomy.[2,3]

Side Effects of Medical Therapy Versus Ablation Complications

Side effects of medical therapy can also influence both the complexity and duration of antiarrhythmic use. Combinations of two or more drugs now are rarely necessary and bring about examinations of whether ablation is an option. Side effects may be transient or permanent or consist of potentially life-threatening proarrhythmias.

Major complications of catheter ablative procedures are reported to occur in approximately 3% to 4% of cases[2] but appear less common than side effects from long-term drug therapy. A significant factor in both ablation success and complication rates is the experience of the operator performing the ablation,[2] stressing the need for a pediatric electrophysiologist to perform these procedures in pediatric-age patients. The tachycardia mechanism dictates potential complications.[4] The decision to balance these risks against medical therapy therefore is dependent upon each center's experience.

Cost Issues in Medical Versus Catheter and Surgical Ablative Therapies

Studies of therapeutic costs can provide analysis of catheter versus surgical costs,[5] but it is difficult to determine the anticipated cost for an individual patient of continued medical therapy. Garson[6] performed a cost analysis of medical therapy, using Wolff-Parkinson-White (WPW) syndrome as a model of chronic disease, with assumptions made regarding costs of drugs, outpatient visits, and hospital stays based on historical data. The study found dramatically reduced rates of mortality, morbidity, and cost for catheter therapy in each instance over medical and surgical therapies.

Regulatory Issues

The only antiarrhythmic agent formally "approved" for use in children is digoxin.[7] The pharmaceutical industry has little financial incentive to perform drug trials in young patients to establish criteria acceptable to the Food and Drug Administration (FDA) when the available market share from pediatrics is so small. Several drugs underwent extensive pediatric evaluation, but the body of this work does not appear in drug package inserts. In 1993, the FDA required pediatric guidelines for any newly released pharmaceutical agent. Although this move was greeted initially with praise, two agents, oral sotalol and intravenous (IV) amiodarone (both with published pediatric data on efficacy, dosing, and safety), were approved and released subsequently without pediatric guidelines in their package inserts. On a practical basis, an accrued volume of experience using antiarrhythmic drugs by the pediatric cardiology community brought about relatively uniform guidelines for dosing, efficacy and safety outside the realm of formal approval by the FDA.

Pharmacokinetics

It is crucial to recognize the fact that each drug has a different profile of absorption, distribution, metabolism, and excretion. These factors play a role in the dose and dosing schedule for each drug, including those of any active metabolites.

Absorption

Drug absorption and distribution are influenced by whether the drug is administered by an oral or IV route. Oral administration and absorption of a drug will depend on the vehicle. A drug given in a solution or suspension is readily available for absorption whereas pill or capsule forms release the active drug slowly. "Long-acting" preparations consist of a cellulose matrix, allowing very slow digestion and absorption over an extended period. Different preparations of the same drug can result in differences in time to peak serum concentration and duration of effect.

Most antiarrhythmic agents have "first-order" oral absorption: the amount absorbed is directly related to the amount in the intestinal tract. For most agents, 75% to 90% may be available for drug action once absorbed. A "first-pass" effect, where absorbed drug is metabolized in the liver or intestinal wall and is unavailable for target site drug action, occurs for some drugs. IV administration of antiarrhythmic drugs results in rapid availability. The phenomenon that a fraction of administered drug is absorbed and active is termed bioavailability.

Some clinical settings may influence the bioavailability of orally administered drugs. Congestive heart failure results in bowel wall edema and decreases absorption. A chronic state of reduced absorption can occur in patients with high central venous pressures and liver enlargement, eg. the patient with single ventricle physiology. Evening administration of drugs can further decrease absorption as the patient sleeps in the supine position. Hepatic congestion can also influence the first pass effect.

Distribution

The two-compartment model works well for most antiarrhythmic drugs. The central compartment consists of the blood volume and tissue of organs with rapid perfusion (essentially part of the "blood volume"). High-perfusion organs include the kidneys, liver, spleen, lungs, and heart. The peripheral compartment consists of low-perfusion tissue: fat, muscle,

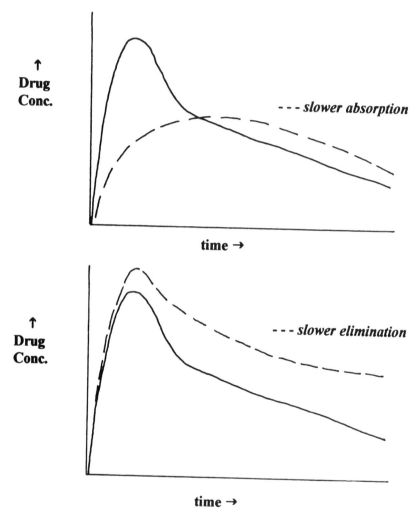

Figure 1. Top: After a single oral dose of drug, there is a rapid rise in drug plasma concentration followed by distribution to the peripheral compartment and slow elimination. Slower absorption of drug (– – –), as may occur because of congestive heart failure or bowel wall edema, results in a later rise of plasma drug levels to a lower peak concentration and slightly prolonged higher level. **Bottom**: In the case of slower elimination (– – –), as may occur with reduced renal function or low cardiac output, there is an appropriate and slightly higher initial peak concentration with a significantly prolonged high level.

and skin. A drug usually equilibrates rapidly in the central compartment and slowly in the periphery. Drugs bound to a high degree in the peripheral compartment (eg, amiodarone) appear to have a larger "volume of distribution" than those highly bound in the plasma (eg, by plasma proteins). The peripheral compartment acts as a reservoir, reversibly transferring drug to the plasma.

Drug distribution depends on several factors: pH, drug size and isomeric form, receptors, competition for binding sites, body composition, protein binding, tissue perfusion, metabolites, and elimination (Figure 1). A curve of drug serum concentration over time generally reflects two phases: the rapid distribution phase to the peripheral compartment (the $t1/2\alpha$) and the slower elimination phase ($t1/2\beta$). The $t1/2$a influences the timing and height of the peak serum concentration and therefore the total dose to be administered. The $t1/2\beta$ affects the dosing schedule.

Age plays a role in differences in drug distribution, particularly for infants, who have a large central compartment and small peripheral compartment. This results in wider fluctuations of serum levels between drug administration, due to a decreased peripheral reserve, and more frequent dosing is necessary. Protein binding is also significantly reduced, reducing the reserve of drug for dissolution and availability.

Metabolism

Drug metabolism affects two issues in antiarrhythmic drug dosing. The first is the age-related change in hepatic metabolism of drugs. Hepatic enzymes with a reduced ability to transform parent compounds to their metabolites can be saturated rapidly, leaving more drug unmetabolized.

The second issue is the active metabolite. This is important for procainamide, quinidine, disopyramide, lidocaine, propafenone, amiodarone, and propranolol. Active metabolites can have an antiarrhythmic effect quite different from the parent drug. A classic example is the procainamide metabolite, N-acetyl procainamide (NAPA). Although procainamide is a Vaughan Williams class IA drug (discussed below), NAPA is classified as a class III drug.

Excretion

Most antiarrhythmic drug excretion is renal. Low cardiac output states and those with selective low renal perfusion (eg, coarctation) will inhibit drug elimination.

"Steady-state" kinetics refers to the amount of drug given being equal to the amount excreted. This state can truly exist only for drugs being given as a continuous IV infusion. Otherwise, the serum concentration of drugs oscillates based on the frequency of administration and the absorption, distribution, and metabolic and elimination characteristics. In practice, a clinical steady state is presumed to be present after five elimination half-lives ($t1/2\beta$) of a drug.

Drug levels are obtained as serum "trough" determinations, prior to the sixth or seventh dose, in order to have meaningful value. A level in the "therapeutic" range implies neither a guarantee of efficacy nor safety. Serum levels do not reflect the drug concentration at the target site. Low serum levels may be correlated with antiarrhythmic efficacy if receptor sites are occupied. Erratic serum concentrations can be found for a number of agents (amiodarone, propafenone, sotalol). Adverse effects, such as blurry vision with class IC drugs, may be more related to peak concentrations. Not all agents warrant routine serum concentration determinations. In general, serum levels are important for the class IA and IC drugs and IV lidocaine. Digoxin levels are helpful if there is poor drug effect, when other drugs that alter the digoxin concentration are also given, in suspected digoxin overdose, or to ascertain compliance.

Pharmacodynamics and Drug Classification Schemes

Pharmacodynamics are the properties of ionic channel and receptor interaction and are similar for children and adults. Situations in which pharmacodynamic principles change, such as hypokalemia and myocardial infarction, are more common in adults, but pediatric correlates exist such as the myocardial scar after congenital heart surgery, which may resemble a myocardial infarction.

The Vaughan Williams antiarrhythmic drug classification scheme is the most widely recognized means of grouping drugs with somewhat similar antiarrhythmic effects.[8] However, the system is far from perfect. Drugs often have effects or metabolites that cross over classes, and drugs in the same class can have very different effects based on ion channel gating characteristics. Interactions with the autonomic nervous system are not considered in the classification. Most importantly, classes are based upon the cellular electrophysiological (EP) responses of normal, in vitro His-Purkinje tissue. This is misleading for in vivo atrial myocardial or atrioventricular nodal (AVN) effects or the effects in diseased tissue.

A meeting in Italy in 1990 resulted in a new proposal for antiarrhythmic drugs based on the desired target mechanism underlying a tachyarrhythmia.[9] Although the "Sicilian Gambit" forced a reconsideration of drug classification schemes, the use of this approach clinically can be cumbersome. Many arrhythmia mechanisms are unknown and the vulnerable target (channels, receptors, use-dependent factors, etc) toward which to direct therapy may be unclear.

Table 1

Classifications of Drug Actions

Mechanism	Arrhythmias	Target	Drugs
Reentry (Na⁺ channel-dependent) Long excitable gaps	Orthodromic SVT	Depress conduction, excitability	Class IA, IC
	Monomorphic VT	Depress conduction, excitability	Class IA, IB, IC
	Type I atrial flutter	Depress conduction, excitability	Class IA, IC
Reentry (Na⁺ channel-dependent) Short excitable gaps	Orthodromic SVT	Prolong refractoriness	Class III
	Atrial fibrillation	Prolong refractoriness	K⁺ channel blockers
	Type II atrial flutter	Prolong refractoriness	K⁺ channel blockers
	Polymorphic VT	Prolong refractoriness	Class IA
	Monomorphic VT	Prolong refractoriness	Class IA
	Bundle branch reentry	Prolong refractoriness	Class IA, Class III
	Ventricular fibrillation	Prolong refractoriness	Class IA, Class III
Reentry (Ca²⁺ channel-dependent)	AV node reentry	Depress conduction, excitability	Ca²⁺ channel blockers
	Verapamil-sensitive VT	Depress conduction, excitability	Ca²⁺ channel blockers
Automaticity Abnormal	Atrial ectopic tachycardia	Hyperpolarize	Muscarinic agonist
		Decrease phase 4	Ca²⁺ or Na⁺ blockers
	Idiopathic VT	Decrease phase 4	Ca²⁺ or Na⁺ blockers
Triggered activity Early afterdepolarizations	Torsades de pointes	Shorten action potential duration	β-blockers
		Suppress early after-depolarizations	
Delayed afterdepolarizations	Digoxin-induced	Suppress delayed after-depolarizations	β, Ca²⁺ block, Mg⁺⁺ Na⁺, β-blockers
		Unload calcium	Adenosine, Ca²⁺ block

Adapted with permission from Reference 9.

The logical extension of the Sicilian Gambit approach is shown in Table 1. Arrhythmias are grouped according to the presumed mechanism, the "target" characteristic of the mechanism, and an appropriate antiarrhythmic agent is then identified.

Vaughan Williams Classification

Class I Agents

The Vaughan Williams classes and representative drugs are shown in Table 2. The class I agents are the "local anesthetics," which block sodium

___ **Table 2** _____

Vaughan Williams Drug Classification

Class IA: Sodium ± potassium blockade, delay repolarization, "antivagal" effects
  Quinidine
  Procainamide
  Disopyramide
Class IB: Sodium channel blockade, shorten repolarization
  Lidocaine
  Mexiletine
  Moricizine
  Phenytoin
  Tocainide
Class IC: Sodium channel blockade, variable effect on repolarization
  Flecainide
  Propafenone
Class II: β-adrenergic blockade, variable selectivity
  Propranolol
  Atenolol
  Metoprolol
  Nadolol
  Esmolol
Class III: Prolong repolarization, calcium blockade, adrenergic blockade
  Amiodarone
  Sotalol
  Bretylium
  Ibutilide
Class IV: Calcium channel blockade
  Verapamil
  Diltiazem
Other agents:
  Adenosine
  Digoxin

channels. They are further subdivided based on their effects on repolarization and effects at faster or slower heart rates.

Class IA Agents

The class IA agents are quinidine, procainamide, and disopyramide. They delay repolarization and have "antivagal" effects and a greater effect at faster heart rates.

Quinidine

Quinidine is the oldest of the local anesthetic drugs. The drug is the D-isomer of quinine and a cinchona derivative (hence "cinchonism" for overdose side effects).

Action. Quinidine is a potent sodium and potassium channel blocker. Sodium channels, predominantly with medium-fast recovery time constants, are blocked during the active state. Quinidine has moderate potassium channel blocking activity as well as low-level effects on α- and muscarinic receptors.

Oral Administration, Kinetics, and Metabolites. Quinidine is administered orally as quinidine sulfate or gluconate. The gluconate form is absorbed slowly with peak levels in 3–4 hours and is given on a q 8-hour schedule. Quinidine sulfate reaches a peak concentration in 1–2 hours and is given every 6 hours. The drug is extensively bound to plasma proteins. Hypoalbuminemia increases serum levels. Higher quinidine levels occur in congestive heart failure due to changes in plasma proteins and vary if bowel wall edema is present. Newborns have more free quinidine than infants or children.[10]

Quinidine is metabolized in the liver by the cytochrome p-450 system to several metabolites; 3-hydroxy quinidine is the most prevalent and most potent of these metabolites. Approximately 20% of the parent drug is excreted unchanged in the urine. Since the drug is a weak base, alkaline urine increases serum levels of quinidine. The drug is poorly removed by dialysis techniques.[11] The elimination half-life of quinidine is 6–8 hours and the "therapeutic" range of quinidine at steady state is 2–6 μg/mL.

Dosing. Quinidine sulfate is given in a dose of 30–60 mg/kg per day, divided into a three or four times daily dose. Quinidine gluconate has 20% less quinidine base and the dose is adjusted upward to compensate. In-hospital initiation of the drug is a necessity due to the propensity for quinidine-induced proarrhythmia.

Side Effects and Interactions. Side effects with quinidine are common, with one third of patients experiencing some difficulty. Not all side effects dictate drug discontinuation. The most common problems are gastrointestinal. The cinchonism of central nervous manifestations includes tinnitus, visual changes, headache, and mental status changes. Other noncardiac side effects include thrombocytopenia, anemia, and agranulocytosis.

Cardiac side effects are those that are expected and those of proarrhythmic effect. The electrocardiogram (ECG) effects seen include prolongation of the PR, QRS, and QT measurements. Bradycardia can appear or be exacerbated, bundle branch blocks may occur, and, with high levels of drug, atrioventricular (AV) block may be seen. The most serious side effect is a drug-induced torsades de pointes (Figure 2), resulting in syncope and potential sudden death.[12] This phenomenon often occurs in the first days of dosing and may be accompanied by low serum potassium levels and by ECG evidence of QT prolongation. The drug can be a negative inotrope and worsen congestive failure in patients with poor ventricular function.

Since quinidine is metabolized by the liver, drugs that increase microsomal enzyme activity, such as phenytoin, phenobarbital, and rifampin, can increase quinidine metabolism. In patients over 5 years old, administration of digoxin with quinidine was shown to increase digoxin levels.[13] Coadministration of warfarin with quinidine can result in prolongation of the prothrombin time. Effects on international normalized ratio (INR) are unknown.

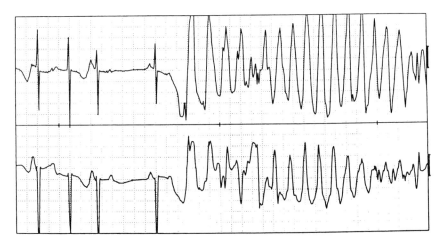

Figure 2. Onset of torsades de pointes VT in a patient taking quinidine. Note the "long–short" sequence before initiation and the T-wave alternans present during sinus rhythm before tachycardia begins.

Procainamide

Procainamide is the most commonly used class IA agent in pediatrics: as a single agent, in conjunction with digoxin, or less often with amiodarone or mexiletine.

Action. Procainamide, like quinidine, is a potent sodium channel blocker (in the active state) and moderate potassium channel blocker. The drug acts to delay repolarization and has greater effect at faster heart rates. There are no effects of the parent drug on α-, β-, muscarinic, or purinergic receptor sites. The membrane effects of procainamide are greater in the presence of infarcted tissue.

Oral Administration, Kinetics, and Metabolites. Procainamide is absorbed rapidly from the gastrointestinal tract, with approximately equal bioavailability of the standard and sustained release (SR) preparations ($\sim$80%). There is minimal protein binding. The drug is transformed in the liver to NAPA, which has mild to moderate class III antiarrhythmic effects. Levels of procainamide and NAPA are based on a genetic capability for hepatic acetylation. The standard formulation has a $t1/2$ of 2.5–4 hours and the SR preparation has a longer $t1/2$ of 6–8 hours.

Procainamide levels generally necessary for clinical antiarrhythmic effect are in the range of 4–8 μg/mL. Plasma therapeutic NAPA levels are similar. The practice of adding the procainamide and NAPA levels is to be discouraged strongly. Procainamide crosses the placenta readily, with a fetal/maternal ratio of approximately 0.80.[14]

Intravenous Administration. After IV administration, procainamide is rapidly distributed. The appearance of NAPA depends on hepatic acetylation.

Dosing. Chronic oral therapy with procainamide utilizes doses in the range of 40–100 mg/kg per day. The dose is divided for administration every 4 hours in small patients. In most patients over 1–2 years of age, dosing every 6 hours is possible and in teenage patients, on an every-8-hour schedule. In the older patient who can swallow the large pills, SR compound is used and administered every 8 hours.

For patients with rare tachycardia episodes, "periodic" procainamide therapy may be possible.[15] In this setting, a patient (usually teenager or adult), ingests a single dose of procainamide of 500–1500 mg at home to terminate sustained tachyarrhythmia.

IV administration of procainamide is more predictable. A loading dose of 7–10 mg/kg, given over 30–45 minutes, is used in patients under 1 year of age. In older patients, this bolus dose is closer to 15 mg/kg, given over

30–45 minutes. The bolus is followed by an infusion of procainamide, starting at 40–50 μg/kg per minute. Infusion rates of up to 100 μg/kg per minute are occasionally necessary in infants. Plasma levels are obtained 4 hours into the infusion.

Side Effects and Interactions.   Side effects are plasma concentration dependent. The most common one is a drug-induced lupuslike syndrome. Fever, pericardial fluid accumulations, arthralgias, and, rarely, hepatic or renal toxicity can be observed. With chronic administration, more than one-half of patients will convert to a positive antinuclear antibody (ANA), but only 20% may show symptoms. A positive ANA is not necessarily an indication to stop the drug if symptoms are absent. A common misperception is that procainamide will elevate digoxin levels. Amiodarone can elevate both procainamide levels and NAPA levels. Cimetidine reduces procainamide renal clearance.

During IV administration procainamide can have negative inotropic effects. Drug-induced ventricular arrhythmia is less common than sinus bradycardia.

Disopyramide

Disopyramide has few therapeutic antiarrhythmic applications in children, mostly due to an unfamiliarity with its effects, lack of significant clinical research with the drug, and difficulties in dosing due to formulation. It took on some degree of use in the setting of vasodepressor syncope.[16]

Action.   Disopyramide has cellular channel effects similar to quinidine, but without the α-receptor effects. It prolongs action potential duration more than the effective refractory period, but these data are based on Purkinje tissue and not on atrial tissue, where disopyramide might have its best pediatric application. Like other antiarrhythmics, disopyramide is available as a mixture of its D- and L-isomers.

Oral Administration, Kinetics, and Metabolites.   Disopyramide is available in standard and SR forms. The standard form is readily available after oral intake, with a peak concentration at 0.5–3 hours. The drug is more protein bound than other antiarrhythmics. Only about 10% of the drug may be biotransformed to N-monoalkylated disopyramide, and this metabolite has fairly weak membrane effects. Scant data are available for the pharmacokinetics of disopyramide in children, but may indicate a short $t^1/_2$ (5 hours). The therapeutic plasma range of disopyramide is 2–5 μg/mL, but, again, there is little pediatric data on the subject in children. Disopyramide crosses the placenta but reaches fetal cord levels less than one-half that of maternal levels.

Dosing. Young infants were given 20–30 mg/kg, those 2–10 years 9–24 mg/kg, and those over 11 years, 5–13 mg/kg per day.[17] The maximum daily adult dose does not exceed 1200 mg. The dosing intervals of the standard and SR preparations are every 6 hours and every 12 hours, respectively.

Side Effects and Interactions. Many patients receiving disopyramide have anticholinergic side effects that limit the drug's clinical utility. Up to 50% of patients have urinary retention, constipation, nausea, anorexia, vomiting, blurred vision, or dry mouth. Exacerbation of AV block, sinus node (SN) disease, and new-onset VT are other side effects.

Digoxin does not influence disopyramide levels. Phenytoin can increase hepatic transformation and atenolol can reduce renal clearance of disopyramide.

Class IB Agents

The class IB agents include lidocaine, mexiletine, moricizine, phenytoin and tocainide. These drugs block fast sodium channels, shorten action potential duration and repolarization, and have amplified effects at faster heart rates.

Lidocaine

Lidocaine is one of the most commonly administered antiarrhythmic drugs, second only to digoxin. It is available only in IV form.

Action. Lidocaine blocks the fast sodium channel and shows use dependence. It has little effect on structures above the His bundle. Shortening of repolarization occurs most in cells with long action potential duration, resulting in an overall homogeneity of repolarization.

Intravenous Administration, Kinetics, and Metabolites. Lidocaine has a rapid distribution phase. Two metabolites, methylglycinexlide and glycinexlide, have sodium channel blocking actions. In congestive heart failure, metabolism is diminished and the dose of lidocaine needs to be reduced. Metabolism may be reduced in neonates.

Kinetics for lidocaine are similar in children and adults, with a $t^1/_2$ of 2 hours and a significant first-pass effect occurs. Therapeutic levels range from 2–5 µg/mL.

Dosing. Lidocaine is given as an IV bolus of 1 mg/kg and may be repeated in 5 minutes. Lidocaine infusions range from 20–50 µg/kg per minute. Low cardiac output dictates a reduction in the infusion rate due to decreased hepatic clearance.

Side Effects and Interactions.   The major adverse reactions with lidocaine are related to the central nervous system (CNS) when plasma levels exceed 6–7 μg/mL[18] and include seizures, apnea, and mental status changes. In patients with atrial tachyarrhythmias or with variable degrees of AV block (especially due to QT prolongation), lidocaine may increase the ventricular response rate.

Since lidocaine undergoes extensive hepatic biotransformation, hepatic flow or microsomal enzyme activity alterations influence lidocaine levels. Lower hepatic flow occurs in congestive failure and with propranolol and cimetidine. Increased microsomal enzyme activity is seen with phenobarbital and phenytoin.

Mexiletine

Mexiletine can be considered an oral congener of lidocaine in many respects. Although its use is not widespread in pediatrics, it may become an important drug in the congenital long QT syndrome (LQTS) due to sodium channel defects.[19]

Action.   Mexiletine is a class IB agent with primary effects on the fast sodium channel. Like lidocaine, its effects are dependent on the state of tissue exposed to the drug, whether healthy or acutely or chronically ischemic. Effects are exaggerated in diseased tissue. In higher potassium states, effects on His-Purkinje tissue are more potent, with profound effects on the sodium channel. Mexiletine also has enhanced effects at rapid stimulation frequencies and suppresses early afterdepolarizations. This latter effect was observed in normal and partially depolarized His-Purkinje tissue.

Oral Administration, Kinetics, and Metabolites.   Mexiletine is rapidly absorbed from the gastrointestinal tract. Cimetidine slows absorption. Hepatic metabolism is extensive, with eight known metabolites, none with significant antiarrhythmic effects. Since metabolism is extensive, alterations in hepatic flow and function have important effects on concentration and elimination. The drug has two enantiomers, D- and L-mexiletine, without known antiarrhythmic differences.

The elimination half-life of mexiletine is relatively long but variable, between 6 and 11 hours. Mexiletine levels are rarely checked, but may help when issues of absorption and metabolism are raised. Levels range from 0.8–2.0 μg/mL.

Mexiletine crosses the placenta, but its use in fetal arrhythmias is rare. We treated one fetus with apparent fetal torsades de pointes VT successfully by maternal mexiletine administration. The fetus proved to have a congenital prolonged QT and intractable VT soon after birth.

Dosing. The starting dose of mexiletine is 2 mg/kg per dose, given every 8 hours. The dose may be increased to 5 mg/kg per dose,[20] and up to 7–8 mg/kg per dose for infants. No loading dose is used.

Side Effects and Interactions. Adverse side effects are common during mexiletine administration, from 20% to 70%. The most common ones are nausea and skin rash. Many of the gastrointestinal complaints can be avoided by giving the drug with food. The skin rash observed is a fine, maculopapular rash, particularly on the dorsum of the hands. Neurological side effects are less common and similar to those of lidocaine. Antacids or cimetidine slow mexiletine absorption. There are no reported interactions with digoxin.

Moricizine

Moricizine was first investigated in the Soviet Union in the 1960s for its phenothiazine effects. These local anestheticlike effects led to its subsequent use as an antiarrhythmic agent.[21] It is rarely used in pediatric practice.

Action. Moricizine blocks fast sodium channels in the inactive state and has voltage- and rate-dependent effects. It also has effects on delayed afterdepolarizations and may be useful in clinical arrhythmias due to abnormal automaticity.[22]

Oral Administration, Kinetics, and Metabolites. Moricizine is absorbed from the intestinal tract in 1–2 hours, is extensively bound to plasma proteins, and is metabolized to more than 30 products in the liver. The elimination half-life is 8 hours. With extensive metabolism, moricizine levels have no relation to effect, implying active metabolites.

Dosing. The dose of moricizine was not well established in children. Available data suggest a starting dose of 200 mg/m^2 per day divided every 8 hours.[22] The maximum is near 600 mg/m^2 per day.

Side Effects and Interactions. As with other class IB drugs, at higher doses, neurological side effects include blurry vision, headache, paresthesias, and tingling. Gastrointestinal symptoms may be alleviated by coadministration with food.

There are no known significant interactions of moricizine with digoxin. As with other Class IB drugs with extensive hepatic transformation, cimetidine may reduce clearance and prolong the elimination half-life.

Phenytoin

Phenytoin was initially used as an anticonvulsive agent but found application in therapy for postinfarction ventricular arrhythmias.[23] The drug is similar to lidocaine in many respects and is predominantly effective in tissue below the His bundle.

Action.   Local anesthetic effects similar to lidocaine are observed. Phenytoin binds predominantly to sodium channels in the inactivated state. High concentrations have some calcium channel blocking effects and influence automaticity. Phenytoin depresses phase 4 depolarization at standard concentrations, explaining the drug's utility for treating digoxin-induced arrhythmias. There are also effects via the CNS, with decreases in sympathetic tone.

Oral Administration, Kinetics, and Metabolites.   Although phenytoin is well absorbed, its peak concentration is delayed from 3–12 hours after administration. Dairy products decrease absorption whereas high protein or fatty diets enhance absorption. The drug is nearly completely metabolized in the liver. A number of drugs impede phenytoin metabolism, including isoniazid, diazepam, methylphenidate, chlorpromazine, chlordiazepoxide, and disulfiram. Phenobarbital and carbamazepine enhance metabolism. No metabolite has significant antiarrhythmic effect. Phenytoin has a unique metabolic feature among the antiarrhythmic agents: it can saturate its metabolism at high doses (>10 mg/kg per day). This is an important issue, as levels rise precipitously with small-dose increases at the saturation point.

Despite more extensive metabolism in young patients, infants have a prolonged phenytoin elimination half-life, up to 24 hours. In patients over 1 year of age, this drops to 8 hours, then rises again in the adult toward 24 hours. The usual therapeutic serum level range is 10–20 μ/mL.

Phenytoin crosses the placenta easily and has a high teratogenic capacity. Its use during pregnancy is contraindicated.[24]

Intravenous Administration.   IV loading with phenytoin must be done carefully due to hypotensive effects. The loading dose is poorly defined, ranging from 1–3 mg/kg over 15–30 minutes, with a maximum daily load of 10–15 mg/kg.

Oral Dosing.   The total oral loading dose is 15 mg/kg, divided every 6 hours. Maintenance doses vary with age, with those beyond the newborn period up to 5–6 years receiving 5–6 mg/kg per day divided every 12 hours.[23] Adults get 300–600 mg/day.

Side Effects and Interactions.   The most frequent side effect of phenytoin is hypotension with IV use. For oral use, side effects are rare with nystagmus and ataxia being the most common. Gingival hyperplasia is exacerbated by poor dental hygiene blood dyscrasias, including aplastic anemia, are reported. Phenytoin has a high teratogenic capacity, leading to "fetal hydantoin syndrome": midline facial clefts, hypertelorism, microcephaly with mental retardation, finger and nail hypoplasia and congenital heart defects in 10%.[25]

One of the more important drug interactions with phenytoin involves warfarin, with an increase in the prothrombin time and INR. Phenytoin may displace verapamil from binding sites and result in increased calcium blockade.

Tocainide

There are no published data on experience with tocainide in children. It is available as an oral preparation in the United States.

Action. Tocainide is similar to lidocaine in its EP effects. Action potential duration and refractory periods are shortened. Blockade of sodium channels with fast time constants occurs, with some frequency dependence. Patients responding to lidocaine are often put on oral tocainide with similar long-term clinical efficacy.

Administration, Kinetics, and Metabolites. Tocanide is available as an enantiomer. The elimination half-life is 10–11 hours. There are no significant metabolites. Peak concentrations are reduced when the drug is taken with a meal, but the total drug absorbed remains unchanged. "Therapeutic" plasma levels are from 3–9 μg/mL.

Dosing. In adult patients, the initial dose is 200 mg three times daily and rarely exceeds 2400 mg/day.[26]

Side Effects and Interactions. Adverse effects are common during tocainide therapy, occurring in up to 50% of patients. The most common noncardiac complaints are nausea, vomiting, dizziness, and paresthesias. Side effects are more frequent when levels exceed 10 μg/mL. Prolongation of the QT interval does not occur, and torsades de pointes is not reported. Pneumonitis occurred.

There are no known significant drug interactions with tocainide.

Class IC Agents

The class IC agents include flecainide, propafenone, and encainide. These drugs are potent sodium channel blocking agents with a variable effect on repolarization and frequency dependence. Encainide was eliminated from clinical use since 1992 due to its proarrhythmic effects. Many studies group the Class IC drugs together, including encainide in the past, but they have different kinetics and metabolites.

Publication of the Cardiac Arrhythmia Suppression Trial (CAST)[24] led to close scrutiny of the use of these agents in pediatrics. As a result, the class IC drugs are among the best understood antiarrhythmic agents in pediatric cardiology. These agents have widespread potential applications.

Flecainide

Flecainide is the most commonly used class IC drug in pediatrics. It was studied extensively[27-29] but remains controversial.[30,31]

Action. Flecainide acetate blocks slow sodium channels in the activated state. It also has some potassium channel blocking traits. Flecainide has a long time constant (taking longer to unbind from sodium channels), a distinction from the class IA drugs. Flecainide may have different effects on His-Purkinje tissue compared to ventricular myocardium. In specialized conduction tissue, refractory periods are shortened and automaticity blunted. In ventricular preparations, action potential duration and refractory periods are prolonged, leading to QRS widening. Both membrane effects and frequency dependence may be diminished in neonatal myocardial cells.

Oral Administration, Kinetics, and Metabolites. After an oral dose, flecainide reaches its peak concentration in 1–2 hours. Milk products block flecainide absorption, and, when patients are put on clear liquid diets, levels can rise substantially.[32] Doses should be reduced by 25% to 30% in this setting.

Flecainide is not extensively metabolized in the liver and is excreted unchanged in the urine. There are two metabolites with weak membrane effects. The elimination half-life varies with age. Newborns can have a half-life as long as 27 hours in the 1st day.[28] Patients under 4–6 months old have a $t_{1/2}$ of 11 hours. In patients age 6 months to 10 years, the $t_{1/2}$ is 8 hours and prolongs to 12 hours in those over 10–11 years.[27]

Flecainide crosses the placenta readily, even in the face of fetal hydrops. Its concentration in the fetus is approximately 70% that of maternal levels.[33] Since there are no significantly active metabolites, the concern of repeated fetal "dosing" from ingestion of amniotic fluid in utero is eliminated.

Intravenous Parameters. IV flecainide is available for use outside the United States. Its dose is 1–2 mg/kg given over 5–10 minutes. A continuous infusion is not used.

Dosing. Flecainide dosing, based on body surface area, correlates better with serum flecainide levels than dosing based on weight.[27] The starting dose in infants is often 80–90 mg/m² per day, divided in a q12 hour sched-ule. The dose for older patients is 100–110 mg/m² per day and gives a reliable trough level of 200–400 ng/mL. There is no loading dose. Older patients, 6 months-10 years, may require q8 hour dosing, due to the change in $t1/2$. Doses can be increased to 200 mg/m² per day, but caution is ad-vised for patients with low levels on high-dose flecainide.[34] Diet changes can result in extensive absorption of the drug, leading to serum levels more in keeping with the dose and a higher risk of adverse effects. A trough level of 200–1000 ng/mL is "therapeutic."

In younger patients unable to swallow pills, a suspension of flecainide must be made. A concentration of 10 mg/mL is common. The suspension should be shaken vigorously to prevent inadvertent administration of too low or too high doses of drug.

Side Effects and Interactions. Side effects of flecainide are related to high levels and administration of the drug to patients with an abnormal heart. The drug is generally safe for those with normal hearts.[30,31] At peak concentration or with overdose, some patients experience blurry vision and oral paresthesia. In patients with paroxysmal SVT, flecainide can result in slow conduction and bring about slower, but incessant SVT.[27] This phe-nomenon is most often observed during the first days of therapy and argues for in-hospital initiation of the drug. Proarrhythmia occurs not infrequently in the patient with an atrial tachyarrhythmia and abnormal anatomy. In addition to the incessant, slower SVTs that may result from flecainide ad-ministration, a narrow QRS tachycardia may become wide due to sustained bundle branch block.

The results of the CAST study,[24] while pointing to a subset of adult, postinfarction patients at risk of serious proarrhythmia on flecainide, have few correlates in the pediatric population. The exception here may relate to the postoperative patient with right ventricular disease, such as tetralogy of Fallot, or left ventricular disease, such as those with surgery for aortic or subaortic stenosis.

A mild negative inotropic effect, especially in adults with already de-pressed function, was reported. In children who present with incessant tachyarrhythmia, control with the drug was often achieved and there were no noted adverse effects on echocardiographic indices of function.[27]

A rise in digoxin levels was reported for adults on flecainide, but this experience was not corroborated in pediatric patients. Flecainide can be used in combination with amiodarone for resistant arrhythmias and with mexiletine for some infant VT due to tumors.

Propafenone

Propafenone's clinical applications are similar to those of flecainide,[35] as are its potential adverse effects in postoperative patients.[36]

Action. Propafenone blocks the sodium channel with a medium range time constant for recovery. Propafenone also has mild β-2 receptor blocking properties. The drug has both voltage- and frequency-dependent effects. There are effects on the slow inward calcium current and delayed outward potassium current, reflecting propafenone's clinical efficacy for control of automatic focus arrhythmias.

Oral Administration, Kinetics, and Metabolites. Propafenone reaches peak concentration 2–3 hours after an oral dose. Increases in the oral dose can overload clearance mechanisms before saturation of the peripheral compartment. Increases in the dose therefore result in markedly increased bioavailability. Propafenone is extensively metabolized in the liver. The major metabolite is 5-OH-propafenone.[37] Patients vary in their ability to oxidatively metabolize the parent drug. In those with extensive metabolism, the half-life of propafenone is on the order of 4 hours. The elimination half-life of 5-OH-propafenone is not known. In patients who are poor propafenone metabolizers, the half-life of propafenone is longer, from 14–16 hours. This has important clinical relevance with respect to dosing schedule and efficacy.

Plasma levels of propafenone have an extremely wide range in clinical studies, from 100–5000 ng/mL. Most patients required levels of at least 150–200 ng/mL for clinical effect. There is no clear relationship between efficacy and level, in part due to the mixed population of metabolizers and nonmetabolizers.

Intravenous Administration. IV propafenone is not commercially available in the United States. After an IV dose, the drug has a distribution half-life of 4–5 minutes and retains clinical effect for up to 1 hour.

Dosing. Oral dosing starts at 150–200 mg/m^2 per day, divided in q 8-hour schedule. Dosing depends to a large extent on the ability of the patient to metabolize propafenone to 5-OH-propafenone. The upper dose is 600 mg/m^2 per day.

The IV dose is 0.2–1.0 mg/kg, given slowly over 5–10 minutes to a maximum of 2 mg/kg total load.[38] There are significant negative inotropic effects, requiring intravascular volume loading. Infusions of 4–10 μg/kg per minute were used.

Side Effects and Interactions. Like flecainide, propafenone should be used with caution, if at all, in patients with a structurally abnormal heart. A higher risk of arrest and sudden death was reported in this subpopulation.[36] Other side effects with oral therapy are also like those of flecainide: blurry vision, paresthesias, and nausea. Rarely, propafenone may cause a lupuslike syndrome.

Conduction system disturbances are relatively common. It is not uncommon for a narrow QRS rhythm during SVT to present with a wide QRS pattern due to bundle branch block. The negative inotropic effects of propafenone are well recognized, especially with IV administration. Unwanted cardiovascular side effects are not related to plasma propafenone levels.

Variable elevation of serum digoxin levels was reported with coadministration with propafenone. Digoxin levels should be monitored periodically.

Class II

The class II agents are the β-adrenergic blockers. A number of agents are available, differing in their β-selectivity, half-lives and "intrinsic sympathomimetic activity." Most "selective" β-blockers are nonselective at higher doses. Sotalol, a drug with mixed β-blocking and class III effects is reviewed in the class III section.

The predominant β-blockers in use in the pediatric age range covered in this section include propranolol, atenolol, metoprolol, nadolol, and esmolol.

Propranolol

Propranolol is the most commonly used β-blocking agent. Propranolol is one of the few antiarrhythmic agents with a commercially available liquid solution. Confusion results because there are two common concentrations: 20 mg per 5 mL and 10 mg/mL. This lack of uniformity results in dosing inaccuracies. The 20 mg per 5 mL preparation is the more common of the two and should be the standard.

Action. Propranolol is the classic nonselective β-blocker. There are membrane effects on the sodium channel. At high concentration, propranolol has weak calcium channel blockade effects. There are no intrinsic sympathomimetic properties. Neonatal tissues are more sensitive to the β-blocking effects than adult tissue.

Oral Administration, Kinetics, and Metabolites. Propranolol is completely absorbed after oral administration, but hepatic metabolism and clearance are so extensive that higher oral doses are needed to reach similar serum concentrations than with the IV preparation. The major metabolite is 4-OH-propranolol. As with most drugs with significant hepatic metabolism, there are wide population variations in degree of metabolism of propranolol, making plasma levels vary just as widely.

In infants, propranolol has a shorter half-life (3–4 hours) than in children over 1–2 years and adults (6 hours).[39] The metabolite has a longer half-life and mild β-blocking effects. Plasma levels of propranolol range from 50–150 μg/mL, but appear useful more as an assay of absorption and compliance than in assessing efficacy.

Propranolol crosses the placenta easily such that fetal levels approximate maternal levels.[40] Fetal hypoglycemia is a concern.

Intravenous Administration. Propranolol is one of the few effective IV antiarrhythmic agents available. The antiarrhythmic effects of IV propranolol are immediate and require careful monitoring.

Dosing. Oral propranolol can be given as a liquid preparation, pill form or SR preparation. The total daily doses are the same, starting from 1–2 mg/kg per day. In infants the total dose is divided in q 6-hour schedule until 4–8 months of age. When young children can swallow pills, a three times daily schedule is often effective. At this stage, once- or twice-a-day SR propranolol could also be considered.

IV propranolol is given as a 0.1–0.2 mg/kg dose over 1–5 minutes. Significant caution is advised, as discussed below.

Side Effects and Interactions. With IV administration, there can be serious bradycardia and hypotension. This is particularly true in the child under one year of age, and the drug probably needs to be avoided in IV form in these young patients. The exception may be in the young child with hypercyanotic spells, where the IV drug may be used with caution.

Propranolol has a number of potential adverse side effects other than bradycardia, AV block, and worsening congestive heart failure. The drug crosses the blood-brain barrier and can cause fatigue, depression, and nightmares. As a β-blocker, it can exacerbate bronchospasm and increase the risk of hypoglycemia. A peripheral vasoreactive condition can cause discoloration and cool extremities.

As with other drugs that are extensively metabolized in the liver, all conditions that influence hepatic flow and biotransformation affect propranolol levels. Coadministration of IV propranolol with calcium channel blockers is contraindicated due to the significant synergistic negative effects on contractility.

Atenolol

Atenolol is a commonly used long acting β-blocker.[41,42] The scored 25- and 50-mg pills can be broken in half while maintaining the SR properties.

Action. Atenolol is a "selective" β-blocker, with primary effects on β-1 adrenergic receptors. It is a competitive antagonist of endogenous catecholaminergic agents. There are no significant intrinsic sympathomimetic or membrane properties of atenolol. The drug is hydrophilic and does not cross the blood-brain barrier.

Oral Administration, Kinetics, and Metabolites. Atenolol reaches peak concentrations 2–3 hours after an oral dose. It can be given once or twice a day with a half-life of up to 9–10 hours. Atenolol has little hepatic transformation and is excreted unchanged in the urine. There are no active metabolites. Plasma levels are not routinely used. Atenolol crosses the placenta, but no reliable data on fetal levels exist.

Dosing. The starting dose of atenolol is 1–2 mg/kg per day, up to 3 mg/kg per day. It can be given as a once- or twice-a-day drug.

Side Effects and Interactions. Since atenolol does not cross the blood-brain barrier, the side effect profile is considerably reduced compared to propranolol. The cardiovascular effects are similar to those of propranolol. Although atenolol is a selective β-1 agent, the risk of bronchospasm is not eliminated completely. Cool extremities can be a common complaint. There are no reported significant drug interactions.

Metoprolol

Metoprolol is a β-blocker with a limited experience of use in pediatrics. It is gaining some favor in the therapy of autonomic dysfunction syndromes.[43]

Action. Metoprolol is a β-1 selective adrenergic blocker. It has no intrinsic sympathomimetic activity and very mild membrane effects. In the United States the drug is available as an oral agent, but the IV preparation is available elsewhere and may be useful for hypertension and thyrotoxicosis, in addition to tachyarrhythmias.

Oral Administration, Kinetics, and Metabolites. Extensive first pass hepatic transformation occurs. The elimination half-life is 3–8 hours. There are no active metabolites. The drug crosses the placenta and is metabolized by the fetal liver.

Dosing. There are no studies of dosing guidelines for metoprolol in children. In adults, a starting dose of 50 mg twice daily may be used and increased to 150–200 mg BID.

Side Effects and Interactions. Insufficient data exist for the side effect profile of metoprolol in children.

Nadolol

Nadolol is available as an oral, SR preparation. It is used in pediatric patients for both SVT and ventricular arrhythmias and for autonomic dysfunction syndromes.[44] It is also used in patients with LQTS.

Action. Unlike atenolol, nadolol is a nonselective β-adrenergic blocking agent. There are no intrinsic sympathomimetic or membrane properties.

Oral Administration, Kinetics, and Metabolites. Nadolol is poorly absorbed but undergoes little hepatic transformation. Peak plasma levels occur 3–4 hours after administration, and the drug is primarily excreted in the urine. The elimination half-life is probably the longest of the SR preparations, on the order of 20–24 hours. There are no active metabolites. There are no data on fetal use.

Dosing. Initial therapy is often recommended at 1 mg/kg per day. Due to its $t^1/_2$, it can be given as a once-daily dose.

Side Effects and Interactions. Nadolol has minimal passage across the blood-brain barrier. The effects on sinus rate and AVN conduction are similar to those of other nonselective β-blocking agents. No significant drug interactions were reported.

Esmolol

Esmolol has come into use recently for therapy of a wide spectrum of tachyarrhythmias,[45] mostly in the postoperative setting, and for control of hypertension, particularly following cardiac transplantation. It may be useful for catheter ablation procedures where AV block is helpful for mapping atrial tachycardias.

Action. Esmolol is an IV β-blocker with relative β-1 cardioselectivity. There are minimal membrane and intrinsic sympathomimetic properties at high dose. The predominant sites of action are the SN and AVN. There are no significant effects on working myocardium or the His-Purkinje system.

Intravenous Administration, Kinetics, and Metabolites. Esmolol distributes rapidly and has an elimination half-life of 7–10 minutes. This characteristic of the drug made it a valuable addition to the pediatric antiarrhythmic armamentarium, as any potentially deleterious effects will be short lived and generally manageable. The drug is metabolized to inactive agents but the metabolism is unaffected by hepatic flow.

Dosing. A loading dose of 500 μg/kg is generally used, given over 1–2 minutes. A maintenance infusion can be used to titrate the desired effect, starting at 50 μg/kg per minute.[46] Additional bolus doses can be administered, with subsequent increases in the infusion rate up to 200 μg/kg per minute.

Side Effects and Interactions. The most frequently cited adverse effect is hypotension during bolus therapy. In small children and those with single ventricle physiology, this effect can be profound, requiring volume and/or inotropic support.

Class III Agents

The class III agents include amiodarone, sotalol, bretylium, and ibutilide. The primary mode of action of all these agents is prolongation of refractoriness. However, there are many other diverse membrane and receptor effects.

Amiodarone

Amiodarone was initially used as an antianginal agent with coronary vasodilating traits. It is a potent agent for control of a variety of tachyarrhythmias.[47,48] Amiodarone was recently released in the United States for IV use, and there is a body of literature for its safety and effectiveness in resistant arrhythmias in children.[49–51]

Action. Amiodarone has many effects in addition to prolonging refractory periods. It is also a sodium channel blocker, showing both voltage and frequency dependence and a noncompetitive α- and β-adrenergic receptor blocker. It inhibits release of presynaptic norepinephrine. Potassium channels show interference of the delayed outward current, accounting for the prolongation of refractoriness.

There are tissue-dependent and age-dependent properties: sodium and calcium channel effects in the SN and AVN. Younger patients show SN effects whereas adults have a more dramatic response in the AVN.

Oral Administration, Kinetics, and Metabolites. Amiodarone is very lipid soluble and is absorbed more slowly than any other oral antiarrhythmic agent. Its peak concentration occurs after 3–7 hours. The drug is metabolized to an active agent, desethylamiodarone, in the liver. Amiodarone and desethylamiodarone are stored in very large volume of distribution in the peripheral compartment. When the drug is discontinued, levels can be significant up to 3 months. Therapeutic levels range from 1.0–2.5 μg/mL but correlate poorly with efficacy due to metabolite action and peripheral storage. Plasma levels are helpful for assessing absorption or compliance.

Although it takes several days to see a clinical effect when initiating therapy, some EP effect can be observed in 1–2 days with standard loading protocols.[52]

Amiodarone crosses the placenta poorly in a 4:1 ratio. The drug is present in low concentration in breast milk, but this is not a contraindication to breastfeeding.

Intravenous Administration. IV amiodarone was studied in a multicenter trial of the drug for resistant, life-threatening pediatric tachyarrhythmias.[51] The drug shows a rapid onset of action, with a clinical effect often occurring during the first dose. The antiarrhythmic effect can persist for 1–6 hours. Amiodarone is mixed in 5% dextrose solution to prevent precipitation. Infusions should be shielded from light.

Dosing. An oral loading protocol, using 10–15 mg/kg per day, is often used for 5–10 days. This dose is usually split in a twice-daily schedule to avoid gastrointestinal side effects. Some centers advocate loading for 3–5 days, using up to 50 mg/kg per day.[53]

Chronic oral therapy after loading is 2–5 mg/kg given once a day. Attempts are made to keep the maintenance dose low to avoid the long term side effects inherent in amiodarone use. Amiodarone is available as a 200-mg tablet. Although this can be broken into halves or quarters or even given on an every-other-day basis, a 10-mg/mL suspension is often made. Controversy exists about the stability of the suspension, and some centers dispense new aliquots weekly. Anecdotal experience indicates that the suspension is stable for at least one month. The contents must be shaken vigorously.

IV dosing of amiodarone should obtain the most immediate effect with the lowest risk of adverse effects. In the largest studies of IV amiodarone to date in young patients, a 5-mg/kg bolus was used and divided into five 1-mg/kg aliquots, each given over 5 minutes.[49,51] No adverse effect was seen in the first 1- to 3-mg/kg bolus, so the drug could be given initially as two 2.5-mg/kg boluses. The average successful load was 6 mg/kg. Infusions of amiodarone were used mostly in those with ventricular tachyarrhythmias, at 10–15 mg/kg per day.

Side Effects and Interactions. Amiodarone has a long list of potential side effects (Table 3). Therefore, interventional techniques for tachyarrhythmias are often considered rather than proceeding with amiodarone therapy. The most common noncardiac side effects with oral amiodarone use are skin photosensitivity, chemical hepatitis, hypothyroidism, hyperthyroidism, and corneal microdeposits. Cardiac side effects include sinus

_____ Table 3 _____

Amiodarone Side Effects

Most common
  Corneal microdeposits
  Photosensitivity
  Hypo- or hyperthyroidism
  Elevated transaminases
Less common
  Pulmonary interstitial fibrosis
  Bradycardia
  AV block
  Paresthesia
  Headache
  Nausea, constipation
  Parotid inflammation
  Epididymitis
  Rash, pruritis, hair loss
With intravenous use
  Hypotension
  Bradycardia
  Pulmonary edema (with high FiO_2)

bradycardia, AV block, and proarrhythmia. Torsades de pointes occurs rarely (<1%). All patients should use high-grade sunblock. Liver and thyroid function tests should be performed at least every 6 months. Amiodarone's high iodine content likely accounts for its effects on thyroid function. Rarely, coadministration of thyroid hormones is necessary but does not seem to interfere with the class III effect. In adult patients on chronic oral amiodarone, irreversible pulmonary fibrosis can occur. This phenomenon was not reported in children. On the other hand, pulmonary function testing was not routinely performed, and the abnormalities may be present but undetected. Many pediatric patients receiving long-term amiodarone therapy are postoperative patients with preexisting abnormalities of pulmonary function.

Hypotension is the predominant side effect with IV therapy. If IV amiodarone is given to a patient receiving high inspired oxygen concentrations, an "adult respiratory distress syndrome" picture may occur.[54]

There are many drug interactions with amiodarone (Table 4). The most frequently cited is digoxin, with digoxin levels rising 25% to 100% with coadministration of amiodarone. The same is true for administration of amiodarone with other antiarrhythmic agents, particularly procainamide, flecainide, quinidine and phenytoin. Excessive increases in prothrombin time and INR were seen with amiodarone therapy for patients on warfarin. Use of β-blockers or calcium channel blockers with amiodarone is controversial, with synergistic effects on SN and AVN function.

_____ **Table 4** _____

Amiodarone Drug Interactions

Digoxin	Increased digoxin levels, 50% to 100%, due to decreased clearance and drug displacement
Quinidine	Increased levels of all, exact basis unknown,
Procainamide	but levels increase 30% to 50%
Phenytoin	
Flecainide	
Warfarin	Increased prothrombin time by >50%, due to decreased clearance
β-blockers and calcium blockers	Increased degree of bradycardia and AV block

Sotalol

Sotalol is available in the United States as a racemic mixture of the D- and L-sotalol enantiomers, and it is being used for a number of difficult-to-control postoperative tachyarrhythmias.[55] Sotalol is often substituted for amiodarone to avoid the amiodarone side-effect profile, but the drugs are quite different in many respects.

Action. Sotalol is a nonselective β-blocker with class III effects. At lower doses β-blockade occurs. The class III effects are present at higher sotalol doses. At higher concentrations, the potassium delayed rectifier current and sodium channel are affected. There are no intrinsic sympathomimetic properties.

Oral Administration, Kinetics, and Metabolism. Sotalol has excellent enteric absorption and peak concentrations are present after 2 hours. The elimination half-life ranges from 7–12 hours and was not studied in children. There are no active metabolites and levels are not clinically helpful. The drug is excreted in the urine. Transplacental passage of the drug occurs, but fetal use is not established.

Dosing. The starting dose is 90–100 mg/m² per day. The drug may be given on a three-times or twice-daily schedule, often based on the response of incessant SVTs. The dose can be increased to 200 mg/m² per day. The smallest unit dose is 80 mg, so suspensions (5 mg/mL is common) must be concocted for small children. An IV preparation is available outside the United States, and doses are in the range of 0.2–1.5 mg/kg.

Side Effects and Interactions. Sotalol has the side-effect profile of β-blockers with mild negative inotropic effects. Unlike other β-blockers, sotalol will prolong the QT interval due to class III effects. The most serious adverse side effect is torsades de pointes, with an incidence approximating that of quinidine-induced torsades.

Bretylium

Bretylium has limited applications in pediatrics.[56] It is used in resuscitative settings for polymorphic VT or monomorphic VT resistant to other standard therapy.

Action. Bretylium has effects in sympathetic ganglia, where it causes an initial release of norepinephrine stores but subsequently prevents further release and reuptake. Bretylium has equal effects on prolongation of action potential duration and repolarization, much like amiodarone.

Intravenous Administration, Kinetics, and Metabolites. The oral form of bretylium has such poor absorption that the drug is effective only as an IV agent. There are EP effects in minutes, allowing attempts at cardioversion or defibrillation. There are no established levels and no significant metabolites. The effects last for 30–120 minutes. Pediatric studies are lacking.

Dosing. The IV dose of bretylium is 5 mg/kg as a rapid push. There are hypotensive effects such that, in hemodynamically stable VT, it should be diluted in 5% dextrose and given slowly. The total dose should not exceed 30 mg/kg. Continuous infusion rates are 15–30 μg/kg per minute.

Side Effects and Interactions. The predominant adverse effect is hypotension, but during resuscitative measures, this is rarely a concern. The hypotensive effect is due to bretylium's peripheral adrenergic blocking properties.

Bretylium may reverse the local anesthetic effect of quinidine and other sodium channel blockers. This explains its use in quinidine-induced torsades de pointes. Although bretylium is used for digoxin-induced arrhythmias, the drug may worsen these rhythms initially due to the early release of norepinephrine. Tricyclic antidepressants block bretylium's synaptic effects.

Ibutilide

Ibutilide is a recently released intravenous class III agent. The drug has not been studied in pediatric patients to date. Adult data are not extensive, focusing primarily on the drug's use in acute termination of atrial fibrillation and flutter.[57]

Action. Action potentials are prolonged, but the mechanism underlying this effect is not understood. Refractoriness is prolonged in both atrial and ventricular myocardial cells. Rather than block potassium currents, as most class III drugs will do, ibutilide activates a slow, inward sodium current.

Intravenous Administration, Kinetics, and Metabolites. The drug has extensive hepatic metabolism. The elimination half-life of ibutilide is approximately 6 hours.

Dosing. Adult studies have used 10–25 μg/kg as a bolus over 10 minutes. The bolus may be repeated in 10 minutes.

Side Effects and Interactions. About 8% of patients develop torsades de pointes VT.[58] AV block can occur. The drug is teratogenic.

Class IV Agents

The class IV agents are the calcium channel blockers. The predominant drug in use is verapamil, with limited experience and applications for nifedipine and diltiazem.

Verapamil

Verapamil is a papaverine derivative available in standard and SR oral preparations and IV preparation. It was introduced as a coronary vasodilator. It is useful for verapamil-sensitive VTs[59] and patients with hypertrophic cardiomyopathy.[55]

Action. Verapamil is a calcium channel blocker and has its greatest influence on the SN and AVN. The drug is an isomeric mixture and binds to calcium channels in the inactive state. Calcium channel blockade is more apparent at faster rates. It is effective in depressing enhanced automaticity and is an α-adrenergic blocker.

Oral Administration, Kinetics, and Metabolites. Verapamil undergoes extensive first-pass metabolism, and less than 25% is bioavailable. Peak levels occur after 2 hours, and the elimination half-life is 4–7 hours. Due to a large volume of distribution, changes in verapamil dosing should be delayed at least 4 days.

There are many metabolites as a result of liver biotransformation. Less than 5% of the drug is excreted unchanged in the urine. None of the metabolites is active. Hepatic dysfunction or low flow has a dramatic effect on prolonging the $t1/2$.

Verapamil is available as a standard and SR preparation. The smallest SR dose is 120 mg, with an elimination half-life of 8–10 hours. In the SR preparation, more verapamil is bioavailable and dosing may be more reproducible. Verapamil levels are not generally useful but range from 0.1 to 0.4 μg/mL.

Transplacental passage is fairly low with a maternal/fetal concentration ratio of approximately 3:1,[60] passing poorly in the presence of hydrops.

Intravenous Administration. IV verapamil has an elimination half-life similar to that of the oral preparation. This has important consequences when adverse effects are encountered in young children (see Side Effects and Interactions).

Dosing. The oral preparation was used with a wide range of reported doses, from 4 to 17 mg/kg per day. The drug is given on a three- or four-times daily schedule. When the SR preparation is used, the total dose is reduced to account for the higher bioavailability. In adults, the dose is 80–120 mg three times daily or 120–240 once a day of SR.

IV verapamil is used for therapy of SVTs or to achieve higher degrees of AV block for the treatment of atrial tachyarrhythmias.

Side Effects and Interactions. With oral verapamil, one of the more common adverse effects is constipation. Headaches, dizziness, rashes, and pruritis also occur. Cardiovascular side effects include bradycardia, AV block, postural hypotension, and worsening of congestive heart failure.

The most significant side effect occurs in young patients with the IV preparation resulting in asystole and cardiovascular collapse.[61] The IV use of the drug should be considered contraindicated in patients under 1 year of age. Verapamil may increase the ventricular response rate of atrial fibrillation in patients with WPW syndrome.

Concomitant use of IV calcium blockers and β-blockers is unwise due to the synergistic negative effects on ventricular function and sinus rate. A mild increase in digoxin levels occurs and a reduction in the digoxin dose is advisable.

Diltiazem

Diltiazem's use in pediatric patients was confined predominantly to control of hypertension.[62] The drug is available in both an oral and IV preparation, but no data are available in children and little data are available from adults to extrapolate.

Action. Diltiazem is a moderately potent blocker of the inward calcium channel. It has no significant sodium channel or α effects.

Administration, Kinetics, and Metabolites. Diltiazem is available in oral and IV forms. After oral administration it is rapidly absorbed, reaching peak levels within 1 hour. There is a wide range of variation in bioavailability due to variations in first-pass metabolism. There are no significant metabolites. The elimination half-life is 3–5 hours.

Therapeutic plasma levels were in the range of 30–270 ng/mL, but there were no data on the clinical utility of levels versus efficacy or side effects.

Dosing.   There are no clear recommendations on the oral dose of diltiazem in children. Adult doses are in the range of 30–120 mg three times a day. IV doses are 0.15–0.45 mg/kg followed by an infusion rate of 0.003 mg/kg per minute.

Side Effects and Interactions.   Chronic oral therapy with diltiazem results in frequent but mild side effects, including headache and postural hypotension. Bradycardia and increased levels of AV block should be anticipated.

Other Agents

The constraints of the Vaughan Williams classification scheme do not permit categories for two widely used agents, adenosine and digoxin.

Adenosine

Adenosine has altered the emergency room therapy of SVT. Adenosine triphosphate is broken down to adenosine and is used in some countries.

Action.   Adenosine is an endogenous purinergic agent. Its EP effects are due to an increase in potassium channel conductance and depression of the slow inward calcium current, resulting in transient AV block and sinus bradycardia. It is also a potent peripheral vasodilator. The EP effects are mediated by an A1-purinergic extracellular receptor, blocked by methylxanthines.

Intravenous Administration, Kinetics, and Metabolism.   The drug is given as a rapid IV bolus. Its effects are seen in 7–20 seconds. An appealing aspect is that its half-life averages 9 seconds. It is therefore a powerful therapeutic and diagnostic agent. Effects are pronounced when the drug is given centrally as opposed to peripherally.

Dosing.   Initial doses of 100–150 μg/kg are given as a rapid bolus, followed by saline flush. The dose may be doubled, up to a maximum of 300 μg/kg or the adult dose of 6–12 mg.[63] An ECG record is essential during adenosine administration to demonstrate atrial tachyarrhythmia.

Side Effects and Interactions. Adenosine may cause transient hypotension, facial flushing, or mild bronchospasm.[64] Ventricular ectopy is not unusual and may be the mechanism of termination of some reciprocating tachycardias, rather than adenosine-induced AV block. Occasionally, atrial fibrillation results from adenosine administration. Aminophylline can interfere with the extracellular actions of adenosine. Dipyridamole and diazepam can inhibit its cellular uptake and potentiate its effects.

Digoxin

Digitalis is the most widely prescribed antiarrhythmic and inotropic agent. The common preparation, digoxin, has its greatest effects on atrial tissue and the AVN.

Action. There are both direct and indirect properties of digoxin. The indirect properties result from autonomic effects mediated by the parasympathetic nervous system. The direct properties of digoxin are due to binding of the drug to the Na-K ATPase transport complex, thereby inhibiting outward flux of sodium ions. The inotropic response of digoxin is due to intracellular calcium loading due to the higher intracellular sodium concentration's enhancement of the Na-Ca pump.

At higher concentrations of digoxin, ventricular automaticity may be enhanced. Debate continues regarding the importance of digoxin's potential effects on accessory pathway refractory periods. A single study showed that digoxin may shorten, lengthen, or leave the antegrade refractory period of accessory pathways unchanged.[65] Sudden death obviously occurs in a small subset of patients with WPW syndrome, and many practitioners believe that the use of digoxin in a patient with overt preexcitation increases this risk.[66]

Oral Administration, Kinetics, and Metabolites. A prolonged distribution phase of 6–8 hours follows oral intake of digoxin due to extensive peripheral binding. Myocardial tissue concentrations of digoxin are higher in children than adults. Peak levels occur in 1–2 hours, and the elimination half-life is long, at 1.5–2 days. Renal dysfunction has a direct influence on extending the half-life. There are no significant metabolites and the majority of the drug is excreted unchanged in the urine.

Therapeutic digoxin levels are in the range of 0.7–2.0 ng/mL. In infants, the presence of a digoxinlike immunoreactive substance may complicate the assay.

Digoxin crosses the placenta readily, with fetal levels approximating maternal levels.[67] Digoxin remains the first-line drug for therapy of fetal SVTs.

Intravenous Administration. The effects of digoxin when used in an IV vehicle are not different from those of the oral preparation. The onset of EP effect is obviously more rapid, on the order of 5–10 minutes.

Dosing. Usually, a total loading dose (TLD) of 30 μg/kg is acceptable, with a slight decrease to 20–25 μg/kg for premature infants. This dose is divided as follows: 50% of the TLD over 15 minutes, followed by two doses at 6-hour intervals of 25% of the TLD each. For IV loading, two thirds to three fourths of the TLD is used, divided in similar fashion. Oral liquid digoxin preparations are available in a 50 μg/mL concentration, whereas IV preparations are available as 100 μg/mL. Because digoxin remains one of the most common drugs prone to prescription error, both the total dose and the volume of dose should be written on all orders.

Maintenance doses of digoxin are 7–10 μg/kg per day. Due to the long half-life of digoxin, the drug can be given on a once-a-day basis.

The dose of digoxin needs to be decreased in patients with renal dysfunction and congestive heart failure. In these states, and when digoxin is coadministered with any other drug, it seems wise to monitor periodic levels. To be meaningful, levels need to be drawn 6 hours after a dose or just prior to a dose.

Side Effects and Interactions. Digoxin toxicity is likely to be seen with levels above 3.0 ng/mL.[68] Effects include proarrhythmic ones, but also include nausea, visual changes and drowsiness. Gynecomastia is a potential side effect with long-term use.

The cardiac manifestations of digoxin toxicity are somewhat age dependent. Younger patients seems to have more SVTs and conduction disturbances, whereas adult patients are prone to ventricular arrhythmias, junctional tachycardia, AV block, and premature ventricular contractions.

Drug interactions with digoxin are illustrated in Table 5. A good rule is that any coadministered antiarrhythmic agent will require a reduction in the digoxin dose.

_____ Table 5 _____

Digoxin Drug Interactions

| | | Mechanism | |
Drug	Change in Digoxin Level	Decreased Absorption	Decreased Clearance
Quinidine	Increase 75% to 100%		X
Amiodarone	Increase 50% to 100%		X
Verapamil	Increase 50% to 100%		X
Antacids	Decrease 25%	X	
Cholestryramine	Decrease 25%	X	
Neomycin	Decrease 25% to 30%	X	
Spironolactone	Increase 30%		X
Indomethacin	Increase 50%		X

_____ Table 6 _____

Recommendations for In-Hospital Drug Initiation

Quinidine
Procainamide
Disopyramide

Flecainide
Propafenone

Sotalol
Amiodarone

Antiarrhythmic Agents in the Ablation Era

The safety and efficacy of radiofrequency ablation procedures made complex drug therapy or use of agents with significant potential side-effect profiles frequently unnecessary. Some drugs, such as quinidine, disopyramide, phenytoin, and moricizine, have either rare applications or significant risk of proarrhythmia that their use becomes limited.

Short-term use of agents such as the class IC drugs or amiodarone are now considered while awaiting ablation or an anticipated resolution of arrhythmia due to natural history considerations. The same may be true for combination therapies, such as class IC drugs with amiodarone, procainamide, and amiodarone and mexiletine with a β-blocker for some ventricular arrhythmias.

Inpatient Versus Outpatient Therapy

Based on the above review of antiarrhythmic agents and published experience, many antiarrhythmic agents warrant initiation in a monitored hospital bed setting, rather than as an outpatient. Table 6 provides recommendations for drugs requiring in-hospital initiation. An Appendix of Drugs follows the references.

References

1. Ludomirsky A, Garson A Jr. Supraventricular tachycardia. In: Gillette PC, Garson A Jr, eds. *Pediatric Arrhythmias: Electrophysiology and Pacing.* Philadelphia: WB Saunders Co; 1990;380–426.
2. Kugler JD, Danford DA, Deal BJ, et al. Radiofrequency catheter ablation for tachyarrhythmias in children and adolescents. The Pediatric Electrophysiology Society. *N Engl J Med* 1994;330:1481–1487.

3. Perry JC, Iverson P, Kugler JD. Radiofrequency catheter ablation of tachyarrhythmias in young patients with structurally abnormal hearts. *Pacing Clin Electrophysiol* 1996;19:579.
4. Schaffer MS, Silka MJ, Ross BA, et al. Inadvertent atrioventricular block during radiofrequency catheter ablation. Results of the Pediatric Radiofrequency Ablation Registry. Pediatric Electrophysiology Society. *Circulation* 1996;94:3214–3220.
5. Case CL, Gillette PC, Crawford FA, et al. Comparison of medical care costs between successful radiofrequency catheter ablation and surgical ablation of accessory pathways in the pediatric age group. *Am J Cardiol* 1994;73:600–601.
6. Garson A Jr. Children with Wolff-Parkinson-White and supraventricular tachycardia: a model cost effectiveness analysis for pediatric chronic disease. *Am J Cardiol* 1993;72:502.
7. *Physicians Desk Reference.* Montvale, NJ: Medical Economics Data Production Co; 1996.
8. Vaughan Williams EM. Classification of antiarrhythmic drugs. In: Sandoe E, Flensted-Jensen E, Olsen KH, eds. *Cardiac Arrhythmias.* Sodertalje, Sweden: Astra; 1970;449–472.
9. Task Force of the Working Group on Arrhythmias of the European Society of Cardiology. The Sicilian Gambit. A new approach to the classification of antiarrhythmic drugs based on their actions on arrhythmogenic mechanisms. *Circulation* 1991;84:1831–1851.
10. Szefler SJ, Pieroni DR, Gingell RL, et al. Rapid elimination of quinidine in pediatric patients. *Pediatrics* 1982;70:370–375.
11. Kim SY, Benowitz NL. Poisoning due to class IA antiarrhythmic drugs. Quinidine, procainamide and disopyramide. *Drug Saf* 1990;5:393–420.
12. Webb CL, Dick M II, Rocchini AP, et al. Quinidine syncope in children. *J Am Coll Cardiol* 1987;9:1031–1037.
13. Marcus FI. Pharmacokinetic interactions between digoxin and other drugs. *J Am Coll Cardiol* 1985;5:82A–90A.
14. Dumesic DA, Silverman NH, Tobias S, et al. Transplacental cardioversion of fetal supraventricular tachycardia with procainamide. *N Engl J Med* 1982;307:1128–1131.
15. Benson DW Jr, Dunnigan A, Green TP, et al. Periodic procainamide for paroxysmal tachycardia. *Circulation* 1985;72:147–152.
16. Milstein S, Buetikofer J, Dunnigan A, et al. Usefulness of disopyramide for prevention of upright tilt-induced hypotension-bradycardia. *Am J Cardiol* 1990;65:1339–1344.
17. Tynan M, Keaton BR, Hayler AM, et al. The dosage of disopyramide in infants and children. *Br J Clin Pract* 1981;35(suppl 11):40–42.
18. Rosen MR, Hoffman BF, Wit AL. Electrophysiology and pharmacology of cardiac arrhythmias. V. Cardiac antiarrhythmic effects of lidocaine. *Am Heart J* 1975;89:526–536.
19. Schwartz PJ, Priori SG, Locati EH, et al. Long QT syndrome patients with mutations of the SCN5A and HERG genes have differential responses to Na+ channel blockade and to increases in heart rate. Implications for gene-specific therapy. *Circulation* 1995;92:3381–3386.
20. Moak JP, Smith RT, Garson A Jr. Mexiletine: an effective antiarrhythmic drug for treatment of ventricular arrhythmias in congenital heart disease. *J Am Coll Cardiol* 1987;10:824–829.
21. Chazov EI, Shugushev KK, Rosenshtraukh LV. Ethmozine. I. Effects of intravenous drug administration on paroxysmal supraventricular tachycardia in the preexcitation syndrome. *Am Heart J* 1984;108:475–482.

22. Evans VL, Garson A Jr, Smith RT, et al. Ethmozine (moricizine HCl): a promising new drug for "automatic" atrial ectopic tachycardia. *Am J Cardiol* 1987; 60:83F–86F.
23. Garson A Jr, Kugler JD, Gillette PC, et al. Control of late postoperative ventricular arrhythmias with phenytoin in young patients. *Am J Cardiol* 1980;46:290–294.
24. The Cardiac Arrhythmia Suppression Trial (CAST) Investigators: Preliminary report: effect of encainide and flecainide on mortality in a randomized trial of arrhythmia suppression after myocardial infarction. *N Engl J Med* 1989;321:406–412.
25. Hanson JW, Smith DW. The fetal hydantoin syndrome. *J Pediatr* 1975;87:285–290.
26. Roden DM, Woosley RL. Drug therapy. Tocainide. *N Engl J Med* 1986;315:41–45.
27. Perry JC, McQuinn RL, Smith RT Jr, et al. Flecainide acetate for resistant arrhythmias in the young: efficacy and pharmacokinetics. *J Am Coll Cardiol* 1989;14:185–191.
28. van Engelen AD, Weijtens O, Brenner JI, et al. Management outcome and follow-up of fetal tachycardia. *J Am Coll Cardiol* 1994;24:1371–1375.
29. Wren C, Campbell RWF. The response of paediatric arrhythmias to intravenous and oral flecainide. *Br Heart J* 1987;57:171–175.
30. Fish FA, Gillette PC, Benson DW Jr. Proarrhythmia, cardiac arrest and death in young patients receiving encainide and flecainide. The Pediatric Electrophysiology Group. *J Am Coll Cardiol* 1991;18:356–365.
31. Perry JC, Garson A Jr. Encainide and flecainide: separating the wheat from the chaff. *J Am Coll Cardiol* 1991;18:366–367.
32. Russell GAB, Martin RP. Flecainide toxicity. *Arch Dis Child* 1989;64:860–862.
33. Perry JC, Ayres NA, Carpenter RJ Jr. Fetal supraventricular tachycardia treated with flecainide acetate. *J Pediatr* 1991;118:303–305.
34. Till J, Herxheimer A. Death of a child with supraventricular tachycardia. *Lancet* 1992;339:1597–1598.
35. Janousek J, Paul T, Reimer A, et al. Usefulness of propafenone for supraventricular arrhythmias in infants and children. *Am J Cardiol* 1993;72:294–300.
36. Erickson C, Perry J, Marlow D, et al. Sudden death during propafenone therapy for atrial flutter in young postoperative heart patients. *Pacing Clin Electrophysiol* 1993;16:939.
37. Kates RE, Yee YG, Winkle RA. Metabolite cumulation during chronic propafenone dosing in arrhythmia. *Clin Pharmacol Ther* 1985;37:610–614.
38. Garson A Jr, Moak JP, Smith RT Jr, et al. Usefulness of intravenous propafenone for control of postoperative junctional ectopic tachycardia. *Am J Cardiol* 1987;59:1422–1424.
39. Pickoff AS, Zies L, Ferrer PL, et al. High-dose propranolol therapy in the management of supraventricular tachycardia. *J Pediatr* 1979;94:144–146.
40. Kleinman CS. Prenatal diagnosis and management of intrauterine arrhythmias. *Fetal Ther* 1986;1:92–95.
41. Trippel DL, Gillette PC. Atenolol in children with ventricular arrhythmias. *Am Heart J* 1990;119:1312–1316.
42. Trippel DL, Gillette PC. Atenolol in children with supraventricular tachycardia. *Am J Cardiol* 1989;64:233–236.
43. O'Marcaigh AS, MacLellan-Tobert SG, Porter CJ. Tilt-table testing and oral metoprolol therapy in young patients with unexplained syncope. *Pediatrics* 1994; 93:278–283.

44. Mehta AV, Chidambaram B. Efficacy and safety of intravenous and oral nadolol for supraventricular tachycardia in children. *J Am Coll Cardiol* 1992;19:630–635.
45. Esmolol Research Group. Intravenous esmolol for the treatment of supraventricular tachyarrhythmia: results of a multicenter, baseline-controlled safety and efficacy study in 160 patients. *Am Heart J* 1986;112:498–505.
46. Trippel DL, Wiest DB, Gillette PC. Cardiovascular and antiarrhythmic effects of esmolol in children. *J Pediatr* 1991;119:142–147.
47. Garson A Jr, Gillette PC, McVey P, et al. Amiodarone treatment of critical arrhythmias in children and young adults. *J Am Coll Cardiol* 1984;4:749–755.
48. Coumel P, Fidelle J. Amiodarone in the treatment of cardiac arrhythmias in children: one hundred thirty-five cases. *Am Heart J* 1980;100:1063–1069.
49. Perry JC, Knilans TK, Marlow D, et al. Intravenous amiodarone for life-threatening tachyarrhythmias in children and young adults. *J Am Coll Cardiol* 1993; 22:95–98.
50. Figa FH, Gow RM, Hamilton RM, et al. Clinical efficacy and safety of intravenous amiodarone in infants and children. *Am J Cardiol* 1993;74:573–577.
51. Perry JC, Fenrich AL, Hulse JE, et al. Pediatric use of intravenous amiodarone: efficacy and safety in critically ill patients from a multicenter protocol. *J Am Coll Cardiol* 1996;27:1246–1250.
52. Escoubet B, Coumel P, Poirer JM, et al. Suppression of arrhythmias within hours after a single oral dose of amiodarone and relation to plasma and myocardial concentrations. *Am J Cardiol* 1985;55:696–702.
53. Mostow ND, Vrobel TR, Noon D, et al. Rapid suppression of complex ventricular arrhythmias with high-dose oral amiodarone. *Circulation* 1986;73:1231–1238.
54. Donica SK, Paulsen AW, Simpson BR, et al. Danger of amiodarone therapy and elevated inspired oxygen concentrations in mice. *Am J Cardiol* 1996;77:109–110.
55. Spicer RL, Rocchini AP, Crowley DC, et al. Hemodynamic effects of verapamil in children and adolescents with hypertrophic cardiomyopathy. *Circulation* 1983;67:413–420.
56. Heissenbuttel RH, Bigger JT Jr. Bretylium tosylate: a newly available antiarrhythmic drug for ventricular arrhythmias. *Ann Intern Med* 1979;91:229–238.
57. Ellenbogen KA, Stambler BS, Wood MA, et al. Efficacy of intravenous ibutilide for rapid termination of atrial fibrillation and atrial flutter: a dose-response study. *J Am Coll Cardiol* 1996;28:130–136.
58. Ibutilide. *Med Lett* 1996;38:38–39.
59. Ohe T, Shimomura K, Aihahra N, et al. Idiopathic sustained left ventricular tachycardia: clinical and electrophysiologic characteristics. *Circulation* 1988; 77:560–568.
60. Wolff F, Breuker KH, Schlensker KH, et al. Prenatal diagnosis and therapy of fetal heart rate anomalies: with a contribution on the placental transfer of verapamil. *J Perinat Med* 1980;8:203–208.
61. Epstein ML, Kiel EA, Victorica BE. Cardiac decompensation following verapamil therapy in infants with supraventricular tachycardia. *Pediatrics* 1985; 75:737–740.
62. Dougherty AH, Jackman WM, Naccarelli GV, et al. Acute conversion of paroxysmal supraventricular tachycardia with intravenous diltiazem. IV. Diltiazem Study Group. *Am J Cardiol* 1992;70:587–592.
63. Overholt ED, Rheuban KS, Gutgesell HP, et al. Usefulness of adenosine for arrhythmias in infants and children. *Am J Cardiol* 1988;61:336–340.
64. Till J, Shinebourne EA, Rigby ML, et al. Clarke B, Ward DE, Rowland E. Efficacy and safety of adenosine in the treatment of supraventricular tachycardia in infants and children. *Br Heart J* 1989;62:204–211.

65. Wellens HJJ, Durrer D. Effect of digitalis on atrioventricular conduction and circus-movement tachycardias in patients with Wolff-Parkinson-White syndrome. *Circulation* 1973;47:1229–1233.

66. Byrum CJ, Wahl RA, Behrendt DM, et al. Ventricular fibrillation associated with the use of digitalis in a newborn infant with Wolff-Parkinson-White syndrome. *J Pediatr* 1982;101:400–403.

67. Kleinman CS, Copel JA, Weinstein EM, et al. In utero diagnosis and treatment of fetal supraventricular tachycardia. *Semin Perinatol* 1985;9:113–129.

68. Smith TW. Digitalis toxicity: epidemiology and clinical use of serum concentration measurements. *Am J Med* 1975;58:470–476.

Antiarrhythmic Drug Properties

Drug	Oral Dose	Dosing Interval	IV Initial and Maintenance	Therapeutic Level	Half-Life (h)	ECG Changes	Side Effects
Class IA							
Quinidine	30–60 mg/kg per d (sulfate)	Divided TID or QID	N/A	2–6 µg/ml	6–8	Increases PR, QRS, QTc	GI upset, tinnitus, thrombocytopenia, anemia, torsades de pointes
Procainamide	40–100 mg/kg per d	q4 h infants, q6–8 in older pts	7 mg/kg infants, 15 mg/kg older patients, infusion 40–80 µg/kg per min	4–8 µg/ml for PA or NAPA. Do not add levels.	Standard 2.5–4 Sustained 6–8	Increases PR, QRS, QTc	Lupus syndrome, arthralgia
Disopyramide	Infants 20–30 mg/kg, 2–10 y 9–24 mg/kg, >11 y 5–13 mg/kg	Divided QID (standard) or BID (sustained)	N/A	2–5 µg/ml	5	Prolongs QRS, QTc	Urinary retention, nausea, constipation, dry mouth, blurry vision, AV block
Class IB							
Lidocaine	N/A	N/A	1 mg/kg, repeated × 4, infusion 20–50 µg/kg per min	2–5 µg/ml	2	Slight decrease in QTc	Seizures, apnea
Mexiletine	2–5 mg/kg per dose	q8 h	N/A	0.8–2 µg/ml	6–11	May decrease QTc in LQT3	Nausea, skin rash
Moricizine	200–600 mg/m² per d	Divided TID	N/A	N/A	8	Slight increase in PR, QRS	Blurry vision, paresthesia, headache
Phenytoin	15 mg/kg load, 5–6 mg/kg maintenance	Load divided q6, maint q12	Load 1–3 mg/kg, maximum daily load 10–15 mg/kg	10–20 µg/ml	Infants = 12–24, >1 y old = 8, adult +24	Slight decrease in QTc	IV: hypotension. Oral: ataxia, nystagmus. Fetal defects.

Drug	Oral dose	Dosing interval	IV dose	Therapeutic level	Half-life (h)	ECG effects	Side effects
Tocainide	200 mg (adult)	BID or TID	N/A	3–9 µg/ml	10–11	Slight decrease in QTc	Nausea, vomiting, dizziness, paresthesias, pneumonitis
Class IC							
Flecainide	80–200 mg/m² per d	Infant, adult: q12, 1–10 y: q8 h	N/A	0.2–1.0 µg/ml	Infant, adult: 12+ 1–10 yrs: 8	Slight increase in PR, QRS, QTc (high dose)	Blurry vision, proarrhythmia (especially in CHD)
Propafenone	150–600 mg/m² per d	Divided q8 h	0.2–1.0 mg/kg, infusion 4–10 µg/kg/min	0.1–5 µg/ml	Depends on metabolism, usually 4–6 h	Increases PR, QRS, QTc	Blurry vision, proarrhythmia (especially in CHD)
Class II							
Propranolol	1–4 mg/kg per d	Infants: q6, child: q8, sustained release: q12	0.1–0.2 mg/kg	50–150 µg/ml	Infants: 3–4 h, >1 y: 6 h	Slow HR, may decrease QTc	Bradycardia, fatigue, AV block, nightmares, hypoglycemia, asthma
Atenolol	1–3 mg/kg per d	QD or BID	N/A	N/A	9–10	Similar to propranolol	Bradycardia, fatigue, asthma
Metoprolol	1–3 mg/kg per d	BID	N/A	N/A	3–8	Similar to propranolol	Not well known
Nadolol	1–2 mg/kg per d	QD	N/A	N/A	20–24	Similar to propranolol	Bradycardia, fatigue, asthma
Esmolol	N/A	N/A	500 µg/kg, then 50–200 µg/kg per min	N/A	7–10 min	Slight decrease HR, increase PR	Hypotension
Class III							
Amiodarone	Load 10–15 mg/kg, maintenance 2–5 mg/kg per d	Load divided q12, maintenance QD	5–6 mg/kg load, infusion 7–10 µg/kg per min	1.0–2.5 µg/kg	>24	Increases PR, QRS, QTc, decrease HR	Thyroid, liver, pulmonary, skin abnormalities, AV block, bradycardia, proarrhythmia

(continues)

Antiarrhythmic Drug Properties

Drug	Oral Dose	Dosing Interval	IV Initial and Maintenance	Therapeutic Level	Half-Life (h)	ECG Changes	Side Effects
Sotalol	90–200 mg/m² per d	Divided TID	0.2–1.5 mg/kg	N/A	7–12	Increase QTc, decrease HR	Torsades de pointes, bradycardia, AV block, negative inotrope
Bretylium	N/A	N/A	5 mg/kg	N/A	4–17 h	None	Hypotension
Ibutilide	N/A	N/A	10–25 µg/kg	N/A	6	Increase PR, marked QTc increase	Torsades de pointes, bradycardia, AV block, teratogenic
Class IV Verapamil	4–17 mg/kg	Standard QID/ TID, sustained QD/BID	0.15 mg/kg	0.1–0.4 µg/ml	4–7	Broad P wave, increase PR	Oral: constipation, headache, bradycardia, CHF. IV: hypotension
Diltiazem	30–120 mg/ dose (Adult)	TID	0.15–0.45 mg/kg, infusion 0.003 mg/ kg per min	0.03–0.27 µg/ ml	3–5	Increase PR, ± decrease HR	
Others Adenosine	N/A	N/A	100–300 µg/kg	N/A	7–10 s	Increase PR, PVC's and VT	Hypotension, bronchospasm, ventricular ectopy
Digoxin	Total 30 µg/kg load (20–25 in premies), Maintenance 5–10 µg/kg	Load divided q8 h Maintenance q12 or QD	IV dose generally 2/ 3 oral dose.	0.7–2.0 ng/ ml	1.5–2 d	Increases PR, depresses ST, some decrease QTc	Nausea, vomiting, visual changes, AV block, atrial and ventricular arrhythmias

N/A, not applicable.

Chapter 11

Emergency Management of Arrhythmias

Michael J. Silka, MD

The electrophysiological (EP) causes and methods for definitive treatment of the various cardiac arrhythmias were discussed in detail in the preceding chapters of this book. The purpose of this chapter is to provide a concise approach to (1) acute evaluation of the pediatric patient with an arrhythmia, (2) basic considerations in diagnostic methods, and (3) emergency treatments. Algorithms for the evaluation and emergency treatment of cardiac arrhythmias that were published by several health care organizations are used as a basis for the recommendations that are presented in this chapter.[1,2]

A fundamental premise of this chapter is that a cardiac arrhythmia is an emergency when it (1) results in significant compromise of end-organ perfusion or (2) has the potential to rapidly degenerate into an arrhythmia that will not sustain cardiac output (eg, asystole or ventricular fibrillation). Thus, a patient with impaired ventricular function and an atrial tachycardia at 180 beats per minute (bpm) may represent an emergency; conversely, a sustained supraventricular tachycardia (SVT) at 220 bpm in a young patient with normal cardiovascular physiology may be relatively well tolerated.

In practice, cardiac arrhythmias resulting in emergencies are encountered most frequently either in an emergency room or in the postoperative cardiac or intensive care unit. Although any type of arrhythmia may be encountered in either setting, the profound physiologic and metabolic changes which occur in the postoperative patient may evoke certain ar-

From Deal B, Wolff G, Gelband H, (eds.). *Current Concepts in Diagnosis and Management of Arrhythmias in Infants and Children*. Armonk, NY: Futura Publishing Co., Inc.; © 1998.

rhythmias infrequently encountered in other settings. For this reason, these arrhythmias will be considered separately.

Cardiac Arrhythmias Requiring Immediate Therapy

Acute and complete cessation of cardiac output in the pediatric patient will occur in three clinical scenarios: asystole, electromechanical dissociation, and ventricular fibrillation or pulseless ventricular tachycardia (VT). As irreversible neurological injury will occur within minutes of cessation of cerebral blood flow, the initial response in any of these settings should be initiation of basic cardiopulmonary resuscitation (CPR).[1,2]

The overall salvage rate in pediatric patients experiencing cardiac arrest remains poor, ranging between 2% and 17%.[3,4] Based on recent data, it would appear that the primary advance required to improve the outcomes of attempted resuscitation in children is in the area of rapid response emergency medical care systems. Clinical studies suggested a higher incidence (19%) of ventricular fibrillation in pediatric patients than previously reported, which may reflect some improvement in emergency response times. This is of critical importance as hospital discharge with no or minimal disability appears more likely when ventricular fibrillation rather than asystole is the initial arrhythmia at the time of attempted resuscitation.[4]

Asystole

Asystole should be the presumed diagnosis when cardiac arrest occurs in the pediatric patient. Following establishment of basic CPR, assisted ventilation (endotracheal intubation or ball-valve-mask) with 100% oxygen should be the first measure initiated. Electrocardiographic (ECG) monitoring may demonstrate an agonal bradycardia, usually a wide QRS complex rhythm with no effective mechanical systole (Figure 1). Either vascular or intraosseous access should be established rapidly. Epinephrine (0.01

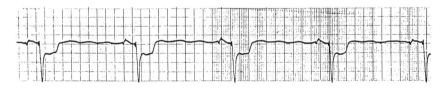

Figure 1. Terminal bradycardia recorded following prolonged attempted resuscitation in a patient with an end-stage dilated cardiomyopathy. Although there was electrical activity (sinus bradycardia at a rate of 28 bpm), no effective cardiac output was associated with this rhythm.

mg/kg) via intravenous or intraosseous routes or (0.1 mg/kg) via endotracheal administration represent standard doses during attempted resuscitative efforts and should be repeated at 3- to 5-minute intervals.

The proposed mechanism of epinephrine during CPR is augmentation of coronary blood flow due to systemic vasoconstriction. There is controversy in the medical literature regarding the potential beneficial or deleterious effects of higher doses of epinephrine during attempted resuscitation, ie, whether increasing the intravenous dose of epinephrine 10 times to 0.1 mg/kg improves overall outcome compared to a standard dose of 0.01 mg/kg.[5,6]

The use of other medications such as atropine, sodium bicarbonate, or calcium may be considered in the patient with asystole; however, the clinician should be aware that there are no scientific or clinical data to support the use of these agents in asystole. The need for a randomized clinical trial utilizing these agents and uniform criteria for reporting pediatric patient outcome was proposed.[7] Transthoracic pacing may be a helpful adjunct to pharmacologic therapy in this acute setting (discussion follows).

Electromechanical Dissociation

Electromechanical dissociation may occur in patients with advanced end-stage ventricular dysfunction or secondary to compromise of venous return (tamponade).[8] Initial resuscitative efforts for the patient with pulseless electrical activity are similar to those for asystole. However, if a reversible cause of electromechanical dissociation is present but not diagnosed, such as pneumothorax or pericardial effusion, resuscitation of the patient is improbable. This is particularly important in the patient with an indwelling central catheter or at risk for a tension pneumothorax. Pericardiocentesis and/or attempted evacuation of the pleural spaces should be performed before resuscitative efforts in such patients are terminated. The one exception to this approach may be the hypotensive patient with proximal aortic dissection and hemopericardium (eg, Marfan's syndrome), in whom pericardiocentesis may result in acute hemodynamic deterioration.[9]

Ventricular Fibrillation

As noted earlier in this chapter, the incidence of ventricular fibrillation in pediatric patients may be somewhat higher than previously reported. A shorter time to first response (initiation of CPR) and the presence of structural cardiovascular disease are factors related to a higher probability of ventricular fibrillation as the presenting arrhythmia when cardiac arrest occurs in a pediatric patient.[4,10]

If ventricular fibrillation is demonstrated during cardiac arrest in a young patient, asystole with artifact or disconnection of an ECG lead should be considered. Basic life support should be continued while this determination is made. However, the success of resuscitation is based on the prompt delivery of electrical defibrillation. Similar considerations and the need for immediate synchronized cardioversion apply in the patient with rapid, pulseless VT (Figure 2).

Current recommendations are for initial defibrillation with an energy of 2 J/kg using the largest paddle size that covers the thorax while maintaining separation from the other paddle.[2,11-13] An electrode gel must be used to reduce impedance at the skin-electrode interface. If the initial 2 J/kg shock is ineffective, defibrillation should be repeated at 4 J/kg, once or twice as necessary. Following three shocks, epinephrine should be administered (0.01–0.1 mg/kg) followed by repeated defibrillation shocks (4 J/kg).

If the above protocols did not terminate ventricular fibrillation, lidocaine (1–2 mg/kg) or Bretylium (5–10 mg/kg) may be administered. However, the use of these agents is based on empiric observations in adult

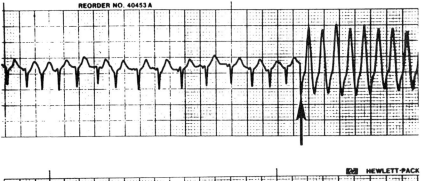

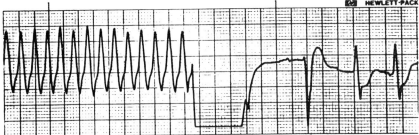

Figure 2. SVT degenerating into pulseless VT followed by the rapid delivery of direct-current countershock. As this rhythm was organized with regular QRS periodicity, the DC shock was delivered synchronized to the QRS complex. Due to multiple episodes of hypotensive tachycardia in this patient, cardioversion-defibrillation electrodes were previously placed.

patients with refractory ventricular fibrillation, with no scientific data to support or refute the use of these medications in pediatric patients.

Emergency Evaluation and Treatment of Bradyarrhythmias

Bradycardia represents an emergency situation in the young patient when associated with compromised end-organ perfusion, most commonly with neurological (syncope) or cardiovascular (hypoperfusion/congestive heart failure) manifestations. The two common settings for bradycardia in young patients are in critically ill patients, where bradycardia represents a failure of normal physiological adaptation, or in patients with cardiovascular disease, where bradycardia represents intrinsic or acquired dysfunction of either the sinus node (SN) or atrioventricular node (AVN)-His Purkinje systems. As the initial treatments of bradycardia in these two settings differ, determination of the etiology of bradycardia is a primary consideration.

Bradycardia in the Critically Ill Patient

In the critically or terminally ill young patient, bradycardia with eventual progression to asystole is the most prevalent terminal cardiac rhythm.[10] In this setting, bradycardia often is a response to hypoxemia-mediated vagal discharge, which results in progressive sinus bradycardia. Progression to high degrees of AV block may also occur if the primary cause is not corrected. Thus, oxygenation and ventilation are the recommended primary treatments for inappropriate bradycardia in the critically ill young patient.[1,2] Vital signs and tissue perfusion should be evaluated following this initial intervention.

Persistent bradycardia resulting in tissue hypoperfusion requires pharmacologic intervention. For acute bradycardia, as with asystole, intravenous or intraosseous epinephrine (0.01 mg/kg) or endotracheal (0.1 mg/kg) are standard recommendations. Isoproterenol may also be used for chronotropic support and is well tolerated as an infusion (0.01–0.1 μg/kg/min). Atropine may be used (0.02 mg/kg intravenous), particularly to prevent vagally-mediated bradycardia during endotracheal intubation. Another important consideration is bradycardia in the patient with neurological injury, where either sinus bradycardia or AV block may be secondary manifestations of increased intracranial pressure.

Bradycardia in the Patient with Structural Cardiovascular Disease

Progressive SN dysfunction is a common and progressive late sequelae of surgical interventions for congenital heart disease. Although bradycardia is most frequently asymptomatic and recognized during the routine post-operative surveillance of these patients, presentation with syncope or progressive congestive heart failure may also occur. These symptoms may be due to either sinus arrest or paroxysmal AV block and require emergent treatment. Clinically, profound bradycardia may be anticipated in the following settings:

1. Following electrical cardioversion of a SVT.
2. During anesthesia induction in the patient with an inherent disorder of AV or distal conduction.
3. During drug- or electrolyte-induced bradycardia.

The initial treatments remain oxygenation and ventilation, with pharmacologic treatment (epinephrine, isoproterenol, or atropine) to follow immediately. Several methods of temporary cardiac pacing may also be of benefit, particularly if rate support is required for several hours or days.

Transcutaneous Transthoracic Pacing. There is limited experience in this mode of pacing the pediatric patient, in which large dispersive electrode patches are applied to the anterior and posterior thorax of the patient. The primary advantages of this method are that emergency pacing may be initiated within 60 seconds and that application of the transthoracic patches does not require interruption of other resuscitative measures. In general, a current of 40–60 mA is required. Most current model defibrillators have the capacity for transthoracic pacing.

The primary limitations of transthoracic pacing are pain in the conscious patient due to chest wall muscle contraction and skin burn or injury at the electrode site. Small burns were reported in neonates within 30 minutes of transthoracic stimulation, indicating the need for careful observation. The use of adult-sized self-adhesive electrodes is appropriate in children over 15 kg in size. There is also a small risk of arrhythmia induction due to the asynchronous mode of pacing.

Transesophageal Pacing. Although transesophageal pacing is most frequently used for the diagnosis and termination of reentrant SVT, it may also be used for profound sinus bradycardia if AV conduction is intact. The distance to insert the catheter to a level adjacent to the posterior left atrium (LA) may be predicted based on body size.[14] For emergency pacing, a 4 French bipolar electrode catheter is utilized. A current of 10–20 mA is generally required for consistent atrial capture, with a pulse width extended to 10 milliseconds when feasible. Esophageal pacing of the ventricle remains unreliable; thus, other methods of pacing are required for AV block (Figure 3).

Temporary Transvenous Pacing. This method of emergency pacing requires placement of a catheter via central venous access. Generally, the

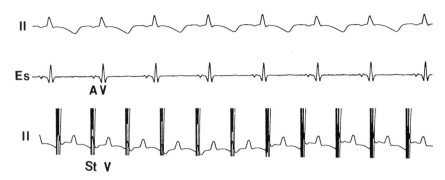

Figure 3. Attempted esophageal ventricular pacing. The two upper tracings are ECG lead II and an esophageal lead recording a small atrial electrogram (A) and a large ventricular electrogram (V). However, the third panel (ECG lead II) demonstrates atrial rather than ventricular pacing from this site, reflecting proximity of the LA to the esophagus.

catheter is positioned at the right ventricular (RV) apex under fluoroscopic guidance. The one exception may be in the post-Fontan patient, where retrograde arterial access to the left ventricle is required. The most common indication for temporary transvenous pacing is the neonate with congenital complete AV block.

Although temporary transvenous pacing may provide reliable and long-term ventricular pacing, there are several limitations in pediatric patients. The first is risk of perforation of the RV. Loss of capture, a friction rub, or pericardial effusion/tamponade may be signs of lead perforation. A second limitation is loss of capture due to lead dislodgment, estimated to occur in 25% of temporary transvenous lead systems.[15] A third is the risk of infection if the catheter is in position for more than 48 hours. The primary indication for temporary transvenous pacing in the patient with bradycardia is to provide a stable heart rate until a permanent lead system may be safely implanted or during anesthesia in a patient with distal conduction system disease.

Epicardial Pacing Wires in the Postoperative Patient. Following open heart surgery, temporary epicardial pacing wires are routinely placed to assist in weaning the patient from cardiopulmonary bypass. In general, these wires are removed 48–72 hours postsurgery, although they may be used for pacing for up to 10 days in the event of transient AV block or profound sinus bradycardia. Although this method of pacing is convenient and quite useful in the immediate perioperative period, exit block may occur suddenly, resulting in severe bradycardia. For this reason, pacing thresholds as well as evidence of infection should be evaluated on a daily basis. If sudden exit block occurs, the pacing output should be set at a maximal value. A second cause of exit block is electrolyte disorder, particularly potassium. Potential treatments for exit block are to reverse the polarity of the pacing wires or to use the skin as a ground if one wire is defective.

Emergency Evaluation and Treatment of Tachyarrhythmias

The initial evaluation of the patient with a sustained tachycardia is similar to that of the patient with profound bradycardia, ie, an assessment of perfusion, respiratory effort, and level of consciousness. Beyond this initial evaluation, the other aspect that must be considered is the potential for the tachycardia to degenerate to an arrhythmia that will not sustain cardiac output, eg, atrial fibrillation in the patient with an accessory AV connection.

Narrow QRS Complex Tachycardias

A number of cardiac arrhythmias may result in a sustained narrow QRS complex tachycardia in young patients (Table 1). The approach to the differential diagnosis of this problem was discussed in Chapter 5.

It is important to emphasize that most but not all episodes of narrow QRS complex tachycardias are due to reentrant SVT in young patients. For example, VT in the newborn characteristically has a relatively narrow QRS complex and may be well tolerated for brief intervals. Second, au-

_____ **Table 1** _____

Narrow QRS Complex Tachycardia: Diagnostic Considerations

Sinus tachycardia
Reentrant SVT with 1:1 AV conduction
   Orthodromic reciprocating tachycardia
   AV nodal reentrant tachycardia
   Permanent form junctional reciprocating tachycardia
Reentrant SVT: variable AV conduction
   Atrial reentrant tachycardia (atrial flutter)
   Atrial fibrillation
Automatic ectopic tachycardia
   Atrial
   Junctional
Ventricular tachycardia
   Newborn
   Fascicular

tomatic atrial and junctional tachycardias are relatively common in young patients and infrequently are responsive to either synchronized direct current (DC) cardioversion or adenosine. Third, the rate of sinus tachycardia may exceed 220 bpm in the febrile, dehydrated infant or following ingestion of a sympathomimetic agent. In general, however, most episodes of narrow QRS complex tachycardia represent some form of reentrant SVT.

The clinical significance of an episode of sustained SVT is related to the age of the patient, rate and duration of the episode of tachycardia, and the presence of associated cardiovascular disease. Thus, an episode of sustained SVT in the older child without structural heart disease primarily will produce palpitations or chest discomfort, usually prompting an evaluation within 2–4 hours; evidence of cardiovascular dysfunction is rarely seen unless persisting for more than 8–12 hours. In contrast, SVT in the newborn may result in more profound clinical deterioration with progressive ventricular dysfunction and pulmonary congestion as the primary clinical manifestations; these symptoms may be the result of prolonged tachycardia that went unrecognized. Cardiovascular collapse was reported in several clinical series analyzing sustained SVT in the newborn infant.[16,17]

SVT in the older patient with structural cardiovascular disease or impaired ventricular function may represent an emergent clinical situation. In these patients, the loss of AV mechanical synchrony and reduced ventricular reserve may result in rapid hemodynamic deterioration during tachycardia.

Therapy for Supraventricular Tachycardia

Therapy for SVT should be initiated after obtaining the diagnosis by ECG recording. Simple vagal maneuvers may be initiated immediately. In the infant, this most commonly is performed as a large icebag applied firmly to the face and forehead for 30–60 seconds or by some form of nasopharyngeal stimulation. A variety of vagal maneuvers, such as breath holding, Valsalva maneuver, or having the patient assume an inverted posture (feet up-head down), may be attempted in the older patient. The overall efficacy of these procedures is generally 30% to 50 % for tachycardias involving conduction over the AVN. Vagal maneuvers are not effective in atrial flutter (AF) or other primary atrial tachycardias, although some transient slowing of AV conduction may be observed, thereby helping in diagnosing the mechanism of tachycardia.

Adenosine replaced most other forms of pharmacologic therapy for acute pharmacologic termination of reentrant SVT involving the AVN. Adenosine is an endogenous nucleoside that produces acute AVN blockade and effectively terminates up to 90% of acute episodes of SVT.[18] The standard recommended dosage is 0.1 mg/kg, which must be delivered rapidly through the hub of the intravenous access due to the very short half-life of this agent; administration via an arterial or umbilical venous line is generally not effective. If not effective, and all problems with intravenous access and rate of administration were excluded, the dosage may be doubled. Potential side effects include shortness of breath, headache, and flushing due to the vasodilatory and bronchoconstrictive effects of adenosine. One must always be prepared for the rare occurrence of ventricular fibrillation[19,20] that may result from adenosine-induced acceleration of the tachycardia with rapid ventricular response; torsades de pointes and antidromic tachycardia using an additional accessory connection were also reported. For these reasons a defibrillator should be on hand at all times adenosine is used. The administration of adenosine may also reveal atrial tachycardia or AF with transient high-grade AV block. In this case, alternative therapies (below) are indicated for arrhythmia termination.

Verapamil (0.1 mg/kg intravenous) also is an effective agent in the treatment of SVT in the older child. However, due to the potential for hypotension in the infant with SVT, verapamil should not be used in this setting and in the presence of profound circulatory compromise.[21] Intravenous digoxin is another form of therapy for SVT. However, digoxin is not indicated as acute therapy in the patient with circulatory compromise due to the delayed onset of effect.

Ibutilide is a new selective class III antiarrhythmic agent that showed some promise in the acute treatment of AF and atrial fibrillation. Conversion efficacy for intravenous ibutilide is 50% to 70% for AF and 30% to 50% for atrial fibrillation.[22,23] Ibutilide prolongs action potential duration and effective refractory period and has a short half-life (10 minutes).[22,24] The standard dose is 0.01–0.02 mg/kg given over 10 minutes and repeated 10 minutes later. There is minimal pediatric experience, although it was effective in several children with AF associated with congenital heart disease in this author's experience. The potential for serious proarrhythmia exists, with QT prolongation and the development of polymorphic VT, with up to 2% of patients requiring cardioversion for this arrhythmia.[24,25]

Two other forms of acute therapy for SVT are electrical. The first is esophageal overdrive pacing, which may be used for both diagnostic and therapeutic purposes. Briefly, a bipolar electrode catheter is positioned at a predetermined distance in the esophagus, with atrial pacing at a cycle length (CL) of 70% to 80% of the tachycardia CL. Placement of the esophageal catheter may also terminate the SVT due to nasopharyngeal stimulation. Success rates as high as 91% for conversion of SVT to sinus rhythm was reported with this technique.[26] However, this method is not universally available, particularly in emergency room settings.

For the infant or child with significant hemodynamic compromise associated with SVT, synchronized DC cardioversion remains the definitive therapy.[13] An initial energy of 0.5 J/kg should be selected. Several impor-

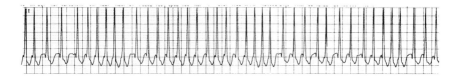

Figure 4. ECG lead II demonstrating a rapid, irregular tachycardia in a patient with prior surgery for congenital heart disease. The primary diagnostic considerations are AF or atrial fibrillation. Due to hypotension, DC cardioversion was performed to restore sinus rhythm.

tant details of cardioversion should be quickly considered prior to performance of this procedure:

1. Synchronization of the device to the patient's ECG should be assured, as shock delivery during the upstroke of the T wave may result in ventricular fibrillation. If ventricular fibrillation does occur, the defibrillator must be changed to the asynchronous mode before a rescue shock will be delivered.
2. The patient should be sedated.
3. Airway control and ventilatory support must be available; the physician must be aware of the potential for prolonged apnea following cardioversion.
4. Use of the largest-sized paddle that avoids contact with the other electrode.

If the initial shock is not effective, the energy should be doubled and the shock repeated. If there is evidence of significant respiratory or circulatory compromise, initiation of assisted ventilation or partial correction of metabolic acidosis may be required before cardioversion is effective. The possibility of an automatic rhythm not responsive to cardioversion should be reviewed when cardioversion fails.

The decision to use vagal maneuvers, adenosine, pacing, or cardioversion is based on the patient's clinical status. The more compromised the patient, the more urgent the need for definitive treatment, ie, synchronized cardioversion. Also, the patient with an irregular tachycardia should be presumed to have AF or atrial fibrillation, which will not respond to vagal stimuli or adenosine (Figure 4).

Wide QRS Complex Tachycardias

Evaluation of the young patient with a wide QRS complex tachycardia requires a brief but systematic evaluation of the patient's vital signs, overall clinical status, and determination of any potential causative factors or associated cardiovascular disease. The differential diagnosis of wide QRS

_____ Table 2 _____

Wide QRS Complex Tachycardia: Diagnostic Considerations

Sinus/supraventricular with bundle branch block*
    Sinus tachycardia
    Atrial tachycardia
        Ectopic automatic
        Atrial reentrant
    Reentrant supraventricular
Sinus/supraventricular with antegrade accessory connection conduction
    Antidromic reciprocating tachycardia
    Atriofascicular tachycardia
    Atrial flutter/fibrillation with AC conduction
Ventricular tachycardia
    Monomorphic
    Polymorphic
    Ventricular flutter/fibrillation (coarse)
    Hyperkalemic ventricular tachycardia ("sine wave")

* Bundle branch block may be preexisting or rate related.

tachycardia is summarized in Table 2. Analysis of the ECG may allow a determination of the mechanism of wide QRS tachycardia[27-30] (Figure 5). VT is present if there is AV dissociation, with the ventricular rate exceeding that of the atrium; other criteria favoring VT include a QRS interval greater than 0.14 seconds and a superior QRS axis. If there is a right bundle branch block (RBBB), VT is more likely if there is a monophasic qR in V_1 and a deep S wave in V_6. If there is a left bundle-branch block (LBBB), VT is more likely if there is a notched S wave and a broad R wave (>30 millisec-

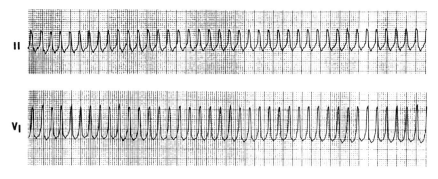

Figure 5. ECG leads II and V_1 demonstrating a regular wide QRS complex tachycardia with an apparent 1:1 P-QRS complex relationship. In this 2-month-old infant, the differential includes both SVT and VT (Table 2); however, a persistent wide QRS complex tachycardia in an infant favors a diagnosis of VT, which was confirmed at EP testing.

onds) in V_1 and V_2 and a Q wave in V_6.[29] Alternatively, AF in a patient with intrinsic bundle branch block may result in a sustained wide QRS complex tachycardia. Other potential causes of a wide QRS complex tachycardia include orthodromic reciprocating tachycardia with either RBBB or LBBB aberrancy or antidromic reciprocating tachycardia with either an AV or atriofascicular connection.[31]

Synchronized DC cardioversion should be the first response to the patient with a sustained wide QRS complex tachycardia resulting in hemodynamic compromise. The same precautionary steps as discussed above with elective cardioversion for narrow QRS complex tachycardias should be employed. In general, an energy of 1–2 J/kg should be used, with the energy doubled if the first shock is not effective.

For the patient with hemodynamically tolerated wide QRS complex tachycardia, a few brief diagnostic measures may be indicated. In the patient with congenital heart disease, AF with bundle branch block should always be a consideration. Thus, adenosine may allow determination of the diagnosis by producing AV block, but precautions should be taken because of the possibility of accelerating the tachycardia and provoking ventricular fibrillation. An esophageal lead may allow determination of a diagnosis of VT with ventriculo-atrial (VA) dissociation (Figure 6); however, 1:1 VA concordance does not allow differentiation between VT with retrograde AVN conduction and reciprocating SVT.

The use of lidocaine for attempted conversion of hemodynamically tolerated VT to sinus rhythm is commonly recommended; however, the efficacy of lidocaine is only approximately 20%. In a recent double-blind crossover study, procainamide was much more effective in the conversion of sustained monomorphic VT to sinus rhythm (78% vs. 20% for lidocaine).[32] The primary efficacy of lidocaine would appear to be in suppression of premature ventricular contractions in the patient at risk for recurrent VT.

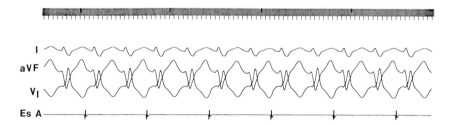

Figure 6. Use of an esophageal ECG (Es A) lead to differentiate SVT from VT. The top three channels are ECG leads I, aVF, and V_1. There are two QRS complexes for each atrial electrogram, which establishes the rhythm as VT at a CL of 350 milliseconds with retrograde 2:1 AV conduction.

Another problem that may confront the clinician is the patient with recurrent episodes of VT. In this scenario, repeated cardioversion may be injurious to ventricular function, and thus other suppressive forms of antiarrhythmic therapy should be utilized. Currently, intravenous amiodarone appears to be a promising agent for the suppression of recurrent VT. Based on limited experience, an initial total intravenous dose of 5 mg/kg (1 mg/kg every 5 minutes) was recommended, followed by a maintenance infusion dose (3–10 µg/kg per minute).[33]

Emergency evaluation and treatment for the young patient with recurrent polymorphic VT may be particularly difficult. If the arrhythmias are related to idiopathic prolongation of the QT interval occurring in the setting of sinus tachycardia, treatment with intravenous β-blockade (0.1 mg/kg) should be the initial step. However, in the setting of bradycardia, rate support with transvenous pacing or isoproterenol infusion

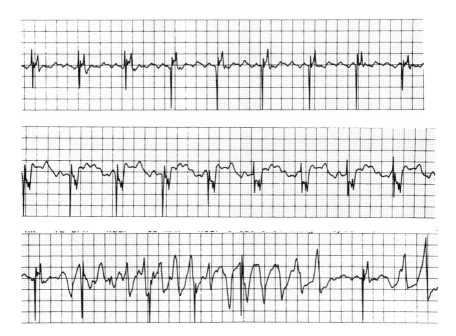

Figure 7. Drug-induced QT prolongation and proarrhythmia. The top ECG (lead II) demonstrates baseline AF with ventricular pacing at a CL of 840 milliseconds. The second ECG demonstrates marked prolongation of both the QRS complex and QT interval following 1.0 mg ibutilide, administered for attempted cardioversion of the AF. The third ECG demonstrates polymorphic VT, with intermittent nonsensing of the ventricular electrogram by the pacemaker during tachycardia. The pacemaker rate was increased to 100 bpm (600-millisecond CL) with complete suppression of ventricular ectopy.

is indicated (Figure 7). Evaluation for any potential ingestion and correction of electrolyte abnormalities should be aggressively pursued; in this setting, intravenous magnesium may be the treatment of choice in a dose of 20–50 mg/kg given intravenously over 2–3 minutes. Additionally, the elimination of any antiarrhythmic or noncardiac drugs with the potential for proarrhythmic effects should be considered[34] (Table 3).

Other possible causes of polymorphic VT include advanced ventricular dysfunction or myocardial ischemia. Periinfarction ventricular arrhythmias are probably underrecognized by pediatric cardiologists, as underscored by a recent report.[35] The primary efforts should be directed toward hemodynamic monitoring and support and the judicious use of antiarrhythmics for suppression of tachycardia.

_____ Table 3 _____

Classes of Medications with Reported Proarrhythmic Potential

Antiarrhythmic
    Class IA, IC
    Class III
Antibiotic
    Erythromycin
    Pentamadine
    Trimethoprim-sulfamethoxazole
Antifungal
    Fluconazole
    Intraconazole
    Ketocomazole
Antihistamine
    Astemizole
    Terfenadine
Central/peripheral nervous system agents
    Haloperidol
    Monoamine oxidase inhibitors
    Phenothinzine derivatives
    Pimozide
    Risperidone
    Tricyclic compounds
Others
    Anesthetics
    Bepridil
    Cisapride
    Indapamide
    Inotropic agents (amrinone, milrinone)
    Probucol

Postoperative Cardiac Arrhythmias

Acute changes in cardiovascular physiology, autonomic tone, and electrolyte balance frequently occur in the acute postoperative cardiac patient. Given these profound alterations, arrhythmias are frequent in these patients.

Bradyarrhythmias commonly occur as a sequelae of surgical intervention, involving either trauma to the SN or distal conduction system. In general, rate support in postoperative patients is provided with epicardial pacing wires, although atrial rate may also be increased with isoproterenol or transesophageal pacing. Acute bradycardia in the postoperative patient may also be a manifestation of respiratory insufficiency, either hypoventilation or tension pneumothorax. Treatment for bradycardia in this setting is based on the correction of the primary problem.

Tachyarrhythmias were discussed in this and several other chapters. Primary atrial tachycardias (flutter) and SVTs require prompt recognition and termination via pharmacologic or electrical means (overdrive pacing or cardioversion).[13,23,25] If there is doubt regarding the diagnosis, electrograms may be recorded from atrial pacing wires to allow evaluation of the ratio of atrial to ventricular depolarizations. This may be performed simply by attaching the two atrial wires to the right and left arm leads of the ECG and evaluating lead I.

Two physical causes of atrial tachycardia in the postoperative patient are catheter-induced ectopy due to mechanical irritation and the presence of an atrial thrombus. The latter deserves consideration in the patient with single ventricle (Fontan) physiology, where sluggish postoperative circulation and abnormalities of the anticoagulation system may predispose to acute thrombus formation, with secondary acute elevation of right atrial pressure resulting in either brady- or tachyarrhythmias.[36] Finally, concurrent use of inotropic agents may result in significant sinus tachycardia, without easily identifiable P waves.

Junctional ectopic tachycardia (JET) is one arrhythmia that occurs predominantly in the acute postoperative cardiac patient. The mechanism of this arrhythmia appears to be enhanced automaticity of tissues in the region of the common His bundle.[37] The ECG characteristics of JET include a narrow or wide complex QRS, the same as during sinus rhythm. There may be AV dissociation by default, due to the ventricular rate exceeding the atrial rate (Figure 8). At times this arrhythmia is well tolerated, with minimal compromise of circulatory dynamics. At other times, however, the rate of tachycardia may exceed 300 per minute, resulting in hypotension and hypoperfusion. In this setting, emergency therapies are mandated.

An important consideration in the treatment of JET is that this is a transient arrhythmia, usually less than 48–72 hours in duration. Thus, the goal in treatment is to maintain organ perfusion by either converting JET

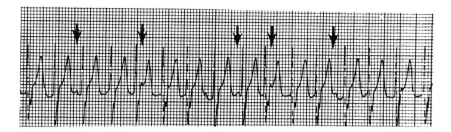

Figure 8. ECG characteristics of JET. There is a narrow QRS complex tachycardia at a CL of 360 milliseconds; there is AV dissociation by default, with the ventricular rate exceeding that of the atrium. Atrial depolarizations (P waves) are indicated by the arrows.

to sinus rhythm or by slowing the ventricular rate to allow adequate cardiac output.

The treatment of JET is controversial, based on differing experience of various institutions. Certain initial steps in therapy appear to be uniform, however. The first is that this arrhythmia is catecholamine sensitive, and reduction or withdrawal of sympathomimetic agents should be an early consideration. The second step is that digoxin, at standard intravenous dosage, may be of some benefit in control of JET and unlikely to result in an adverse effect. Beyond these initial steps, there is some controversy. The use of intravenous procainamide (15 mg/kg) over 60 minutes is often effective in slowing the rate of JET, if not resulting in tachycardia termination; diltiazem may also be effective. A recent study[37] also suggested similar benefit with intravenous amiodarone, at an initial dose of 5 mg/kg over 30–60 minutes. The goal is to at least slow the rate of tachycardia, either to allow adequate diastolic filling to maintain cardiac output or to institute overdrive atrial pacing to restore AV synchrony. The primary problem with either procainamide or amiodarone is potential depression of myocardial function with further provocation of hypotension and hypoperfusion.

The use of cooling blankets to result in central hypothermia is another modality that can be used for the control of JET resulting in hemodynamic compromise.[38] In general, the goal is to reduce the core temperature, while maintaining perfusion of critical organs. A final treatment that was proposed is the use of catheter ablation of the JET focus.[39] Although there are few reports of this treatment, permanent AV block and the need for permanent cardiac pacing should be anticipated with this approach.

The use of paired ventricular pacing was revisited recently and appears to provide a very effective therapy for JET.[40] This technique results in halving the effective heart rate since the second beat of the pair does not produce a mechanical systole. Waldo and associates[41] originally described the technique for management of JET in a postoperative child in 1976.

There are several potential causes of a wide QRS complex tachycardia in the postoperative patient. Several of these were already discussed, such as SVT or AF with aberrant conduction or VT. Another potential cause of VT in the postoperative patient is hyperkalemia. This electrolyte abnormality most frequently occurs in the hypoperfused, oliguric patient where cellular breakdown and metabolic acidosis may result in sudden increase in serum potassium to values greater than 7.0 mEq/L. The characteristic wide complex tachycardia of hyperkalemia is a "sine-wave" QRS morphology at rates greater than 200 bpm.[42] As with other acute tachyarrhythmias, recognition of the etiology of the arrhythmia is the basis for effective treatment. Acute treatment methods include hyperventilation, intravenous NaHCO$_3$, and calcium.

Conclusions

The appropriate emergency treatment of any arrhythmia begins with an accurate assessment of the EP mechanism involved. The wide array of pharmacologic agents available improved our ability to safely manage most critical arrhythmias. However, it is the ultimate responsibility of the clinician to be familiar with both the beneficial actions and potential adverse effects of any treatment modality used and to be prepared to respond rapidly and appropriately in such settings.

References

1. Guidelines for cardiopulmonary resuscitation and emergency cardiac care. Emergency Cardiac Care Committee and Subcommittees, American Heart Association. *JAMA* 1992;268:2251–2281.
2. Chamides L, Hazinski MF, eds. *Textbook of Pediatric Advanced Life Support*, Vol 7. Dallas: American Heart Association; 1994:1–12.
3. Eisenberg M, Bergner L, Hallstrom A. Epidemiology of cardiac arrest and resuscitation in children. *Ann Emerg Med* 1983;12:672–674.
4. Mogayzel C, Quan L, Graves JR, et al. Out-of-hospital ventricular fibrillation in children and adolescents: causes and outcomes. *Ann Emerg Med* 1995;25:484–491.
5. Dieckmanm RA, Vardis R. High-dose epinephrine in pediatric out-of-hospital cardiopulmonary arrest. *Pediatrics* 1995;95:901–913.
6. Hoekstra JW, Griffith R, Kelley R, et al. Effect of standard-dose versus high-dose epinephrine on myocardial high-energy phosphates during ventricular fibrillation and closed-chest CPR. *Ann Emerg Med* 1993;22:1385–1391.
7. Zaritsky A. Pediatric resuscitation pharmacology. Members of the Medications in Pediatric Resuscitation Panel. *Ann Emerg Med* 1993;22:445–455.
8. Herlitz J, Estrom L, Wennerblom B, et al. Survival among patients with out-of-hospital cardiac arrest found in electromechanical dissociation. *Resuscitation* 1995;29:97–106.
9. Isselbacher EM, Cigarroa JE, Eagle KE. Cardiac tamponade complicating proximal aortic dissection. Is pericardiocentesis harmful? *Circulation* 1994;90:2375–2378.

10. Walsh CK, Krongrad E. Terminal cardiac electrical activity in pediatric patients. *Am J Cardiol* 1983;51:557–561.
11. Gutgessel HP, Tacker HA, Geddes LA, et al. Energy dose for ventricular defibrillation in children. *Pediatrics* 1976;58:898–901.
12. Atkins DL, Sirna S, Kieso R, et al. Pediatric defibrillation: importance of paddle size in determining transthoracic impedance. *Pediatrics* 1988;82:914–918.
13. Kerber RE. Transthoracic cardioversion of atrial fibrillation and flutter: standard techniques and new advances. *Am J Cardiol* 1996;78(suppl 8A):22–26.
14. Benson DW Jr, Sanford M, Dunnigan A, et al. Transesophageal atrial pacing threshold: role of interelectrode spacing, pulse width, and catheter insertion depth. *Am J Cardiol* 1984;53:63–67.
15. Silver MD, Goldschlager N. Temporary transvenous cardiac pacing in the critical care setting. *Chest* 1988;93:607–613.
16. Gikonyo BM, Dunnigan A, Benson DW Jr. Cardiovascular collapse in infants: association with paroxysmal atrial tachycardia. *Pediatrics* 1985;76:922–926.
17. Deal BJ, Dick M, Beerman L, et al. Cardiac arrest in young patients with Wolff-Parkinson-White syndrome. *Pacing Clin Electrophysiol* 1995;18:815. Abstract.
18. Camm AJ, Garratt CJ. Drug therapy. *N Engl J Med* 1991;325:1621–1629.
19. Mulla N, Karpawich PP. Ventricular fibrillation following adenosine therapy for supraventricular tachycardia in a neonate with concealed Wolff-Parkinson-White syndrome treated with digoxin. *Pediatr Emerg Care* 1995;11:238–239.
20. Ben-Sorek ES, Wiesel J. Ventricular fibrillation following adenosine administration. A case report. *Arch Intern Med* 1993;153:2701–2702.
21. Epstein ML, Kiel EA, Victorica BE. Cardiovascular decompensation following verapamil therapy in infants with supraventricular tachycardia. *Pediatrics* 1985;75:737–740,
22. Stambler BS, Wood MA, Ellenbogen KA, et al. Efficacy and safety of repeated intravenous doses of ibutilide for rapid conversion of atrial flutter or fibrillation. The Ibutilide Repeat Dose Study Investigators. *Circulation* 1996;94:1613–1621.
23. Ellenbogen KA, Clemo HF, Stambler BS, et al. Efficacy of ibutilide for termination of atrial fibrillation and flutter. *Am J Cardiol* 1996;78(suppl 8A):42–45.
24. Roden DM. Ibutilide and the treatment of atrial arrhythmias. A new drug "almost unheralded" is now available to US physicians. *Circulation* 1996;94:1499–1502.
25. Kowey PR, VanderLugt JT, Luderer JR. Safety and risk/benefit analysis of ibutilide for acute conversion of atrial fibrillation/flutter. *Am J Cardiol* 1996;78(suppl8A):46–52.
26. Dick M II, Scott WA, Serwer GS, et al. Acute termination of supraventricular tachyarrhythmias in children by transesophageal pacing. *Am J Cardiol* 1988;61:925–927.
27. Kindwall KE, Brown J, Josephson ME. Electrocardiographic criteria for ventricular tachycardia in wide complex left bundle branch block morphology tachycardias. *Am J Cardiol* 1988;61:1279–1283.
28. Brugada P, Brugada J, Mont L, et al. A new approach to the differential diagnosis of a regular tachycardia with a wide QRS complex. *Circulation* 1991;83:1649–1659.
29. Andries EW, Brugada J, Brugada P. An algorithm for diagnosing wide QRS complex tachycardia. *Prim Cardiol* 1992;18:29–46.
30. Steurer G, Gursoy S, Frey B, et al. The differential diagnosis on the electrocardiogram between ventricular tachycardia and preexcited tachycardia. *Clin Cardiol* 1994;17:306–308.
31. Benson DW Jr, Smith WM, Dunnigan A, et al. Mechanisms of regular, wide QRS tachycardia in infants and children. *Am J Cardiol* 1982;49:1778–1788.

32. Gorgels APM, van den Dool A, Hofs A, et al. Comparison of procainamide and lidocaine in terminating sustained monomorphic ventricular tachycardia. *Am J Cardiol* 1996;78:43–46.

33. Perry JC, Fenrich AL, Hulse E, et al. Pediatric use of intravenous amiodarone: efficacy and safety in critically ill patients from a multicenter protocol. *J Am Coll Cardiol* 1996;27:1246–1250.

34. Martyn R, Somberg JC, Kerin NZ: Proarrhythmia of nonantiarrhythmic drugs. *Am Heart J* 1993;126:201–205.

35. Johnsrude CL, Towbin JA, Cecchin F, et al. Postinfarction ventricular arrhythmias in children. *Am Heart J* 1995;129:1171–1177.

36. Gewellig M, Wyse RK, de Leval MR, et al. Early and late arrhythmias after the Fontan operation: predisposing factors and clinical consequences. *Br Heart J* 1992;67:72–79.

37. Raja P, Hawker RE, Chaikitpinyo A, et al. Amiodarone management of junctional ectopic tachycardia after cardiac surgery in children. *Br Heart J* 1994;72:261–265.

38. Pfammatter JP, Paul T, Ziemer G, et al. Successful management of junctional tachycardia by hypothermia after cardiac operations in infants. *Ann Thorac Surg* 1995;60:556–560.

39. Case CL, Gillette PC. Automatic atrial and junctional tachycardias in the pediatric patient: strategies for diagnosis and management. *Pacing Clin Electrophysiol* 1993;16:1323–1335.

40. Kohli V, Young ML, Perryman RA, et al. Paired ventricular pacing is the primary therapy for management of postoperative junctional ectopic tachycardia. Personal communication.

41. Waldo AL, Krongrad E, Kupersmith J, et al. Ventricular paired pacing to control rapid ventricular heart rate following open heart surgery. Observations on ectopic automaticity. Report of a case in a four-month-old patient. *Circulation* 1976;53:176–181.

42. Dittrich KL, Walls RM. Hyperkalemia: ECG manifestations and clinical considerations. *J Emerg Med* 1986;4:449–455.

_____ *Chapter 12* _____

Ablation Therapy

Edward P. Walsh, MD

Introduction

Like many advances in medicine, the concept of transcatheter ablation in cardiac tissue was inspired, at least in part, by a clinical accident. The case in point involved a diagnostic intracardiac electrophysiology (EP) study reported from Paris in 1978, during which a patient received a conventional direct current (DC) cardioversion to treat an induced ventricular tachycardia (VT).[1] When the external thoracic shock was delivered, energy somehow diverted through the His bundle catheter causing inadvertent complete heart block. Clever minds seized upon the therapeutic potential of this phenomenon so that by 1980 ablation with DC energy directed through an electrode catheter was used for intentional interruption of atrioventricular (AV) conduction in select patients with intractable atrial arrhythmias.[2,3] Indications for DC ablation were gradually extended over the ensuing decade, but the risk of acute and late complications with this rather traumatic energy form were significant, resulting in very restricted use in both the adult[4–6] and pediatric populations.[7–9] A major technological advance occurred in 1985, when Huang and associates[10] reported results of animal experiments with radiofrequency (RF) current as a safer and more focal method of ablating cardiac tissue. This alternate energy form was used for cardiac ablation in adult patients by 1987,[11,12] in pediatric patients by 1990,[13,14] and quickly grew to be a preferred technique for the management of many tachyarrhythmias.

This chapter is a general overview of RF ablation (RFA) in the pediatric age group, concentrating on those technical and clinical features that may

From Deal B, Wolff G, Gelband H, (eds.). *Current Concepts in Diagnosis and Management of Arrhythmias in Infants and Children.* Armonk, NY: Futura Publishing Co., Inc.; © 1998.

differ between children and adults. Fortunately, the data available regarding pediatric ablation are quite extensive, due largely to the foresight of Dr. John Kugler, who in 1991 initiated the multicenter Pediatric RF Ablation Registry, which currently includes information from 46 contributing centers involving over 4000 procedures. These data, along with published single-center experiences from Boston Children's Hospital and elsewhere, provide the framework for discussion in this chapter. In-depth analysis of RF biophysics and complex mapping techniques are beyond the scope of this text, but the interested reader is referred to several comprehensive reviews of these topics for details.[15-18] The basic concept of RFA is the application of unmodulated sinusoidal waveforms at relative high frequency (300–750 kHz) via an electrode catheter to achieve tissue heating, creating a thermal injury. The selective delivery of well-circumscribed lesions to a specific target such as an accessory connection (AC) results in tissue destruction and loss of electrical conduction.

Technical Considerations in Pediatric Patients

Cardiac ablation procedures involve the following stages: (1) preablation analysis of cardiac structure and function, with attention to details of congenital heart defects and prior cardiac surgery; (2) maintenance of appropriate sedation and anticoagulation; (3) vascular access for the requisite number of electrode catheters within the constraints of vessel caliber and cardiac chamber size; (4) compulsive mapping and proper positioning of the ablation catheter at the target site; and (5) delivery of RF energy while minimizing collateral damage to normal myocardium. Technical details of each stage will be discussed individually.

Radiofrequency Ablation in Congenital Heart Disease

Roughly 20% of pediatric RFA procedures involve patients with congenital cardiac defects,[19] and the proportion is likely to rise as this technology is extended to more children and young adults with late postoperative atrial and ventricular reentrant tachycardias. It cannot be overemphasized that the precise cardiac anatomy, and specific details of any past cardiac surgery, must be clarified before ablation is attempted. This is particularly true in cases of AV discordance and canal defects, where the normal AV conduction tissues may be displaced far from the standard position (Figure 1), or may even involve complex "slings" of His-Purkinje fibers between two separate AV nodes (AVN).[20] Thanks primarily to the elegant pathological work of Anderson and Becker,[21,22] it is possible to decipher the expected location of the normal conduction system with reasonable accuracy even in the most anatomically complex hearts. These pathological

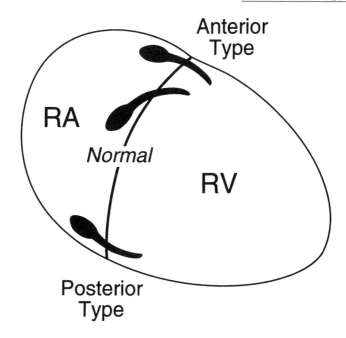

Figure 1. Diagrammatic view (right anterior oblique projection) of the proximal AV conduction system, showing variation in location for the compact node and His bundle in certain congenital heart defects. The anterior location is usually encountered in patients with L-transposition (corrected transposition) of the great vessels. The posterior location is typical for AV canal defects. For a detailed discussion of conduction system anatomy, see References 20–24.

studies now supplemented by in vivo mapping experience from both the operating room[23] and catheterization laboratory.[24] For any patient with complex anatomy, information of this sort should be reviewed prior to ablation in an effort to insure correct localization of the His bundle and thereby minimize the risk of accidental damage to normal AV conduction.

ACs presently account for the majority of ablation procedures performed in patients with congenital heart disease.[24,25] The indication in most cases involves symptomatic reciprocating tachycardia, but AC ablation is also performed for some asymptomatic or mildly symptomatic children as a prelude to cardiac surgery when the impending operation might involve patching or vascular redirection that could limit future catheter access to an arrhythmia focus. Although ACs were described in association with nearly all varieties of structural cardiac malformations, the incidence is clearly highest among patients with Ebstein's anomaly and "corrected" transposition of the great arteries.[26] In these particular defects, ACs are typically found along the embryological tricuspid valve ring. Clear deline-ation of AV valve anatomy (using transthoracic, transesophageal, or intra-cardiac echocardiography) and precise localization of the AV groove (by angiography or specialized coronary artery electrode catheters) will maxi-mize the chance of successful ablation.[27,28]

More recently, RFA was extended to patients with congenital heart defects who developed late postoperative reentrant tachycardias, including atrial muscle reentry ("flutter") of the type that occurs in tachy-brady syn-drome and some monomorphic VTs (eg, following tetralogy of Fallot re-pair). Current data would suggest that these arrhythmias involve macro-reentry circuits that are largely defined by a combination of fixed anatomic obstacles (such as caval orifices, septal defects, or valve rings) and surgical scars (including atriotomy or ventriculotomy incisions, caval cannulation sites, patch margins, and anastomotic suture lines). As will be discussed later in this chapter, effective RFA in these cases entails elimination of a critical isthmus of tissue that is usually accomplished by creating a line of conduction block between two of the aforementioned anatomic or surgical boundaries. Thus, not only must the anatomy of the cardiac defect be well understood, but details of all surgical incisions and patch locations must be ascertained from review of old operative notes. High-quality imaging with echocardiography and angiography are again important, as is clear comprehension of the unusual atrial anatomy that accompanies such sur-gical repairs as the Mustard, Senning, or Fontan operations.

Sedation and Anticoagulation

RFA procedures in younger patients are performed under general an-esthesia at many centers,[19] primarily to minimize the risk of abrupt patient movement at times of RF applications and complex catheter manipulation (eg, transseptal puncture). In addition, the ventilator cycle for an intubated patient can be held during RF energy delivery as a means of improving catheter tip stability over the target site. Since many children are quite sensitive to any manipulation near the neck and facial area, general anes-thesia also simplifies vascular access to the subclavian or jugular veins. In most instances, the use of a general anesthetic does not seem to interfere in a significant way with tachycardia induction or mapping. When isofluo-rane and propofol were tested specifically for this in a group of pediatric patients undergoing ablation for ACs and AVN reentry, there were no de-monstrable effects on EP measurements.[29] The exceptions may be arrhyth-mias caused by automatic foci, such as ectopic atrial tachycardia and right ventricular outflow tract (RVOT) tachycardia, where the focus may become quiescent under deep levels of anesthesia. It may be advisable in these situations to rely on lighter levels of titrated intravenous sedation.[30]

There is wide institutional variation regarding anticoagulation policy during and after RFA. Embolic events were indeed reported in association with ablation procedures in both children and adults, but fortunately remain quite rare.[31,32] All would agree that systemic heparinization is mandatory during left-heart procedures, as well as any right-heart procedure in a patient with congenital heart disease and intracardiac shunting. Most would also advocate heparin use during uncomplicated right-heart procedures involving multiple venous catheters. Standard intravenous doses of 100 units per kilogram (maximum 5000 units) are usually given at the completion of vascular access or after completion of the transseptal puncture, with additional doses given throughout the case guided by frequent measurements of activated clotting time.[33] The decision to continue anticoagulation beyond the acute procedure is more controversial, since it is unclear if the risk of emboli truly extends beyond the time that catheters are in the heart.[34] Opinions range from no postablation anticoagulation to a very aggressive policy of coumadin for up to 6 months. Most centers adopted some intermediate plan, perhaps using overnight heparin infusions and/or low-dose aspirin for a few weeks after the procedure.

Vascular Access and Catheter Choice

Smaller vascular caliber and smaller cardiac chamber size strongly influence the number and size of catheters chosen for ablation procedures in children. One must often be content with a reduced number of diagnostic electrode catheters, but this should not detract from study quality if some technical shortcuts are used, including (1) use of a multipolar catheter that combines His bundle recording from proximal electrodes and right ventricular (RV) pacing from the distal electrode pair; (2) use of a multipolar coronary sinus (CS) electrode that combines mitral ring recording from distal electrodes and atrial pacing from the proximal electrode pair; and (3) positioning of an esophageal lead for left atrial (LA) stimulation and recording. These steps make it possible to perform even the most complex ablations with only two or three catheters when necessary. For some arrhythmia targets that offer reliable diagnostic markers on the surface electrocardiogram (ECG) (eg, manifest preexcitation from an AC or incessant ectopic atrial tachycardia), successful mapping and ablation may be possible with a single intravascular catheter (Figure 2).

Ablation catheters are currently available in sizes 5–8 French, with distal electrode tips varying from 3–8 mm in length (Figure 3). Although RF lesion size cannot be controlled precisely with current technology, there is a general correlation between lesion dimensions and the surface area of the ablation electrode tip. Thus, a 5-French device with a 3-mm

with RFA in both adult and pediatric patients attests to the general safety of such intracardiac lesions. However, there is still limited long-term follow-up on the technique as well as unanswered questions regarding whether immature myocardium reacts in the same fashion as mature tissue. Studies of RF lesions in a developing sheep model, for example, suggested that RF scars in the atrium or ventricle of young lambs may expand with time and that the lesion border can be quite irregular with extension of fibrotic tissue into surrounding myocardium.[40] The significance of these animal findings for a young child undergoing ablation is uncertain, but they do emphasize the need for judicious patient selection and careful follow-up. An additional concern arises from the smaller cardiac dimensions in young children, which lessens the margin of error whenever RF lesions are made near the AVN and other vital structures. For all these reasons, it is prudent to minimize nonproductive RF applications and pinpoint the lesion to the arrhythmia target site as exactly as possible.

The most obvious means of focusing the RF lesion is compulsive mapping technique. Details of precision mapping will be presented later in this chapter during discussion of individual arrhythmia mechanisms, but it is not uncommon to encounter sites during ablation that are still not effective despite ideal electrogram characteristics, resulting in the need for some number of "test" applications before the target is finally eliminated. There are several methods for reducing the damage done during these unsuccessful trials. First, the duration of the application can be limited. For most tachycardias, it was widely observed that a properly positioned ablation catheter eliminated the target within 5 seconds or so of initiating RF delivery. Thus, there is usually little to gain with extended RF applications beyond 5–10 seconds if the desired end point is not reached,[41] and, in fact, the likelihood of transient arrhythmia interruption (with late recurrence) may be higher with unproductive lesions of long duration. The second variable that can be manipulated to minimize cardiac damage is temperature. Now that many commercial ablation systems are being designed with thermistors at the catheter tip, low-temperature RF applications (eg, 50°C) can be delivered that may serve as an ancillary mapping tool. In a series of pediatric patients undergoing AC ablation, it was recently shown that 50° applications could cause reversible AC interruption (Figure 4) and accurately predicted the site of permanently successful ablation when the temperature was subsequently increased to 70°.[42] All these techniques have the potential not only to reduce unnecessary myocardial damage but also to refine map quality and thus maximize the chance of permanently successful ablation. When combined with the use of small catheter tips as mentioned earlier, the risk for ablation in a very small child should be reduced.[43]

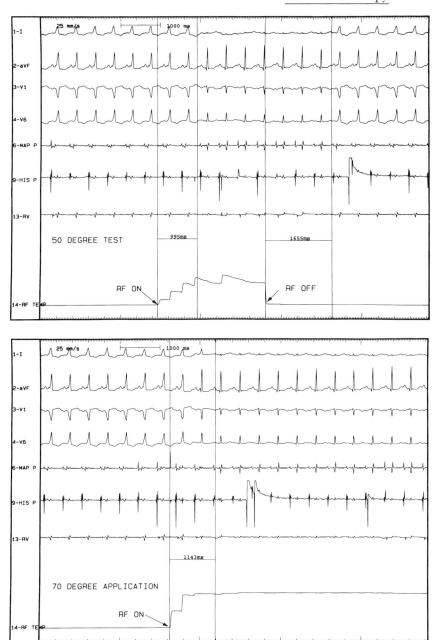

Figure 4. Low-temperature mapping during successful RFA for WPW syndrome. In **A,** a 50° test application is begun, with disappearance of preexcitation at 995 milliseconds. The lesion is immediately terminated and the δ wave returns within 1655 milliseconds. The RF generator was then reset for 70° (**B**), and a long duration application permanently eliminated the accessory connection.

_____ **Table 1** _____

Targets for Radiofrequency Ablation Procedures

Well-established procedures
  Atrial ectopic (automatic) tachycardia
  Type I atrial flutter
  Complete AV node interruption for refractory atrial tachycardia
  Junctional ectopic (automatic) tachycardia
  AV node reentry
    Fast pathway modification
    Slow pathway modification
  Accessory connections
    WPW syndrome
    Concealed accessory connection
    Mahaim fiber
    PJRT
  VT
    RVOT (automatic) tachycardia
    Idiopathic left VT
    Bundle branch reentry

Newer procedures
  Atrial fibrillation
  Intra-atrial reentry (postoperative congenital heart defects)
  Double AV nodes in complex congenital heart disease
  VT
    Reentry after congenital heart disease surgery
    Reentry after myocardial infarction

Specific Arrhythmias

Table 1 catalogs the current arrhythmia mechanisms that seem to be suitable targets for RFA. Comprehensive discussion of each tachycardia can be found elsewhere in this text; this chapter will focus primarily on mapping technique and current results for ablation.

Automatic Ectopic Atrial Tachycardia

Automatic atrial tachycardia (AAT) is an uncommon disorder that is caused by a single atrial focus of abnormal automaticity outside the sinus node. Although the abnormal focus can be located anywhere within the right atrium (RA) or LA, there is a general trend in children toward localization near either the pulmonary veins or the RA appendage.[44] The precise etiology is unknown.

This arrhythmia is insidious. Symptoms may be absent or minimal until a point is reached where a secondary cardiomyopathy arises from the sustained rapid rates. If AAT is detected early before ventricular dysfunction has developed, there is a role for medication trials and close follow-up in these patients, since some may go on to have spontaneous resolution of tachycardia.[45,46] When medications are ineffective or ventricular function is already compromised, catheter ablation is now the preferred management option at many centers. The acute success rate exceeds 90%, but perhaps the most remarkable benefit of permanent AAT eradication is prompt recovery of ventricular function in individuals with secondary myopathy, which can usually be observed within a few weeks of the procedure.[47]

Mapping for this disorder is based primarily on activation sequence during sustained AAT, looking for the electrical epicenter of atrial depolarization. As the mapping/ablation catheter is moved along the atrial endocardial surface, local electrogram timing is indexed against the onset of the P wave on the surface ECG. Locations with activation that precede the P wave by at least 20 milliseconds are investigated in more detail, until the earliest possible electrograms are identified as potential sites for ablation (Figure 5). There do not appear to be reliable electrogram characteristics apart from activation time that predict successful ablation sites. Although a split or fractionated signal may be identified in some cases, the electro-

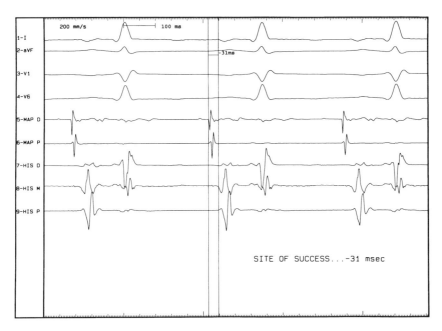

Figure 5. Mapping during ectopic atrial tachycardia in a teenage boy with a focus near the left upper pulmonary vein. The map/ablate catheter (MAP) is located at the site of successful ablation and reveals a local atrial signal that preceded the onset of the P wave on surface ECG by 31 milliseconds.

gram at the AAT focus in the majority of young patients is generally normal appearing in all aspects except its timing.[30] At ideal sites, the electrogram was observed to precede the P wave by 20–60 milliseconds (mean 40 milliseconds). Mapping is naturally most efficient when the patient is in incessant tachycardia, but this is not always easy to insure. Because AAT is not inducible with standard programmed stimulation, one must rely on the intrinsic automaticity of the focus, which may be quite unpredictable. Even among patients who demonstrated incessant tachycardia up to the time of an attempted ablation, the focus can become quiescent during the procedure, possibly as a result of sedation and/or mechanical trauma from the catheter tip. An infusion of isoproterenol is often (but not always) effective in restoring automaticity for such patients.[30]

An AAT focus responds promptly when an RF application is delivered from a properly positioned catheter. In most instances there is abrupt tachycardia termination within 5 seconds or less of beginning the lesion, while in other patients there may be transient acceleration of tachycardia rate over a few seconds followed by abrupt cessation within 10 seconds or less.[44,48] Both patterns of termination are optimistic indicators of permanently successful ablation, but it should be emphasized that prolonged acceleration without termination after 10 seconds probably indicates that the lesion is slightly off target and should not be continued for fear of inducing transient suppression of AAT with almost certain late recurrence.

Intraatrial Reentrant Tachycardia (Flutter)

Prevention of recurrent atrial flutter (AF) after surgery for congenital heart disease remains one of the most difficult challenges faced by pediatric electrophysiologists. Conventional therapy with medications[49,50] or pacing[51] was so unreliable that ablation is now being tested aggressively as an alternate management option. The early results for ablation are encouraging, but by no means perfect. Acute success rates are reported in the range of 70%,[52,53] although late flutter recurrence (with the same or different circuits) remains problematic, particularly in postoperative Fontan patients. The risk of recurrence is still being defined, but is probably on the order of at least 40%.[53A]

These are technically demanding procedures that require sophisticated mapping with entrainment pacing,[17] along with detailed imaging of atrial anatomy. Unlike common type I AF[54,55] encountered in adult patients (where the proper site for RF application is almost always located between the posterior tricuspid valve and the region of inferior vena cava), AF after congenital heart surgery can involve complex circuits related to a variety of surgical scars or anatomic boundaries. Fortunately, most of the circuits reported to date seem to be restricted to regions within the RA, usually involving tissue along or somewhere anterior to the crista terminalis (CT). Catheter access to a site of interest is thus straightforward in patients who underwent repair of relatively simple defects such as atrial or ventricular septal defect (VSD) or tetralogy of Fallot. The same can be said for patients who underwent old-style Fontan procedure involving an atriopulmonary connection, although the anatomic distortion that accompanies marked RA dilation in this setting is a problem unto itself. For postoperative Mustard or Senning patients, a retrograde approach back through the tricuspid valve is often necessary to reach the critical portions of the RA. For the newer style Fontan patients with a "lateral tunnel," access to RA tissue is obviously difficult unless a fenestration or baffle leak is present.

To understand ablation for this disorder, it is helpful to first examine a simplified model of muscle reentry. Figure 6 shows a diagrammatic circuit of atrial macroreentry that is maintained primarily by the altered conduction that occurs along the edge of an atriotomy scar. In this model, note that there is a narrow corridor or isthmus along the upper CT, bounded by the superior vena cava (SVC) orifice and the cranial end of the incision. Located within the isthmus is a "zone of slow conduction" having a medial entrance site and a lateral exit site. Tachycardia will be eliminated in this model if conduction through the isthmus is blocked completely by one or more RF applications delivered in a linear fashion between the SVC and the scar. In practice, it is seldom this simple. Among the many pitfalls is difficulty achieving a sufficiently high density of simultaneous atrial recording sites to allow construction of an accurate map for the entire circuit. This problem can be addressed to a limited extent with the use of many multipolar catheters or novel catheter designs[56] but is far from solved (Figure 7). In addition, a given patient may have two reentry circuits that are seemingly different but utilize just one narrow corridor (in either the clockwise or counterclockwise directions) or several different circuits that are widely separated within the atrium. The notion of the slow conduction zone is also more complicated in reality. These areas are not always easy to identify, may vary in both size and degree of conduction delay, and are not necessarily located in the narrowest isthmus of the circuit. Finally, the biophysics of creating true lines of conduction block over relatively large distances in the atrium with conventional catheters still requires technological refinement. Considering all these difficulties, the current success rate for flutter ablation is surprisingly good.

Mapping begins with simple recording during sustained intraatrial reentry, looking at local electrogram timing. These data usually allow one to construct a crude picture of the general direction of the circuit and are most useful when the tachycardia cycle length (CL) is relatively

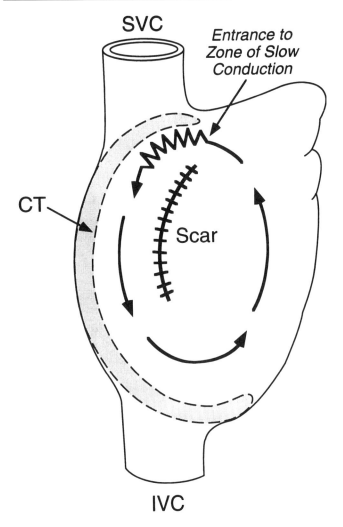

Figure 6. Diagrammatic model of an intraatrial macroreentrant tachycardia of the type that may occur after surgery for congenital heart defects. This circuit is supported by the corridor of conduction defined between the CT and an atriotomy scar (Scar). The corridor is most narrow at the cranial end of the scar near the SVC. In this example, conduction time is prolonged through the narrow isthmus, creating a so-called "zone of slow conduction." See text for details. CT = crista terminalis, SVC = superior vena cava, IVC = inferior vena cava.

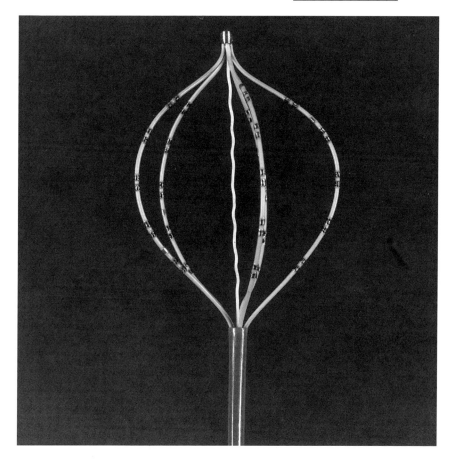

Figure 7. "Basket" catheter (Cordis-Webster Inc, Baldwin Park, Calif) of the type now in human clinical trials for mapping within the RA. The catheter is delivered through a 10-French sheath, and is then expanded within the atrium by retracting a central pull wire, thereby coaxing the five spokes to conform to the three-dimensional geometry of the atrial endocardium. By recording simultaneously from all 50 electrodes (10 per spoke), rapid activation sequence mapping is possible for complex tachycardias such as AF.

long with a P-wave onset that is discrete enough to mark the beginning of electrical systole. Apart from activation timing, the electrograms are also scrutinized for fractionation and split potentials that are often indicators of incisional scars and slow conduction zones. These data are then combined with anatomic information to generate an idea of the most likely site(s) for effective lines of block.

The ablation catheter is moved to an area of interest, where entrainment pacing is performed to verify that the local tissue is indeed part of the circuit[57] and to check the position relative to a slow conduction zone (Figure 8). Multiple RF applications are then made between the two edges of the corridor to eliminate tachycardia. The atrial CL may initially lengthen when the line of block is first begun, but reentry should stop entirely (Figure 9) when all conduction through the isthmus is finally interrupted.[52] While many other tachycardias discussed in this chapter involve discrete foci that stop promptly with a single correctly positioned RF lesion, the technique for flutter ablation typically involves multiple prolonged applications while slowly dragging the catheter tip across the entire isthmus.

Whether RFA will eventually supplant medical therapy in this condition is uncertain. At the very least, however, the experience with catheter therapy will help pinpoint the most likely "hot spots" after specific operations and thereby guide modifications in surgical technique that could ultimately prevent the occurrence of this tachycardia.

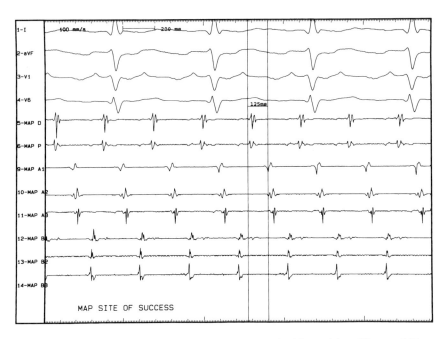

Figure 8. Mapping during atrial reentrant tachycardia (flutter) in a 17-year-old boy status post-Fontan operation. The atrial CL is 312 milliseconds, and conducts in a 2:1 fashion. Shown are surface ECG recordings (I, aVf, V1, V6), along with atrial electrograms from the map/ablate catheter (MAP D and MAP P) and other multipolar RA electrodes. MAP D is located in the region of successful ablation where local activation precedes the onset of the flutter wave on surface ECG by 125 milliseconds. Based on entrainment characteristics, this region was thought to represent the entrance area to a zone of slow conduction.

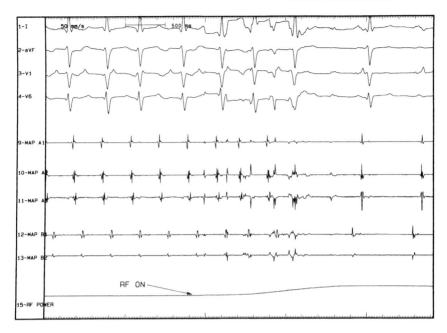

Figure 9. The same patient shown in Figure 8 during RF application for AF. There is some electrical artifact present when the RF generator is first activated, but it is still noted that the atrial tachycardia stops abruptly less than 2 seconds into the application. Following a series of linear applications across this area, flutter could no longer be induced.

Accessory Connections

Wolff-Parkinson-White (WPW) syndrome and other varieties of ACs rightly earned their title as the "Rosetta Stone of Electrophysiology."[58] More was learned from them regarding the physiology and treatment of reentrant tachycardia than perhaps any other form of cardiac electrical pathology, and this is especially true for the technique of catheter ablation. ACs currently account for 75% of ablation procedures in children,[19] an experience that helped refine our mapping skills, knowledge of ablation biophysics, and clinical judgment.

The acute success rate for AC ablation with RF energy exceeds 90% in most clinical series.[59-61] The Pediatric RF Ablation Registry currently reports a slightly lower 89% overall success rate, but this figure reflects the learning curves of more than 40 contributing centers, as well as a high number of complex patients with concomitant anatomic heart defects.

In classic WPW syndrome, the AC is capable of conduction in either an antegrade or retrograde direction, and is manifest during sinus rhythm as a δ wave on surface ECG. Mapping starts with review of the 12-lead ECG, which can serve as a rough indicator of AC location based on δ-wave polarity and QRS axis. Multiple algorithms evolved for this purpose,[62-64] but in practice none has perfect predictive value, perhaps reaching only about 70% accuracy when used prospectively.[65] Nonetheless, this first approximation from the ECG is important in young patients since it may influence the catheter approach for the procedure, such as whether a CS electrode is absolutely needed or whether a transseptal puncture might have to be done. Once catheters are in place, formal mapping commences along the AV groove during preexcited sinus rhythm, looking for the site of earliest ventricular activation along the valve ring as an indicator of the ventricular insertion for the AC. Next, the atrial insertion is identified by looking for the site of earliest retrograde atrial activation during either rapid ventricular pacing or sustained orthodromic tachycardia. Besides localizing the AC on the basis of atrial and ventricular signals, it may also be possible to identify a separate discrete electrical potential that is thought to arise from the AC itself. The electrogram at a promising ablation site should reflect the rapid conduction through an AC by containing nearly continuous atrial and ventricular activity with little isoelectric time in between and ideally should include an AC potential (Figure 10). The electrogram must also reflect good catheter tip position along the true AV groove by containing sharp atrial and ventricular signals that are both easily seen at standard amplification, with the ventricular component roughly twice as large as the atrial component.[66] When all these features are present, an RF application can be attempted, and, if localization was indeed accurate, AC conduction should be interrupted within a few seconds of beginning the lesion (Figure 11). Ablation for a "concealed" (retrograde conducting only) AC is performed in a manner identical to that used for WPW syndrome, except that mapping of the ventricular insertion during antegrade preexcitation is obviously not possible.

AC location strongly influences the rates of acute success, late recurrence, and potential complications with this procedure. There is good news and bad news at every possible locus. For LFW ACs, as an example, the acute success rate is clearly high (nearly 100%) and recurrence is less likely, but the catheter approach (whether transseptal or retrograde) can be technically demanding; occasionally, the AC has an epicardial location not easily ablated from an endocardial approach. In addition, there exists a very small risk of systemic emboli whenever the catheter is in the left heart. Right free-wall (RFW) ACs, on the other hand, are more easily reached from a standard venous approach, but it may be surprisingly difficult to maintain stable catheter contact along the lateral tricuspid valve ring, resulting in a lower success rate and a higher recurrence rate. Septal ACs are also easily reached, but can be difficult to map and eliminate owing to the complex anatomy of the septal space and the risk of injury to the normal conduction system. Expanded clinical experience, as well as technical mod-

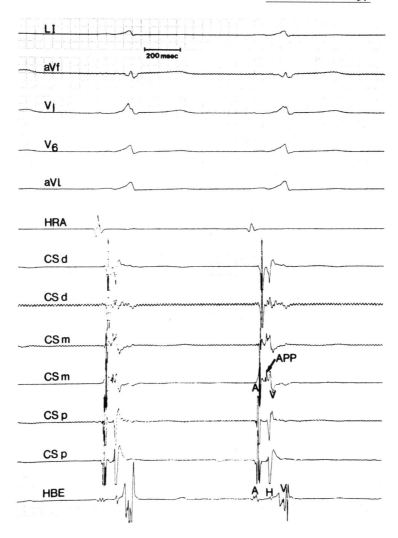

Figure 10. Surface ECG recordings (I, aVf, V1, V6, aVl) and intracardiac electrograms recorded during preexcited sinus rhythm in a patient with a left posterior-lateral AC. The connection is localized by the CS electrode to the middle recording pairs (CSm). The electrogram at this site contains nearly continuous electrical activity, with early registration of ventricular activation that precedes the onset of the δ wave on surface ECG. There is, in addition, a sharp high frequency signal between atrial (A) and ventricular (V) activity that likely represents an AC potential (APP).

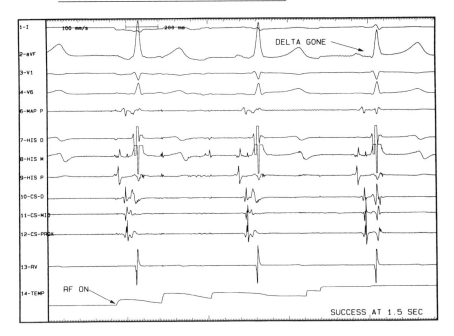

Figure 11. Surface ECG leads and intracardiac electrograms during a successful RF application in a patient with WPW syndrome (left lateral AC). Within 1.5 seconds of beginning the application, the δ wave (best seen in ECG lead aVf) is no longer present, and the short local A-V time on both the CS catheter and proximal mapping/ablate catheter (MAP P) normalize. Following a full 40-second lesion at this site, the AC was permanently eliminated.

ifications in catheter delivery (eg, specialized long vascular sheaths to improve tissue contact during right-sided ablation), overcame or minimized many of these problems, but it still seems fair to say that no AC can be taken for granted, regardless of location.

There are two less conventional, but no less important, ACs that are potential targets for RFA. The first of these is the so-called Mahaim fiber, now understood to represent a long insulated AC running from the right anterolateral AV groove down to the anterior wall of the RV, where it approximates or possibly joins the terminal portion of the right bundle branch near the moderator band.[67] Mahaim fibers are characterized by relatively slow decremental conduction that is confined to the antegrade direction only. Mapping depends primarily on a painstaking search for a discrete Mahaim potential[68] that typically can be traced for some distance along the length of the fiber over the RV anterior wall. Successful interruption was observed with ablation at either the atrial end, the ventricular end, or some midway point but must always involve a site where a high-quality Mahaim potential is recorded (Figure 12). The second atypical con-

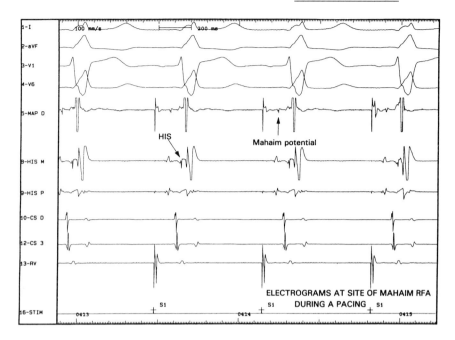

Figure 12. Discrete potential recorded at the site of successful elimination of a Mahaim fiber. The atrium was being paced along the anterolateral RA to accentuate the degree of preexcitation. The Mahaim potential is clearly different in timing from the normal His bundle recording.

nection is the slowly conducting concealed AC responsible for the permanent form of junctional reciprocating tachycardia (PJRT). These retrograde conducting ACs are usually found in the posterior septal area[69] and can be responsible for incessant reentrant tachycardia, eventually leading to a secondary cardiomyopathy. Mapping of a PJRT AC is based on identification of the earliest atrial activation during sustained tachycardia (Figure 13) and demonstration of a discrete AC potential.[70] Effective elimination can be achieved with a properly positioned RF application along the AV groove at the atrial insertion site.

Atrioventricular Nodal Reentrant Tachycardia

Catheter therapy for AVN reentry accounts for about 10% to 25% of RF procedures in pediatric practice,[19,71] compared to nearly 50% in most adult series. Clearly, AVN reentrant tachycardia (AVNRT) is more of a management issue in the adult age group, but it may still be a source of highly symptomatic tachycardia for some young patients.

The EP of the AVN area is extremely complex. Our current working model for AVNRT is a rather simplistic view incorporating two so-called

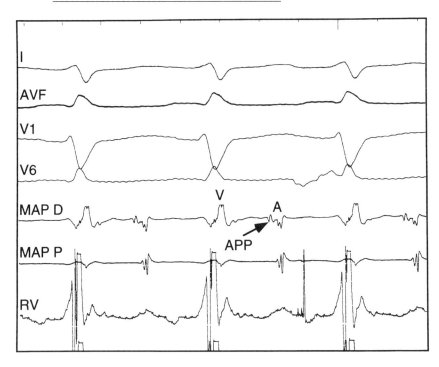

Figure 13. Surface ECG recording (I, aVf, V1, V6) and intracardiac electrograms recorded during orthodromic reciprocating tachycardia in a patient with PJRT. Note the long VA interval, which is characteristic of this disorder. The distal electrode pair of the mapping catheter (MAPd) is located at the site of successful RFA. Atrial activity (A) at this site precedes the surface P wave, and, in addition, there is a discrete sharp potential just prior to the atrial activity which may be a potential (APP) from the PJRT connection itself.

"pathways" (one "fast" and one "slow") that support reentry based on differences in their conduction velocity and refractoriness. The two pathways are also distinguished by their anatomic location (Figure 14), with the fast pathway typically described toward the anterior-superior portion of the AVN at the apex of Koch's triangle and the slow pathway more inferiorly at the base of Koch's triangle anterior to the CS.[72] While this model may be perfectly adequate for understanding tachycardia and guiding treatment for most patients, it must be remembered that there has yet to be convincing demonstration of discrete anatomic correlates for these pathways in humans. There are also some subtle but important variations in position of the nodal pathways, particularly the fast pathway, that may increase the degree of difficulty and risk for an ablation in certain patients.[73] Since the potential consequences of a misdirected RF application near the AVN are profound, these procedures require very clear anatomic knowledge of the

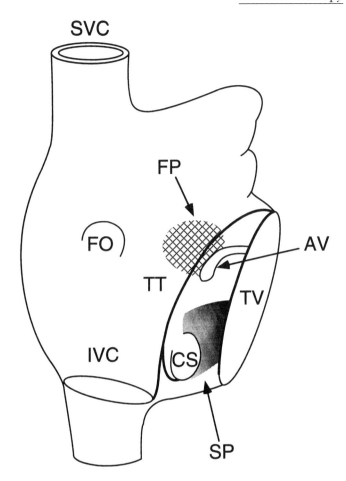

Figure 14. Schematic representation of the triangle of Koch and proximal AV conduction system. The compact node (AV) is located in the apical third of the triangle. The usual target region for successful elimination of slow pathway (SP) conduction is indicated by light shading. The usual region for fast pathway (FP) interruption is indicated by cross hatching. CS = ostium of coronary sinus, FO = fossa ovale, IVC = inferior vena cava, TT = tendon of Todaro, TV = septal leaflet of tricuspid valve.

Koch's triangle region and an open mind about the true nature of the "black box" that causes AVNRT.

Ablation procedures for AVNRT entail modification of nodal EP by eliminating or attenuating conduction through one pathway, while preserving AV conduction through the remaining pathway. The methodology evolved rapidly. Originally, the fast pathway was targeted with RF applications made along the anterior-superior aspect of the AVN that usually eliminated reentry and resulted in first-degree heart block as normal antegrade conduction was diverted to the slow pathway. These procedures were quick to perform, and the success rate was high (better than 95%), but there was a concerning incidence of inadvertent high-grade AV block (3% to 8%) that could necessitate pacemaker implantation.[74] Fast pathway modification was largely abandoned in favor of the slow pathway approach. Although slightly more tedious in terms of mapping and total procedure time, the success rate for the slow pathway approach is every bit as high, the PR interval remains physiological after ablation, and the incidence of inadvertent high-grade AV block appears to be less (1% to 2%) in most series.[75]

The slow pathway is mapped using a combination of anatomic landmarks and electrogram characteristics.[76] To begin, the boundaries of the triangle of Koch are defined by the fluoroscopic location of the His bundle

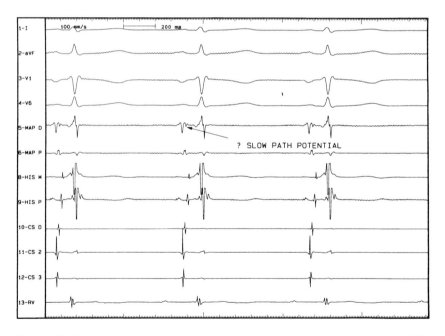

Figure 15. Mapping during sinus rhythm in a teenage girl with recurrent AVNRT. Shown are surface ECG leads (I, aVf, V1, V6) along with intracardiac electrograms from the map/ablate catheter (MAP D and MAP P), His bundle area (HIS), coronary sinus (CS), and right ventricle (RV). The mapping catheter is located at the site of successful slow-pathway ablation, toward the basal region of Koch's triangle, and anterior to the CS. The signal is remarkable for a complex atrial component that contains a somewhat discrete secondary spike (→) that may represent a slow-pathway potential.

recording catheter, the CS electrode, and the edge of the tricuspid valve. The tip of the ablation catheter is then moved into the basal portion of the triangle to rest on atrial tissue anterior to the CS along the tricuspid valve rim. Signals recorded during normal sinus rhythm from a well-positioned catheter should contain a dominant ventricular component, with a smaller but sharp atrial component that is frequently fractionated or otherwise complex (Figure 15). Often, it is also possible to record a sharp discrete signal that is thought to reflect a potential from the slow pathway itself.[76] Identification of the slow pathway potentials may be difficult in some individuals so that many procedures are done on the basis of favorable anatomic information alone.[77]

Applications of RF energy are usually made during normal sinus rhythm, while watching to insure that fast pathway conduction is not jeopardized and also looking for appearance of junctional automaticity during the lesion.[78] Mild to moderate junctional acceleration [90–150 beats per minute (bpm)] is a desirable observation during the application and usu-

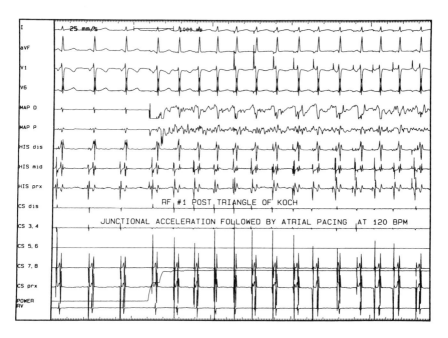

Figure 16. Tracings from a teenager with recurrent AVNRT at the moment of RFA. The application was performed in the region of the slow-pathway during sinus rhythm and resulted in almost immediate junctional acceleration to moderate rates of about 110 bpm. Atrial pacing at 120 bpm began shortly thereafter which made it easier to monitor the integrity of the fast-pathway during the remainder of the lesion. The slow-pathway was successfully eliminated with a single 45-second application.

ally indicates that the catheter tip is well situated in the area of the slow pathway (Figure 16). However, rapid junctional acceleration (above 150 bpm) can be a more ominous sign, indicating the potential for damage to the compact AVN, and is usually an indication to stop the lesion and reposition the catheter elsewhere. After each application, AVN physiology is reexamined to see if the targeted pathway was eliminated. The ideal end point is elimination of all slow pathway activity and well-preserved (or even enhanced) fast pathway conduction. However, it may sometimes be adequate to achieve partial damage to the slow pathway to the point that it can still conduct single beats but is incapable of supporting more than a single echo beat or so of reentry.[79] The risk of AVNRT recurrence may be slightly higher when single echoes remain, but it is probably an adequate end point in cases where any additional lesions would need to be made uncomfortably close to the compact AVN.

Ablation for AVNRT in a young population is feasible and is associated with a high rate of success. However, most data regarding AVNRT ablation in the Pediatric RF Ablation Registry involved teenagers, with few procedures done in younger children. What is difficult to measure, therefore, is whether the risk of heart block is higher in a smaller child where the dimensions of Koch's triangle are reduced. Uncertainty of this type resulted in a general tendency to restrict AVNRT ablation during the preteen years to those highly symptomatic children who failed at least one trial of pharmacologic control.

Ventricular Tachycardia

Among the several possible mechanisms for VT in young patients, three specific forms were identified as suitable targets for RFA. The overall experience remains quite small in comparison to the number of patients undergoing ablation for supraventricular mechanisms. In the Pediatric RF Ablation Registry, for instance, only about 2% of total procedures involved a ventricular arrhythmia, but the results thus far are encouraging.

The first type of VT to consider is the RVOT variety, which is thought to be caused by an automatic or triggered focus within the infundibular region. It is loosely associated with the diagnosis of RV dysplasia in some older patients,[80] but in the vast majority of cases there is no demonstrable cardiac pathology. This form of VT is generally hemodynamically stable but under catecholamine stimulation may degenerate. It may cause significant symptoms in some individuals and may lead to a secondary myopathy in those who spend large portions of the day at rapid rates. Medical therapy is sometimes successful, but patients who do not respond to drugs or who have depressed ventricular function may be good candidates for RFA. Localization of the focus is quite similar to the technique described earlier for AAT, involving activation sequence mapping throughout the RV, looking for sites (Figure 17) where the local electrogram precedes the onset of the QRS on surface ECG by 20–60 milliseconds.[81] Also similar to AAT, accurate mapping depends on a high level of spontaneous activity at the automatic focus, and these procedures can be frustrating if the focus becomes quiescent before mapping is complete. Activation sequence data may be supplemented by "pace mapping" from the ablation catheter tip electrode, trying to find a location where the paced QRS morphology matches exactly the QRS morphology of spontaneous tachycardia on 12-lead ECG. Applications of RF current at ideal sites should terminate VT within a few seconds of beginning the lesion. Small series described ablation of RVOT foci in a young population with very acceptable records of safety and success.[82]

The second type of VT amenable to RF therapy is the uncommon disorder of idiopathic left VT, sometimes referred to as Belhassen's tachycardia.[83] It usually occurs in patients with an otherwise normal heart and

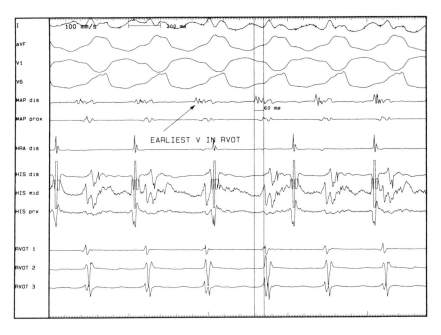

Figure 17. Mapping during sustained automatic VT arising from the RVOT in a 14-year-old boy with moderately depressed ventricular function from nearly incessant tachycardia. Shown are surface ECG leads (I, aVf, V1, V6) along with intracardiac electrograms from the map/ablate catheter (MAP), RA (HRA), His bundle area (HIS), and a reference catheter in the RVOT. Retrograde V-A dissociation is present. The map catheter is located at the site of successful ablation and shows local electrical activation that precedes the onset of the surface QRS by 60 milliseconds.

is distinguished by its QRS appearance of right bundle-branch block morphology and superior axis. These ECG findings correlate well with intracardiac mapping data that have localized this arrhythmia near the left posterior fascicle along the ventricular septum. A retrograde arterial approach for the ablation catheter is usually necessary when treating this arrhythmia. Mapping concentrates on localization of a discrete sharp potential that precedes the QRS during tachycardia (Figure 18) and is probably of Purkinje fiber origin.[84] An RF application at such a site should terminate VT promptly and prevent reinduction.

Macroreenetrant VT of the type seen late after repair of congenital heart defects is the third form of VT to be treated with RFA and is probably the most clinically important. Published experience thus far is limited to case reports and small institutional series[85–87] involving patients after repair

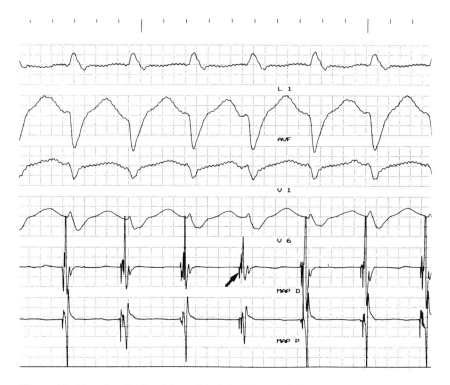

Figure 18. Mapping during idiopathic left VT in a child with paroxysmal VT but an otherwise normal heart. Shown are surface ECG leads (I, aVf, V1, V6) along with intracardiac recordings from the distal and proximal map/ablate catheter (MAP D and MAP P). The catheter is located at the site of successful RFA and reveals an early electrogram that precedes the onset of the surface ECG but is most notable for a discrete sharp initial deflection (→) that probably is recorded from Purkinje tissue along the left posterior fascicle.

of tetralogy of Fallot or VSDs. There are many technical features in common with AF mapping, beginning with the need for clear definition of all anatomic electrical boundaries and surgical scars. Once VT is induced with programmed stimulation, the circuit is mapped using a combination of ventricular activation sequence, entrainment pacing, and identification of possible zones for slow conduction (Figure 19). This information can also be supplemented by standard pace mapping in sinus rhythm, trying to recreate the exact QRS morphology of clinical VT with pacing from the ablation catheter tip. Electrical data are then combined with knowledge of the anatomic substrate to identify candidate sites within the circuit that could be interrupted with RF lesions. Several applications delivered in a linear fashion may be necessary before conduction through a potential narrow isthmus is blocked completely. Acute success rates seem optimistic in this condition (as high as 93% in a recently reported[88] series of 16 pa-

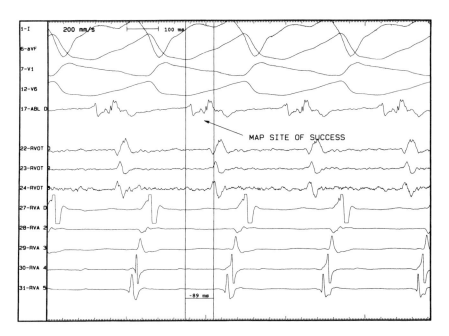

Figure 19. Mapping during sustained monomorphic VT in a young man with repaired tetralogy of Fallot. Shown are surface ECG leads (I, aVf, V1, V6), along with intracardiac signals from the mapping/ablation catheter (ABL D) and other multipolar catheters at the RV apex (RVA) and RVOT. The VT involves a macroreentrant circuit in the outflow tract region and was well tolerated with a CL of 303 milliseconds. The ablation catheter is located in the posterior RV outflow tract at the site of the successful RF application, where the local signal is notable for an electrogram onset, which precedes the QRS by 89 milliseconds, and displays a long duration of fractionated activity. This site was suspected to represent the mid portion for a zone of slow conduction.

tients), but longer follow-up and expanded clinical experience is still needed to determine the risk of late VT recurrence. If the data suggest a high probability for permanent eradication of VT in this population, it is likely that ablation will largely replace drug therapy, and may even obviate the need for defibrillator implant in some individuals.

Complications/Tachycardia Recurrence

Balanced against the impressive rates for acute success of RFA are the issues of procedural complications and late tachycardia recurrence. Neither of these problems are trivial.

Complications

Beyond the routine hazards of cardiac catheterization, ablation in both adults and children entails additional risks related to the need for complex catheter manipulation and creation of the RF lesion itself. These include cardiac perforation, valve injury, coronary artery injury, damage to AV conduction, and systemic embolic events. Perhaps the best data to review in this regard come from the original publication of the Pediatric RF Ablation Registry,[71] which provided a detailed discussion of all complications encountered during the initial 725 procedures reported between January 1991 and September 1992 from 24 contributing centers. Patient ages in this study ranged from 3 weeks to 21 years with a mean of 12 years. There was an acute complication rate of 3.7%, with late complications in 1.1%, for a total of 4.8%. Of these, a serious event that seemed to have a direct relation to the ablation catheter occurred in 1.4% of cases (second- or third-degree AV block in seven, valve damage in two, and cardiac perforation in one). In addition, there were four patient deaths reported, including one that occurred in the laboratory, and three late sudden events. None of these deaths involved "routine" patients; all had either congenital heart defects or cardiomyopathy, and three of the four were less than 4 years of age. Not surprisingly, small patient size (less than 15 kg) was an independent risk factor for a complication of any sort. Bear in mind that these data represent a relatively early phase of the clinical experience with RFA in children, when most centers were climbing a steep portion of the learning curve. Both this initial Registry report and subsequent Registry experience[89] clearly indicate that the complication rate falls as a center gains more experience with the technique. Nevertheless, despite many technical improvements and vastly expanded procedure volume, a small risk of serious untoward events still exists with RFA procedures in all age groups.

There are, in addition, some undefined long-term concerns that will only be clarified with protracted follow-up, such as the issue of radiation exposure.[90] Depending on the tachycardia mechanism, the mean fluoroscopy time reported in the early Pediatric RF Ablation Registry experience[71] ranged from 46 minutes (for AVNRT cases) to 80 minutes (for RFW ACs). This value shortened with more experience to the point where the mean fluoroscopy time is currently about 40 minutes for all Registry patients, which compares quite favorably to fluoroscopy time for other types of interventional catheterization. Furthermore, many laboratories are now equipped with "pulsed" fluoroscopy units that can decrease the x-ray exposure to about one quarter the levels emitted by conventional imaging systems. Long-term consequences of the RF lesion itself is another undefined concern, particularly for very young children. Follow-up thus far did not indicate a potential for late arrhythmogenicity or other difficulties from an ablation site, but this will require further scrutiny.

Tachycardia Recurrence

Recurrence of tachycardia after an acutely successful ablation procedure remains a source of intense frustration for all concerned. As listed in Table 2, many factors contribute to this problem, and these factors vary in relevance depending on the type of arrhythmia being ablated. The exact recurrence risk is difficult to determine, since few patients undergo repeat EP studies late after an ablation. Short-term freedom from clinical events may not necessarily prove that a cryptic substrate (eg, concealed AC) is truly gone in a patient who had infrequent tachycardia episodes. Conversely, a fair number of patients, particularly teenagers, tend to complain of periodic palpitations after RFA, which often turns out to be only an

_____ Table 2 _____

Factors Influencing Arrhythmia Recurrence after Ablation

Difficulties with catheter tip position
  Inaccurate map (off target)
  Catheter dislodgment during application
  Inadequate contact/pressure
  Mechanical catheter trauma interrupts or suppresses target
Nature of the target
  Right-sided or septal location of accessory pathways
  Epicardial location of accessory pathway
  Distorted cardiac anatomy (eg, Ebstein's anamoly)
  Arborized/trangential/multiple accessory pathways
  Difficulty maintaining automaticity from an atrial or ventricular focus
  Multiple arrhythmia mechanisms
Biophysical issues
  Inadequate tissue heating (despite good catheter tip temperatures)
  High impedence (low energy delivery due to coagulum on catheter tip)
  Lesion too small or discontinuous (during flutter or VT ablation)

enhanced awareness of sinus tachycardia rather than arrhythmia. Fortunately, a few detailed clinical series[91–93] are available with postablation EP data, and these studies provide a fairly accurate recurrence risk for the more common arrhythmia mechanisms of roughly 6% to 10%. The risk seems to be "low" (1% to 20%) after procedures for LFW ACs and AVNRT,[71,91] "intermediate" (5% to 40%) for RFW ACs[71,91] and ectopic atrial foci,[71,94] and "high" (40% or more) after procedures for postoperative AF.[95] In most cases, if a tachycardia substrate is going to recur, it usually does so within 3 months of the procedure,[91] although late recurrences continue to be reported by the Pediatric RF Ablation Registry.

There was initial optimism that recurrence would be reduced significantly once temperature monitoring was available on ablation catheters. This technology, now in wide clinical use, helped somewhat, but the problem was not conquered, as evidenced by the results of a recent multicenter trial that found no significant difference in electrode tip temperature between permanently successful ablation sites and those with later recurrence.[91] Temperature monitoring still plays a major role in RFA procedures in terms of improving map quality[42] and preventing coagulum formation from overheating[96] but is clearly not the entire solution to the problem of tachycardia recurrence.

Indications for Ablation in Pediatric Patients

Indications for catheter ablation in pediatric patients vary widely from institution to institution, but there are a few areas of clear consensus. All centers, for instance, consider the infant to be a special case with ablation procedures reserved for life-threatening or truly refractory tachycardia.[97] Apart from the technical issues of vascular access and a potentially increased complication risk, there are important natural history considerations that tend to dampen enthusiasm for an invasive procedure at this age. Spontaneous and complete resolution of AC conduction was demonstrated to occur in nearly one third of affected children within 12 months of birth,[98,99] and there seems to be a high rate of spontaneous disappearance for AAT during this time as well.[26] Except for very special circumstances,[43,100] palliation with medical therapy is generally preferred[101] during infancy to allow every opportunity for a natural cure.

After age 12 months, it becomes less likely that any of the common arrhythmia substrates (such as ACs and AVNRT) will regress spontaneously. Ablation becomes a more realistic management option at this point, with the final decision based upon such variables as patient age/weight, severity of symptoms, family attitude, and the preference of the primary physician. Figure 20 shows a simplified patient selection scheme of the type in effect at Boston Children's Hospital, which relies primarily on age and symptom status. The infant category, as indicated, is unique. Between ages 1 and 4

Indications for RF Ablation

	Infant	Patient Age Group 1-4 yrs (<15kg)	5-13 yrs (>15kg)	>13 yrs
Mild Sx	-	-	±	+
MOD Sx	-	±	+	+
Severe Sx	±	+	+	+
(Myopathy)	±	+	+	+
(CHD)	±	+	+	+

Figure 20. Patient selection guidelines for RFA, showing the general scheme in effect at Boston Children's Hospital. Each young patient must be evaluated on a case-by-case basis, but symptom status and age, as shown here, are the key variables in the final decision. Besides the severity of symptoms (Sx) during tachycardia, the presence of tachycardia-induced cardiomyopathy (Myopathy) or congenital heart disease (CHD) must also be factored into such decisions. +, usually indicated; ±, indicated in some patients; —, usually not indicated.

years (when the average weight is less than 15 kg and the complication rate may be higher), ablation is usually reserved for severely symptomatic children and those whose condition is complicated by congenital heart disease or a tachycardia-induced myopathy. Moderately symptomatic children in this age category will sometimes be considered suitable candidates if their arrhythmia control is dependent on potent medications including class Ic or class III agents. For those who are doing well on relatively benign therapy such as β-blocker or calcium channel blocker, ablation is usually deferred until a later age.

Indications become more liberal in the 5- to 13-year age range. Although most centers would still refrain from ablation in a child with mild symptomatology, it may be a very reasonable alternative to any sort of chronic medical therapy, including the more benign agents. The risks of the procedure do not appear to be significantly higher than average in this age group[71] when ablation is performed at experienced pediatric centers using appropriate technical modifications and with the availability of qualified pediatric anesthesia and nursing support. For the teenage and young adult age group, RFA is typically offered to all symptomatic patients, including those with only mild difficulty who may simply wish to be free of tachycardia for participation in competitive athletics and other strenuous activities. As many as 30% of the Pediatric RF Ablation Registry patients[71] fell into this type of low-risk group where the prime indication for the procedure was "patient choice."

Balancing the risk and benefit of RFA in children is a complex equation that must be solved on a case-by-case basis. Despite more than 6 years of experience with the technique, some clinical scenarios (eg, whether to ablate an asymptomatic patient with WPW syndrome) defy our ability to make this calculation with any authority.[102,103] Indications for ablation will thus continue to evolve as technical advances are introduced and expanded follow-up data become available. The value of a multicenter Registry in helping to answer these questions is immeasurable.

References

1. Vedel J, Frank R, Fontaine G, et al. Bloc auriculo-ventriculaire intra-Hisien definitif induit au cours d'une exploration endoventriculaire droite. *Arch Mal Coeur Vaiss* 1979;72:107–112.
2. Gallagher JJ, Svenson RH, Kasell JH, et al. Catheter technique for closed-chest ablation of the atrioventricular conduction system. *N Engl J Med* 1982;306:194–200.
3. Scheinman MM, Morady F, Hess DS, et al. Catheter-induced ablation of the atrioventricular junction to control refractory supraventricular arrhythmias. *JAMA* 1982;248:851–855.
4. Scheinman MM, Evans-Bell T, Executive Committee of the Percutaneous Cardiac Mapping and Ablation Registry. Catheter ablation of the atrioventricular junction: a report of the Percutaneous Cardiac Mapping and Ablation Registry. *Circulation* 1984;70:1024–1029.
5. Warin JF, Haissaguerre M. Fulguration of accessory pathways in any location: report of seventy cases. *Pacing Clin Electrophysiol* 1989;12:215–218.
6. Fisher JD, Brodman R, Kim SG, et al. Attempted nonsurgical ablation of accessory pathways via the coronary sinus in the Wolff-Parkinson-White syndrome. *J Am Coll Cardiol* 1984;4:685–694.
7. Gillette PC, Garson A Jr, Porter CJ, et al. Junctional automatic ectopic tachycardia: new proposed treatment by transcatheter His bundle ablation. *Am Heart J* 1983;106:619–623.
8. Silka MJ, Gillette PC, Garson A Jr, et al. Transvenous catheter ablation of a right atrial automatic ectopic tachycardia. *J Am Coll Cardiol* 5:999–1001, 1985.
9. Bromberg BI, Dick M II, Scott WA, et al. Transcatheter electrical ablation of accessory pathways in children. *Pacing Clin Electrophysiol* 1989;12:1787–1796.
10. Huang SK, Jordan N, Graham A, et al. Closed-chest catheter desiccation of the atrioventricular junction using radiofrequency energy: a new method of catheter ablation. *Circulation* 1985;72:389. Abstract.
11. Lavergne T, Guize L, LeHeuzey JY, et al. Closed-chest atrioventricular junction ablation by high-frequency energy transcatheter desiccation. *Lancet* 1986; 2:858–859.
12. Borggrefe M, Budde T, Podczeck A, et al. High frequency alternating current ablation of an accessory pathway in humans. *J Am Coll Cardiol* 1987;10:576–582.

13. VanHare GF, Velvis H, Langberg JJ. Successful transcatheter ablation of congenital junctional ectopic tachycardia in a ten-month-old infant using radiofrequency energy. *Pacing Clin Electrophysiol* 1990;13:730–735.
14. Dick M II, O'Connor BK, Serwer GA, et al. Use of radiofrequency current to ablate accessory connections in children. *Circulation* 1991;84:2318–2324.
15. Nath S, DiMarco JP, Haines DE. Basic aspects of radiofrequency catheter ablation. *J Cardiovasc Electrophysiol* 1994;5:863–876.
16. Haines DE, Watson DD. Tissue heating during radiofrequency catheter ablation: a thermodynamic model and observations in isolated perfused and superfused canine right ventricular free wall. *Pacing Clin Electrophysiol* 1989; 12:962–976.
17. Stevenson WG, Sager PT, Friedman PL. Entrainment techniques for mapping atrial and ventricular tachycardias. *J Cardiovasc Electrophysiol* 1995;6:201–216.
18. Jackman WM, Friday KJ, Yeung-Lai-Wah JA, et al. New catheter technique for recording left free-wall accessory atrioventricular pathway activation. Identification of pathway fiber orientation. *Circulation* 1988;7:598–611.
19. Walsh EP. Radiofrequency catheter ablation for cardiac arrhythmias in children. *Cardiol Rev* 1996;4:200–207.
20. Walsh EP, Saul JP, Triedman JK, et al. Ablation of the "second conducting system": Mahaim fibers, and "double AV nodes" in congenital heart disease. *Circulation* 1994;90:100. Abstract.
21. Davies MJ, Anderson RH, Becker AE. *The Conduction System of the Heart*. London: Butterworths; 1983.
22. Anderson RH, Becker AE, Arnold R, et al. The conducting tissues in congenitally corrected transposition. *Circulation* 1974;50:911–923.
23. Dick M II, Norwood WI, Chipman C, et al. Intraoperative recording of specialized atrioventricular conduction tissue electrograms in 47 patients. *Circulation* 1979;59:150–160
24. Levine JC, Walsh EP, Saul JP. Radiofrequency ablation of accessory pathways associated with congenital heart disease including heterotaxy syndrome. *Am J Cardiol* 1993;72:689–693.
25. VanHare GF, Lesh MD, Stanger P. Radiofrequency catheter ablation of supraventricular arrhythmias in patients with congenital heart disease: results and technical considerations. *J Am Coll Cardiol* 1993;22:883–890.
26. Saul JP, Walsh EP, Triedman JK. Mechanisms and therapy of complex arrhythmias in pediatric patients. *J Cardiovasc Electrophysiol* 1995;6:1129–1148.
27. Seward JB, Packer DL, Chan RC, et al. Ultrasound cardioscopy: embarking on a new journey. *Mayo Clin Proc* 1996;71:629–635.
28. Lesh M, VanHare GF, Chien W, et al. Mapping in the right coronary artery as an aid to radiofrequency catheter ablation of right sided accessory pathway. *Pacing Clin Electrophysiol* 1991;14:671. Abstract.
29. Lavoie J, Walsh EP, Burrows FA, et al. Effects of propofol or isoflurane anesthesia on cardiac conduction in children undergoing radiofrequency catheter ablation for tachydysrhythmias. *Anesthesiology* 1995;82:884–887.
30. Walsh EP. Transcatheter ablation of ectopic atrial tachycardia using radiofrequency current. In: Huang SK, ed. *Catheter Ablation for Cardiac Arrhythmias*. Armonk, NY: Futura; 1994;421–443.
31. Thakur RK, Klein GJ, Yee R, et al. Embolic complications after radiofrequency catheter ablation. *Am J Cardiol* 1994;74:278–279.
32. Epstein MR, Knapp LD, Martindill M, et al. Embolic complications associated with radiofrequency catheter ablation. Atakr Investigator Group. *Am J Cardiol* 1996;77:655–658.

33. Bowers J, Ferguson JJ III. The use of activated clotting times to monitor heparin therapy during and after interventional procedures. *Clin Cardiol* 1994; 17:357–361.
34. Saul JP, Epstein MR, Triedman JK, et al. Embolic complications associated with RF ablation procedures. Does the risk extend beyond the procedure? *Pacing Clin Electrophysiol* 1995;18:819. Abstract.
35. Schluter M, Kuck KH. Radiofrequency current for catheter ablation of accessory atrioventricular connections in children and adolescents. Emphasis on the single-catheter technique. *Pediatrics* 1992;89:930–935.
36. Minich LL, Snider AR, Dick M II. Doppler detection of valvular regurgitation after radiofrequency ablation of accessory connections. *Am J Cardiol* 1992; 70:116–117.
37. Saul JP, Hulse JE, De W, et al. Catheter ablation of accessory atrioventricular pathways in young patients: use of long vascular sheaths, the transseptal approach, and a retrograde left posterior parallel approach. *J Am Coll Cardiol* 1993;21:571–583.
38. Swartz JF, Fisher WG, Tracy CM. Ablation of left-sided atrioventricular accessory pathways via the transseptal atrial approach. In: Huang SKS, ed. *Radiofrequency Catheter Ablation of Cardiac Arrhythmias*. Armonk, NY: Futura; 1994;251–275.
39. Hagen PT, Scholz DG, Edwards WD. Incidence and size of patent foramen ovale during the first 10 decades of life: an autopsy study of 965 normal hearts. *Mayo Clin Proc* 1984;59:17–20.
40. Saul JP, Hulse JE, Papagiannis J, et al. Late enlargement of radiofrequency lesions in infant lambs. Implications for ablation procedures in small children. *Circulation* 1994;90:492–499.
41. Laohaprasitiporn D, Walsh EP, Saul JP, et al. Dynamics of catheter tip temperature are not better than time alone for prediction of permanently successful radiofrequency lesions. *Pacing Clin Electrophysiol* 1995;18:832. Abstract.
42. Cote JM, Epstein MR, Triedman JK, et al. Low-temperature mapping predicts site of successful ablation while minimizing myocardial damage. *Circulation* 1996;94:253–257.
43. Erickson CC, Walsh EP, Triedman JK, et al. Efficacy and safety of radiofrequency ablation in infants and children <18 months of age. *Am J Cardiol* 1994;74:944–947.
44. Walsh EP, Saul JP, Hulse JE, et al. Transcatheter ablation of ectopic atrial tachycardia in young patients using radiofrequency current. *Circulation* 1992;86:1138–1146.
45. Mehta AV, Sanchez GR, Sacks EJ, et al. Ectopic automatic atrial tachycardia in children: clinical characteristics, management and follow-up. *J Am Coll Cardiol* 1988;11:379–385.
46. Naheed ZJ, Strasburger JF, Benson DW Jr, et al. Natural history and management strategies of automatic atrial tachycardia in children. *Am J Cardiol* 1995;75:405–407.
47. Fishberger SB, Colan SD, Saul JP, et al. Myocardial mechanics before and after ablation of chronic tachycardia. *Pacing Clin Electrophysiol* 1996;19:42–49.
48. Perry JC, Fenrich AL, Legras MD, et al. Acceleration of atrial ectopic tachycardia as a guide to successful radiofrequency ablation. *Pacing Clin Electrophsyiol* 1993;16:2007–2011.
49. Weindling SN, Saul JP, Triedman JK, et al. Recurrent intra-atrial reentry tachycardia following congenital heart disease surgery. The search for an optimum therapy. *Circulation* 1995;92:764. Abstract.

50. Long B, Wren C, Brodherr-Herberlein S, et al. Atrial tachycardia following congenital heart surgery. *Pacing Clin Electrophsyiol* 1996;19:580. Abstract.
51. Rhodes LA, Walsh EP, Gamble WJ, et al. Benefits and potential risks of atrial antitachycardia pacing after repair of congenital heart disease. *Pacing Clin Electrophysiol* 1995;18:1005–1016.
52. Triedman JK, Saul JP, Weindling SN, et al. Radiofrequency ablation of intraatrial reentrant tachycardia after surgical palliation of congenital heart disease. *Circulation* 1995;91:707–714.
53. Kalman JM, VanHare GF, Olgin JE, et al. Ablation of 'incisional' reentrant atrial tachycardia complicating surgery for congenital heart disease. Use of entrainment to define a critical isthmus of conduction. *Circulation* 1996; 93:502–512.
53A. Triedman JK, Bergau DM, Saul JP, et al. Efficacy of radiofrequency ablation for control of intraatrial reentrant tachycardia in patients with congenital heart disease. J Am Coll Cardiol 1997;30:1032–1038.
54. Kirkorian G, Moncada E, Chevalier P, et al. Radiofrequency ablation of atrial flutter. Efficacy of an anatomically guided approach. *Circulation* 1994;90:2804–2814.
55. Steinberg JS, Prasher S, Zelenkofske S, et al. Radiofrequency catheter ablation of atrial flutter: procedural success and long-term outcome. *Am Heart J* 1995;130:85–92.
56. Jenkins KJ, Walsh EP, Colan SD, et al. Multipolar endocardial mapping of the right atrium during cardiac catheterization: description of a new technique. *J Am Coll Cardiol* 1993;22:1105–1110.
57. Stevenson WG, Khan H, Sager P, et al. Identification of reentry circuit sites during catheter mapping and radiofrequency ablation of ventricular tachycardia late after myocardial infarction. *Circulation* 1993;88:1647–1670.
58. Gallagher JJ. Forward. In: Benditt DG, Benson DW, eds. *Cardiac Preexcitation Syndromes.* Boston: Martinus Nijhoff; 1986;XI–XIII.
59. Jackman WM, Wang XZ, Friday KJ, et al. Catheter ablation of accessory atrioventricular pathways (Wolff-Parkinson-White syndrome) by radiofrequency current. *N Engl J Med* 1991;324:1605–1611.
60. Calkins H, Langberg J, Sousa J, et al. Radiofrequency catheter ablation of accessory atrioventricular connections in 250 patients. Abbreviated therapeutic approach to Wolff-Parkinson-White syndrome. *Circulation* 1992;85:1337.
61. VanHare GF, Witherell CL, Lesh MD. Follow-up of radiofrequency catheter ablation in children: results in 100 consecutive patients. *J Am Coll Cardiol* 1994;23:1651–1659.
62. Arruda M, Wang X, McClelland J, et al. ECG algorithm for predicting sites of successful radiofrequency ablation of accessory pathways. *Pacing Clin Electrophysiol* 1993;16:865. Abstract.
63. Fitzpatrick AP, Gonzales RP, Lesh MD, et al. New algorithm for the localization of accessory atrioventricular connections using a baseline electrocardiogram. *J Am Coll Cardiol* 1994;23:107–116.
64. Chiang CE, Chen SA, Teo WS, et al. An accurate stepwise electrocardiographic algorithm for localization of accessory pathways in patients with Wolff-Parkinson-White syndrome from a comprehensive analysis of delta waves and R/S ratio during sinus rhythm. *Am J Cardiol* 1995;76:40–46.
65. Triedman JK, Dindy C, Rhodes LA, et al. Utility of ECG preexcitation mapping prior to transcatheter ablation. *Circulation* 1994;90:589. Abstract.
66. Calkins H, Kim YN, Schmaltz S, et al. Electrogram criteria for identification of appropriate target sites for radiofrequency catheter ablation of accessory atrioventricular connections. *Circulation* 1992;85:565–573.

67. Klein LS, Hackett FK, Zipes DP, et al. Radiofrequency catheter ablation of Mahaim fibers at the tricuspid annulus. *Circulation* 1993;87:738–747.

68. Okishige K, Strickberger SA, Walsh EP, et al. Catheter ablation of the atrial origin of a decrementally conducting atriofascicular accessory pathway by radiofrequency current. *J Cardiovasc Electrophysiol* 1991;2:465–475.

69. Ticho BS, Saul JP, Hulse JE, et al. Variable location of accessory pathways associated with the permanent form of junctional reciprocating tachycardia and confirmation with radiofrequency ablation. *Am J Cardiol* 1992;70:1559–1564.

70. Ticho B, Saul JP, Walsh EP. Radiofrequency catheter ablation for the permanent form of junctional reciprocating tachycardia. In: Huang SK, ed. *Catheter Ablation for Cardiac Arrhythmias.* Armonk, NY: Futura; 1994;397–409.

71. Kugler JD, Danford DA, Deal BJ, et al. Radiofrequency catheter ablation for tachyarrhythmias in children and adolescents. The Pediatric Electrophysiology Society. *N Engl J Med* 1994;330:1481–1487.

72. Kadish A, Goldberger J. Ablative therapy for atrioventricular nodal reentry arrhythmias. *Prog Cardiovasc Dis* 1995;37:273–293.

73. Trohman RG, Pinski SL, Sterba R, et al. Evolving concepts in radiofrequency catheter ablation of atrioventricular nodal reentry tachycardia. *Am Heart J* 1994;128:586–595.

74. Langberg JJ, Harvey M, Calkins H, et al. Titration of power output during radiofrequency catheter ablation of atrioventricular nodal reentrant tachycardia. *Pacing Clin Electrophysiol* 1993;16:465–470.

75. Langberg JJ. Comparison of the anterior and posterior approach for ablation of atrioventricular nodal reentrant tachycardia. In: Huang SKS, ed. *Radiofrequency Catheter Ablation of Cardiac Arrhythmias.* Armonk, NY: Futura; 1994:229–237.

76. Jackman WM, Beckman KJ, McClelland JH, et al. Treatment of supraventricular tachycardia due to atrioventricular nodal reentry, by radiofrequency catheter ablation of slow-pathway conduction. *N Engl J Med* 1992;327:313–318.

77. Kalbfleisch SJ, Strickberger SA, Williamson B, et al. Randomized comparison of anatomic and electrogram mapping approaches to ablation of the slow pathway of atrioventricular node reentrant tachycardia. *J Am Coll Cardiol* 1994;23:716–723.

78. Jentzer JH, Goyal R, Williamson BD, et al. Analysis of junctional ectopy during radiofrequency ablation of the slow pathway in patients with atrioventricular nodal reentrant tachycardia. *Circulation* 1994;90:2820–2826.

79. Baker JH, Plumb VJ, Epstein AE, et al. Predictors of recurrent atrioventricular nodal reentry after selective slow pathway ablation. *Am J Cardiol* 1994;73:765–769.

80. Ritchie AH, Kerr CR, Qi A, et al. Nonsustained ventricular tachycardia arising from the right ventricular outflow tract. *Am J Cardiol* 1989;64:594–598.

81. Klein LS, Shih HT, Hackett FK, et al. Radiofrequency catheter ablation of ventricular tachycardia in patients without structural heart disease. *Circulation* 1992;85:1666–1674.

82. O'Connor BK, Case CL, Sokoloski MC, et al. Radiofrequency catheter ablation of right ventricular outflow tachycardia in children and adolescents. *J Am Coll Cardiol* 1996;27:869–874.

83. Gaita F, Giustetto C, Leclercq JF, et al. Idiopathic verapamil-responsive left ventricular tachycardia: clinical characteristics and long-term follow-up of 33 patients. *Eur Heart J* 1994;15:1252–1260.

84. Nakagawa H, Beckman KJ, McClelland JH, et al. Radiofrequency catheter ablation of idiopathic left ventricular tachycardia guided by a Purkinje potential. *Circulation* 1993;88:2607–2617.

85. Burton ME, Leon AR. Radiofrequency catheter ablation of right ventricular outflow tract tachycardia late after complete repair of tetralogy of Fallot using the pace mapping technique. *Pacing Clin Electrophysiol* 1993;16:2319–2325.

86. Goldner BG, Cooper R, Blau W, et al. Radiofrequency catheter ablation as a primary therapy for treatment of ventricular tachycardia in a patient after repair of tetralogy of Fallot. *Pacing Clin Electrophysiol* 1994;17:1441–1446.

87. Biblo LA, Carlson MD. Transcatheter radiofrequency ablation of ventricular tachycardia following surgical correction of tetralogy of Fallot. *Pacing Clin Electrophysiol* 1994;17:1556–1560.

88. Gonska BD, Cao K, Raab J, et al. Radiofrequency catheter ablation of right ventricular tachycardia late after repair of congenital heart defects. *Circulation* 1996;94:1902–1908.

89. Danford DA, Kugler JD, Deal B, et al. The learning curve for radiofrequency ablation of tachyarrhythmias in pediatric patients. Participating members of the Pediatric Electrophysiology Society. *Am J Cardiol* 1995;75:587–590.

90. Lindsay BD, Eichling JO, Ambos HD, et al. Radiation exposure to patients and medical personnel during radiofrequency catheter ablation for supraventricular tachycardia. *Am J Cardiol* 1992;70:218–223.

91. Calkins H, Prystowsky E, Berger RD, et al. Recurrence of conduction following radiofrequency catheter ablation procedures: relationship to ablation target and electrode temperature. The Atakr Multicenter Investigators Group. *J Cardiovasc Electrophysiol* 1996;7:704–712.

92. Langberg JJ, Calkins H, Kim YN, et al. Recurrence of conduction in accessory atrioventricular connections after initially successful radiofrequency catheter ablation. *J Am Coll Cardiol* 1992;19:1588–1592.

93. Chen X, Kottkamp H, Hindricks G, et al. Recurrence and late block of accessory pathway conduction following radiofrequency catheter ablation. *J Cardiovasc Electrophysiol* 1994;5:650–658.

94. Walsh EP, Saul JP, Triedman JK, et al. Natural and unnatural history of ectopic atrial tachycardia: one institution's experience. *Pacing Clin Electrophsyiol* 1994; 17:746. Abstract.

95. Triedman JK, Bergau DM, Saul JP, et al. Midterm outcome of ablative therapy for atrial reentrant tachycardia in patients with congenital heart disease. *Pacing Clin Electrophysiol* 1996;19:579. Abstract.

96. Calkins H, Prystowsky E, Carlson M, et al. Temperature monitoring during radiofrequency catheter ablation procedures using closed loop control. Atakr Multicenter Investigators Group. *Circulation* 1994;90:1279–1286.

97. Kugler JD. Radiofrequency catheter ablation for supraventricular tachycardia. Should it be used in infants and small children? *Circulation* 1994;80:639–641.

98. Benson DW Jr, Dunnigan A, Benditt DG. Follow-up evaluation of infant paroxysmal atrial tachycardia: transesophageal study. *Circulation* 1987;75:542–549.

99. Perry JC, Garson A Jr. Supraventricular tachycardia due to Wolff-Parkinson-White syndrome in children: early disappearance and late recurrence. *J Am Coll Cardiol* 1990;16:1215–1220.

100. Case CL, Gillette PC, Oslizlok PC, et al. Radiofrequency catheter ablation of incessant, medically resistant supraventricular tachycardia in infants and small children. *J Am Coll Cardiol* 1992;20:1405–1410.

101. Weindling SN, Saul JP, Walsh EP. Efficacy and risks of medical therapy for supraventricular tachycardia in neonates and infants. *Am Heart J* 1996;131:66–72.

102. Deal BJ, Dick M, Beerman L, et al. Cardiac arrest in young patients with Wolff-Parkinson-White syndrome. *Pacing Clin Electrophysiol* 1995;18:815. Abstract.

103. Klein GJ, Prystowsky EN, Yee R, et al. Asymptomatic Wolff-Parkinson-White. Should we intervene? *Circulation* 1989;80:1902–1905.

The Evolving Surgical Management of Pediatric Arrhythmias

Constantine Mavroudis, MD
Carl L. Backer, MD
and Barbara J. Deal, MD

Introduction

Surgical therapy for atrioventricular (AV) arrhythmias underwent marked changes over the last 15–20 years due to technologic improvements and imaginative research.

The initial hallmark studies by Sealy[1] paved the way for Cox,[2] Guiraudon,[3] and others[4–7] to apply surgical ablative techniques to cure many types of AV arrhythmias, the most common of which were arrhythmias due to accessory connections (AC)—both manifest [Wolff-Parkinson-White (WPW) syndrome] and nonmanifest (concealed) AV nodal (AVN) tachycardias resulting from perinodal pathways, ectopic atrial tachycardias, and some types of atrial flutter (AF).[8] The results were excellent as the probability of success approached 100% and the mortality reduced to 0% to 1%[9–11] (Tables 1 and 2).

The introduction of transcatheter radiofrequency (RF) ablation dramatically changed the management of these arrhythmias.[12–14] As a result, the primary treatment for these atrial arrhythmias is RF ablation, reserving surgery for those unlikely cases of failed RF ablation or in those growing

From Deal B, Wolff G, Gelband H, (eds.). *Current Concepts in Diagnosis and Management of Arrhythmias in Infants and Children.* Armonk, NY: Futura Publishing Co., Inc.; © 1998.

_____ Table 1 _____

Pediatric Arrhythmia Surgery at Duke University (1981–1985), Washington University (1985–1991), and Children's Memorial Hospital (1988–1991)*

Diagnosis	DU/WU	CMH
WPW	62 (67%)	6 (55%)
CBT	19 (20%)	2 (18%)
AAT	2 (2%)	1 (9%)
PJRT	1 (1%)	—
JET	1 (1%)	—
MF	2 (2%)	—
AVN	3 (3%)	1 (9%)
VT	3 (3%)	1 (9%)

* A total of 100 patients underwent surgery for 104 arrhythmias. AAT, automatic atrial tachycardia; AVN, atrioventricular node reentry; CBT, concealed bypass tract; JET, junctional ectopic tachycardia; MF, Mahaim fibers; PJRT, permanent junctional reciprocating tachycardia; VT, ventricular tachycardia; WPW, Wolff-Parkinson-White syndrome.

Reproduced with permission from Reference 26.

cases where concomitant open heart surgery is required, such as mitral valve repair, redo Fontan procedures, etc.

The introduction of the Maze procedure,[15] principally used for adult patients with refractory atrial fibrillation, resulted in further research and

_____ Table 2 _____

Outcome of Arrhythmia Surgery in Children

	DU/WU (n = 90)	CMH (n = 10)
Arrhythmia terminated	88 (98%)	9 (90%)
Complications		
Complete heart block	3 (3%)	—
Postpericardiotomy syndrome	17 (19%)	—
Bleeding	2 (2%)	1 (10%)
False aneurysm	—	1 (10%)
Death	6 (7%)	—

Reproduced with permission from Reference 26.

modifications[16,17] to allow therapeutic applications to Fontan patients with troubling and life-threatening atrial arrhythmias. The clinical impact of these new procedures is now under investigation with promising short-term results.[18,19]

These technological advances and clinical applications increased the scope of therapeutic interventions and resulted in close consultation between cardiologists and cardiac surgeons to better serve their patients.

The purpose of this chapter is twofold. The first is to review the now seldom used surgical ablation techniques that may be required in those cases where RF ablation failed. The second is to document the new surgical ablation techniques that were recently applied to control atrial fibrillation (Maze procedure) and atrial arrhythmias (flutter) that are primarily associated with Fontan patients.

Surgical Ablation for Wolff-Parkinson-White Syndrome/Concealed Bypass Tracts

The surgical techniques that were developed to treat the various anatomic variants of WPW/concealed connections are noteworthy not only because of the relevance to present-day needs in the event of failed RF ablation but also because of the advances that gave rise to the surgical procedures to treat atrial fibrillation and AF.

Intraoperative Mapping

Intraoperative epicardial and/or endocardial mapping is always performed at the time of surgery to confirm the catheterization findings and to assess the immediate postoperative result. The purpose is to establish the mechanism of the tachycardia, localize the anatomic connection, and determine whether multiple AC exist. The atrial activation sequence is determined during ventricular pacing and induced supraventricular tachycardia (SVT), and the ventricular activation is assessed during atrial pacing if the patient has manifest preexcitation. At our institution, we used combinations of hand-held electrodes as well as multiple electrodes on bands to achieve intraoperative mapping results. At Washington University, Cox and associates[20] utilized a digital acquisition system with a maximum capacity of 256 channels. A band containing 16 bipolar electrodes is placed around the AV groove, thereby permitting recording of simultaneous electrocardiograms (ECGs) from the entire AV groove (Figure 1). This system expedites intraoperative mapping and allows for identification of multiple connections (Figure 2) without the need for manipulating the heart in any way, obviating the need for cardiopulmonary bypass for this part of the operation. Once the mapping is completed and analyzed, the ablative part of the operation can be performed.

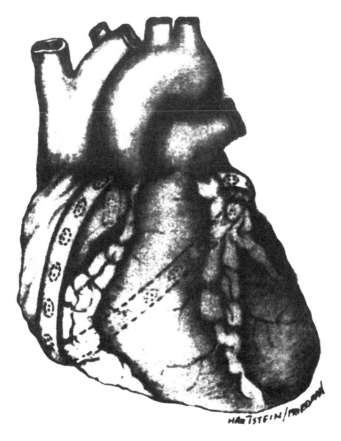

Figure 1. After the band electrode was moved to the atrial side of the AV groove, reciprocating tachycardia is induced and a retrograde atrial map is performed. Reproduced with permission from Reference 91.

Surgical Principles

The general goal of surgical therapy for the WPW syndrome/concealed bypass tract is to divide or cryoablate AC that are responsible for the reentry phenomenon and clinical tachycardia. The two surgical techniques that were developed are the endocardial and epicardial techniques (Figure 3). The endocardial technique[2,20,22] requires cardiopulmonary bypass and is performed within the right atrium (RA) or left atrium (LA), depending on the anatomic location of the bypass tract. The epicardial technique[23–25] may or may not require cardiopulmonary bypass, depending on the location of the bypass tract and is performed on the epicardial surface of the heart at the AV junction by dividing the atrial end of the connection. Ex-

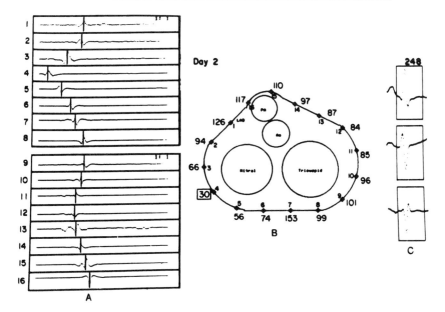

Figure 2. A: Hard copy of the terminal display showing activation sequence of the 16 electrodes contained in the band. This is an antegrade ventricular preexcitation map with the band placed on the ventricular side of the AV groove; the electrode showing earliest activation (electrode 4) is located at the site of the ventricular insertion of the AC. **B** and **C:** Hard copy of the terminal display showing activation sequence of the base of the ventricles during stable antegrade preexcitation. The designated window is displayed on the right side of the screen. The activation sequence is related to a sketch of the base of the heart, and the earliest site of ventricular activity during stable antegrade preexcitement is enclosed in a box. Adapted with permission from Reference 91.

cellent results were achieved by both techniques, the choice being surgeon and institution dependent.

Left Free-Wall Accessory Connections

Ablation of left free-wall (LFW) AC is usually performed by the endocardial technique from within the LA utilizing cardiopulmonary bypass and cardioplegic arrest. The exposure is through a left atriotomy usually performed at the interatrial (Sondergaard's) groove similar to that for mitral valve repair/replacement. After proper exposure, a curvilinear incision parallel to and 2 mm away from the posterior mitral annulus is made, extending from the left fibrous trigone to the posterior septum (Figure 4A and B). A dissection plane is then developed between the fat pad of the AV groove and the superior portion of the left ventricle (LV) extending to the epicardial reflection throughout the entire length of the initial incision

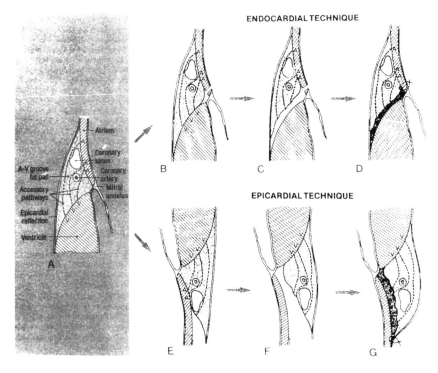

Figure 3. Diagrammatic representation of a cross-section of the posterior left heart. The different depths at which LFW connections can be located in relation to the mitral annulus and epicardial reflection are shown (**A**). **B–D**: The endocardial surgical technique. **E–G**: The epicardial technique. Reproduced with permission from Reference 92.

(Figure 4C and D). The dissection is completed by extending the ends of the incision and the dissection, "squaring off" to the mitral annulus to divide any AC that might be located at the juxtaannular area.[20] This dissection exposes the entire LFW space to the respective boundaries, thereby ensuring division of any or all AC. The endocardial incision is then sutured to complete the procedure (Figure 4E).

The epicardial approach (Figure 5) for LFW AC requires upward and rightward cardiac retraction for proper exposure, which more often than not results in severe hemodynamic instability. As a result, most surgeons employing this technique prefer to use cardiopulmonary bypass, despite the fact that no intracavitary exposure is required for this technique. Once exposure is achieved, the epicardial reflection of the atrium is entered and a plane of dissection is established between the AV groove fat pad and the atrial wall. Coronary sinus (CS) tributaries often require ligation and division, and care must be taken to avoid coronary artery injury. The dissection

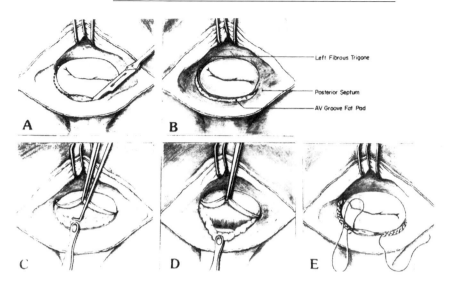

Figure 4. Endocardial technique for dividing LFW AC in the WPW syndrome. Adapted with permission from Reference 2.

plane is extended to the level of the posterior mitral valve annulus and carried slightly onto the top of the posterior LV. This maneuver divides the atrial end of all AC in this area except for those that lie immediately adjacent to the mitral valve annulus. If present, these juxtaannular connections can be interrupted by a cryosurgical probe that is placed at the level of the mitral valve annulus. The atrial epicardial reflection is then reapproximated by suture technique. Both techniques have their respective advantages and disadvantages,[20,23] which can be applied selectively, depending on the anatomic circumstances governing the operation. Anatomic variation may be especially important in the case of simultaneous repair of congenital heart disease and ablation of AC. The surgeon should be familiar with both techniques.

Posterior Septal Accessory Connections

The endocardial approach to posterior septal connections is through the RA. Normothermic cardiopulmonary bypass is usually used with certain precautions, which include closure of any intracardiac shunts before right atriotomy. Preoperative evaluation may not always confirm the presence of a patent foramen ovale. Care then is taken to fibrillate the heart shortly after cardiopulmonary bypass and before RA entry in order to check for, and close, a patent foramen ovale. This maneuver will ensure that no air is introduced to the LV during a beating cardiac cycle. After complete

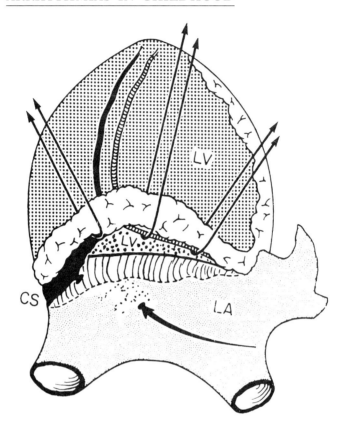

Figure 5. The epicardial approach to LFW AC. A schematic
of the LV viewed from an operative position. The fat pad is
mobilized and the AV junction exposed. CS, coronary sinus;
LA, left atrium; LV, left ventricle. Reproduced with permission
from Reference 25.

patent foramen ovale closure, the heart can be defibrillated and the operation continued. After completion of the endocardial mapping, a supraannular incision is made 2 mm above the posterior medial tricuspid
valve annulus, beginning at least 1 cm posterior to the His bundle (Figure
6). The supraannular incision is extended counterclockwise onto the posterior RA free wall. This incision provides exposure to the posterior septal
space near the LV and the epicardial reflection at the posterior right ventricle (RV) near the crux of the heart. The posterior septal space fat pad
is then dissected away from the top of the posterior ventricular septum
while the heart is beating or during hypothermic cardioplegic arrest, depending on the vascularity of the dissection plane and the preference of
the surgeon.

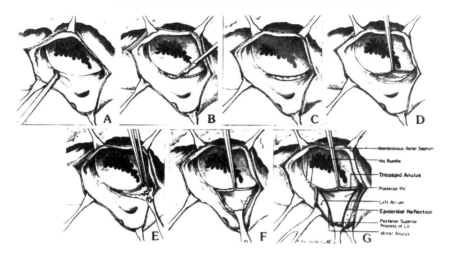

Figure 6. Endocardial technique for surgical division of posterior septal AC in the WPW syndrome. The junction of the posterior medial mitral and tricuspid valve annuli forms an inverted V at the posterior edge of the central fibrous body, and the fat pad comes to a point at the apex of that V. The apex of the V is always posterior to the His bundle, although the distance between the apex of the V and the His bundle may vary. As long as the dissection in this region remains posterior to the central fibrous body, the His bundle will not be damaged. After the anterior point of the fat pad is gently dissected away from the apex of the V (ie, away from the posterior edge of the central fibrous body), the mitral valve annulus comes into view at the point where it joins the tricuspid valve to form the central fibrous body. Adapted with permission from Reference 2.

The epicardial approach to posterior septal AC is very similar to that for the LFW connections except of course for the location. The posterior septal AC are divided by developing a dissection plane between the fat pad and the top of the posterior ventricular septum, following the mitral annulus over to the posterior superior process of the LV, and following the epicardial reflection from the posterior RV, across the crux, onto the posterior LV. Cryolesions are placed at regular intervals around the annulus to ensure complete division of all AC.

Right Free-Wall Accessory Connections

The epicardial dissection for right free-wall (RFW) AC can be performed without cardiopulmonary bypass in the majority of cases. An incision is made in the epicardium, establishing a dissection plane between the RA wall and the AV groove fat pad to the tricuspid valve annulus (Figure 7) throughout the entire length of the RA free wall. Cryolesions at appropriate intervals can ensure complete AC ablation.

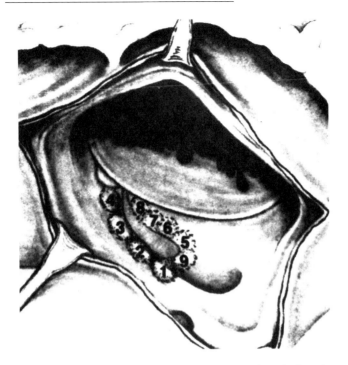

Figure 8. Cryolesions are placed in positions 1 to 4, then in positions 5 to 8, and finally in position 9. During the application of cryothermia at positions 7 and 8, prolongation of the AV intervals begins to occur. Reproduced with permission from Reference 93.

cryolesion since it may be too close to the AVN. After a short period of recovery, the cryoablation may continue until all the lesions were placed and remapping confirmed the success of the procedure.

Other Forms of Supraventricular Tachycardia

Other forms of SVT that are often incessant include automatic atrial tachycardia, atrial reentrant tachycardia, the permanent form of junctional reciprocating tachycardia, and junctional ectopic tachycardia. These arrhythmias, due to their incessant nature, can lead to severe but essentially reversible cardiomyopathy[34–36] and ought to be treated aggressively with RF ablation or with surgery in the case of failed catheter ablation.[37–39]

Some authors had good results with simple cryoablation and excision of automatic foci when found.[7,35,39] Others[40] experienced recurrences because of the multiple ectopic foci that are associated with these arrhythmias.

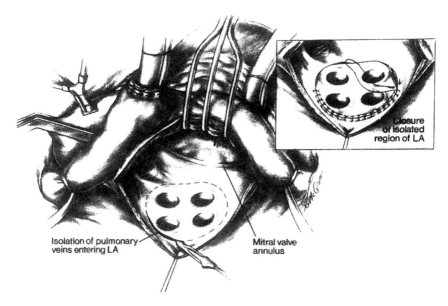

Figure 9. Isolation of an arrhythmogenic focus adjacent to the pulmonary veins. LA, left atrium. Reproduced with permission from Reference 94.

This led surgeons to apply more extensive techniques such as pulmonary vein isolation (Figure 9), LA isolation (Figure 10), RA isolation (Figure 11), and His bundle cryoablation with pacemaker insertion in difficult cases. In general, refractory cases are rare and require an individualized treatment plan for accurate diagnosis and ablation.

We successfully operated on two children with primary atrial tachycardia. One 11-year-old girl had paroxysmal sinoatrial (SA) reentry tachycardia since infancy, refractory to virtually all antiarrhythmic therapy. Two attempts at RF catheter ablation were unsuccessful, thought to be due to the wide area in the superior RA with early activation mapping. At surgery, repeat activation mapping indicated additional involvement of the posterior LA. Resection of the posterolateral RA was performed, with an encircling incision around the pulmonary veins. She had no recurrence of the atrial reentrant tachycardia in 4 years, but developed late sinus bradycardia requiring an atrial pacemaker 3 years postoperatively. Another 10-year-old girl had triggered atrial tachycardia near the perimeter of a secundum atrial septal defect (ASD). At the time of ASD closure, cryoablation of the medial rim of the atrial defect was performed. Postoperatively she had no inducible SVT, with no recurrences during 2 years of follow-up.

Some patients develop VT after remote repair of congenital heart disease—especially in those patients with repaired tetralogy of Fallot. In patients with coexistent hemodynamic abnormalities, surgical excision and/or cryoablation in the region of the RV outflow tract, generally with pulmonary valve insertion, appears to be a safe, effective therapy with favorable results reported.[46-50] We recently performed resection of the VT focus in the RV outflow tract together with pulmonary valve replacement and pulmonary arterioplasty with good results in two adult patients with postoperative tetralogy of Fallot. Surgical intervention for other forms of refractory VT was rarely reported in children. RV dysplasia was managed by disengagement of the RV wall,[51] but fell out of favor due to resultant RV failure. Idiopathic VT is sometimes amenable to discrete cryoablation following endocardial mapping. Patients with refractory tachycardia, including those with long QT syndrome, may benefit from implantation of an automatic implantable cardioverter defibrillator.[52]

Atrial Flutter and Atrial Fibrillation

The comprehensive approach to unravel the causative mysteries of SVT through anatomic discovery, physiological experimentation, surgical intervention, and RF ablation was one of the great therapeutic success stories for a particular cardiac disease. This success, in turn, led to a comprehensive study of atrial fibrillation and AF with the idea that a safe, effective, and reliable therapeutic intervention can be developed. To this end, Boineau[53] and Cox and associates[54-56] introduced the idea and confirmed through experimentation that clinical AF/fibrillation can be thought of as a continuum, extending from a single, microreentrant circuit of right-sided AF at one end to multiple simultaneous macroreentrant circuits over the entire surface of the RA and LA. In subsequent studies Ferguson and Cox and associates[57] suggested that AF was dependent on anatomic obstacles on the right and left sides of the heart which include the superior and inferior vena caval (IVC) orifices, the annuli of the AV valves, and the pulmonary veins. Atrial fibrillation, conversely, was found to be independent of any anatomic obstacles, making this arrhythmia different from the other SVTs as well as VT. More important to sustaining atrial fibrillation are factors such as number of wavelets, surface area of tissue, and intraatrial size, volume, and pressure.[56] These factors are present to various degrees in patients dependent upon the presence or absence of concomitant disease (acquired vs. congenital vs. nonstructural heart disease).

In order to more clearly define operative cure for atrial fibrillation, a four-part definition was developed by Cox[58] and Ferguson[57] that includes

(1) elimination of the clinical arrhythmia, (2) maintenance of SA nodal tissue as the driving impulse for the heart, (3) maintenance of intact AV conduction, and (4) restoration of atrial transport function. The evaluation of past and future procedures to treat atrial fibrillation will be based on the above definition.

The Maze Procedure

The Maze procedure is designed to reduce or eliminate the critical number of reentrant circuits available to maintain the fibrillatory process (Figure 12). The initial[15] (Figure 13) and subsequent modifications[60] (Fig-

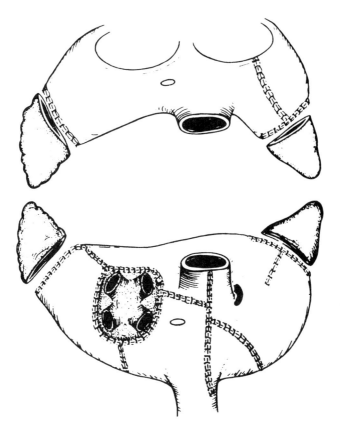

Figure 12. The completed Maze procedure (original) for cure of atrial fibrillation as viewed from the posterior aspect. Reproduced with permission from Reference 97.

Table 4

Surgery for Atrial Fibrillation*

Author	Oprn	Atrial Fibrillation Disease	Eliminates Reentrant Circuits	Decrease Fibrillatory Mass	Surgical Technique (Side)	Tech Diff	SR	Eliminates AF	Restores ATF	Number of Patients
Cox[61]	1	Idiopathic	Y	N	L, R	3+	Y (100%)	Y (99%)	Y (80%)	75
McCarthy et al[66]	1	Idiopathic	Y	N	L, R	3+	Y (100%)	Y (99%)	Y (80%)	14
DeFauw[67]	2	Idiopathic	N	Y	L, R	1+	Y	N	N	21
Brodman et al[68]	3	Rheumatic	Y	N	L	2+	Y	N	Y	1
Hioki et al[69]	4	Rheumatic	Y	N	L, R	3+	Y	Y	Y	1
Kawaguchi et al[63]	5	Rheumatic	Y(?)	N(?)	L, R	2+	Y (92%)	Y (92%)	Y	51
Sueda et al[70]	6	Rheumatic	Y	Y	L	2+	Y (85%)	Y (85%)	Y (82%)	13
Shyu et al[64]	7	Rheumatic	N	Y	L, R	1+	Y (64%)	Y (64%)	Y (64%)	22
Itoh et al[71]	1	Rheumatic	Y	N	L, R	3+	Y (100%)	Y	Y	15
Graffigna et al[72]	8	Rheumatic	N	Y	L	1+	Y (70%)	N	N	100
Blitz et al[73]	1	HOCM	Y	N	L, R	3+	Y†	Y	Y	1
Bonchek et al[74]	1	ASD	Y	N	L, R	3+	Y	Y	Y	1

Oprn = Operation; 1 = Maze procedure; 2 = corridor procedure; 3 = left-sided maze procedure only; 4 = maze with modification to pulmonary vein isolation; 5 = unspecified modification to maze procedure; 6 = pulmonary vein isolation + areas of isolation; 7 = L and R compartmentalization procedure; 8 = left atrial isolation procedure. Idiopathic, primary atrial fibrillation in the absence of valvular disease in the majority of patients; rheumatic, almost all patients with underlying valvar disease and concomitant valve surgery; HOCM = hypertrophic obstructive cardiomyopathy; ASD, atrial septal defect; L, left; R, right; Tech Diff, technical difficulty of antiarrhythmic portion of the operative procedure; SR, patients in sinus rhythm late postoperatively; AF, atrial fibrillation; ATF, late atrial transport function.
Reproduced with permission from Reference 8.

Recurrent Atrial Tachycardia
in Fontan Patients

Evolving technical modifications of the Fontan operation led to improved survival.[75–78] Greater survival and longevity uncovered the expected high incidence of atrial arrhythmias, estimated to occur in approximately 30% to 50% of patients, which account for significant morbidity and mortality.[79,80] Developmental risk factors for atrial arrhythmias in Fontan patients include age at initial operation, type of atriopulmonary artery connection, perioperative arrhythmias, duration of follow-up, and resultant unfavorable hemodynamics. Drug therapy,[40] antitachycardia pacemakers,[81] and transcatheter ablation[82–84] had variable impact on arrhythmia control. This led us to pursue a program of intraoperative intracardiac cryoablation, mostly in conjunction with procedures to rectify stenoses, create or complete total cavopulmonary artery anastomosis, and address AV valve dysfunction. In most cases, the clinical arrhythmia was the primary indication for the operation.

Patient Selection

We selected 13 patients who underwent Fontan revision for management of recurrent atrial arrhythmias with hemodynamic abnormalities. Recurrent atrial reentry tachycardia refractory to medical therapy was present in nine patients. One patient had recurrent atrial fibrillation or AF and one patient had profound atrial bradycardia with intermittent tachycardia. Symptoms during tachycardia were low output or shock in eight, and syncope in three. Prior antiarrhythmic therapy with a mean of 2.3 drugs per patient was unsuccessful in the patients with atrial reentry tachycardia. All but 1 patient had marked limited physical activity: 12 patients were considered to be in NYHA class 3–4. One patient suffered a stroke 2 months prior to surgical revision.

Significant associated hemodynamic abnormalities were present in 12 of 13 patients, including RA-to-pulmonary artery obstruction, severe RA dilatation, and residual right-to-left shunts. One patient had excellent hemodynamic findings, but his life-threatening tachycardia circuit was localized to the ''red'' atrium. All patients, excluding the patient with atrial fibrillation, underwent preoperative electrophysiological (EP) mapping studies.

Cryoablation Technique

All patients underwent resternotomy and complete dissection without incident. An RA reference electrode was sutured near the RA/superior vena caval (SVC) junction. Epicardial mapping was performed during in-

duced atrial tachycardia after cannulation but before cardiopulmonary bypass. Endocardial atrial mapping was repeated following institution of
warm cardiopulmonary bypass in those patients who did not have residual
shunting (Figure 14). We identified three major anatomic sites as follows
thought to be critical to the tachycardia circuit (Figure 15): area 1 shows
the area between the CS os and the IVC os, as well as the area between the
AV valve annulus and the IVC os; area 2 shows the lateral atriotomy, which
corresponded to the length of the crista terminalis (CT); and area 3 shows
the region at the superior limbus corresponding to the prior ASD patch.
Cryoablation lesions were delivered by a 15-mm diameter probe (Frigitron-
ics, Shelton, Conn) at −60°C for 90 seconds for each lesion. All patients
had cryoablation lesions placed in area 1. In those selected patients requiring further therapy in areas 2 and 3, cryoablation lesions were linearly
placed to connect these areas with an anatomic orifice, ie, vertical lesions
along the CT from the SVC to the IVC or lesions to connect the superior
limbus to the SVC. In those patients who required takedown of the atrial

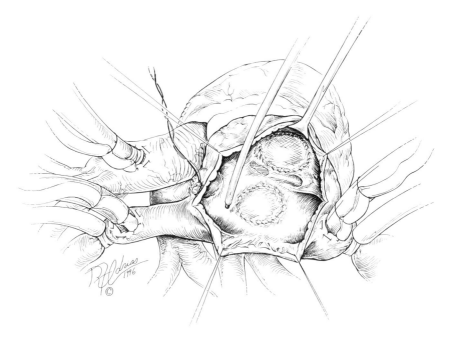

Figure 14. Diagrammatic representation of an open RA view in an atriopulmonary
Fontan patient, without residual atrial shunts, who has been placed on normothermic aortobicaval cardiopulmonary bypass en route to EP mapping and arrhythmia circuit cryoablation, cavopulmonary artery conversion, and atrial antitachycardia pacemaker placement. An RA bipolar wire served as the reference electrode
and electrical pathway for arrhythmia stimulation. A hand-held electrode is used to
perform the EP mapping.[16] Reproduced with permission from Reference 18.

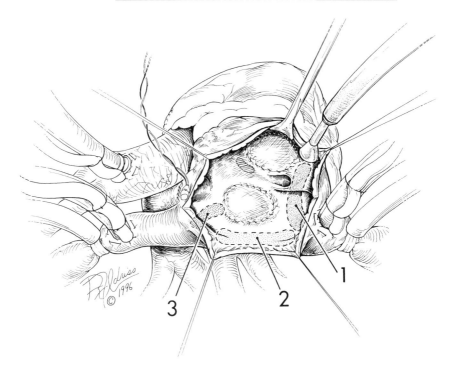

Figure 15. Diagrammatic representation of an open RA view (see Figure 14). There were three major areas where tachycardia localized. **Area 1**: the area between the CS os and the IVC os, as well as the area between the AV valve annulus and the IVC os; **area 2**: the lateral atriotomy which corresponded to the length of the CT; and **area 3**: the region at the superior limbus corresponding to the prior ASD patch. Reproduced with permission from Reference 18.

partition, aortic cross-clamping and blood cardioplegia were used to gain access to the systemic side of the circulation to complete the cryoablation procedure. This was especially appropriate in those patients whose CS and tricuspid valve were partitioned to the pulmonary venous return atrium and systemic ventricle (Figure 15). In all cases, the goal of therapy was to interrupt all potential connections for the atrial arrhythmia circuit.

Pacemaker Implantation

An atrial antitachycardia pacemaker (Intertach II, Intermedics, Inc) was implanted in 11 of 13 patients. Standard transvenous endocardial leads were inserted at the time of atriotomy using a transmural technique.[85,86] The lead was positioned in a remnant of the anatomic RA that is part of the pulmonary venous circuit, necessitating chronic anticoagulation.

Anatomic Revisions

The goal of therapy for those atriopulmonary Fontan patients with arrhythmia and/or obstructive anatomic indications for reoperation is conversion to total cavopulmonary artery connections, arrhythmia circuit cryoablation, and atrial antitachycardia pacemaker placement. There are basically three types of anatomic connections: atrial compartmentalization with RA-to-pulmonary artery anastomosis, classical right Glenn operation and an atrial-to-left pulmonary artery anastomosis, and a total cavopulmonary artery reconstruction.

The conduct of the operation is similar for all patients. Following aortobicaval cardiopulmonary bypass, intraoperative EP mapping, and arrhythmia circuit cryoablation, the patient is cooled in preparation for total cavopulmonary artery conversion and atrial antitachycardia pacemaker placement.

For those patients with atriopulmonary anastomoses, a standard total cavopulmonary artery connection is accomplished using a lateral tunnel or

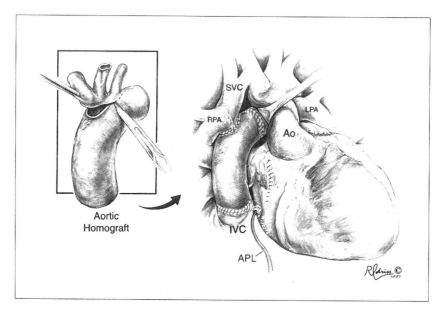

Figure 16. Diagrammatic representation of a total cavopulmonary artery extracardiac conversion in a patient with an established classic right Glenn/RA-to-left pulmonary artery Fontan connection. An aortic homograft was used to connect the left pulmonary artery with the IVC using the favorable curve of the ascending and transverse arch of the homograft. The Glenn anastomosis was connected side-to-side to the homograft to complete the reconstruction. A transmural bipolar steroid-eluting atrial lead (Medtronic, Inc, Minneapolis) is placed in the LA appendage for antitachycardia pacemaker placement. Reproduced with permission from Reference 18.

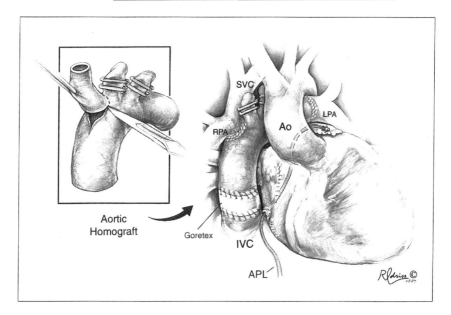

Figure 17. Total cavopulmonary artery extracardiac Fontan conversion (see Figure 16). Occasionally, the aortic homograft may require a Gore-Tex graft extension (composite graft) to connect the left pulmonary artery with the IVC. The Glenn anastomosis can be connected to the homograft as appropriate. Reproduced with permission from Reference 18.

an extracardiac technique.[75–78] Extensive pulmonary artery reconstruction, when necessary, is performed at that time. In those patients with a right Glenn procedure and an atrial-to-left pulmonary artery anastomosis, more creative pulmonary artery reconstructions are required (Figures 16 and 17). Under cardioplegic arrest, left-side procedures are performed such as prosthetic atrial patch resection, valvular reconstructions, completion of cryoablative lesions, the lateral tunnel reconstruction (when elected), transmural atrial wire placement (Figure 17) for the antitachycardia pacemaker (Intertach II, Intermedics, Inc),[85] ventricular vent placement, atrial wall reduction, and atriorrhaphy. The atrial pacemaker lead is placed in the red atrium using the transmural technique reported by Hoyer and associates.[86] This is followed by de-airing, aortic cross clamp removal, rewarming, vent removal, and extracardiac IVC connection if and when elected. Separation from cardiopulmonary bypass is followed by transesophageal echocardiographic assessment.

Discussion

We had no surgical mortality and only one case of transient surgical heart block in a patient with corrected transposition. During mean follow-up of 2.5 years, 11 of 13 patients remain off all antiarrhythmic medications. One patient had recurrent SVT 4 weeks postoperatively, with one recurrence in the next 23 months on procainamide. One patient with incessant SVT associated with low output preoperatively developed a slow asymptomatic atrial tachycardia 21 months postoperatively, responding to β-blocker therapy. In the 11 patients with antitachycardia pacemakers, four had tachycardia detected and terminated by the pacemaker in the first 3 months postoperatively only, with no subsequent recurrences. All patients are currently in NYHA class 1–2.

We believe that the presence of recurrent or life-threatening atrial arrhythmias in the postoperative Fontan population should prompt a comprehensive cardiac catheterization and an EP study to assess their hemodynamic status. In our experience, echocardiography alone may not detect significant residual abnormalities. Conversion to a total cavopulmonary connection with arrhythmia circuit cryoablation can be accomplished with low morbidity and mortality. As previous studies showed,[87–90] Fontan conversion to total cavopulmonary artery connection alone is not effective therapy for atrial arrhythmia control. We believe that Fontan conversion to total cavopulmonary artery connection, surgical mapping, and arrhythmia circuit cryoablation, combined with antitachycardia pacing, will significantly improve the outcome in this troublesome population. In addition, we speculate that prophylactic cryoablation in area 1 at the time of initial Fontan procedure may favorably impact the development of atrial tachycardia.

References

1. Cobb FR, Blumenschein SD, Sealy WC, et al. Successful surgical interruption of the bundle of Kent in a patient with Wolff-Parkinson-White syndrome. *Circulation* 1968;36:1018–1029.
2. Cox JL, Gallagher JJ, Cain ME. Experience with 118 consecutive patients undergoing operation for the Wolff-Parkinson-White syndrome. *J Thorac Cardiovasc Surg* 1985;90:490–501.
3. Guiraudon G, Fontaine G, Frank R, et al. Encircling endocardial ventriculotomy: a new surgical treatment of life-threatening ventricular tachycardias resistant to medical treatment following myocardial infarction. *Ann Thorac Surg* 1978;26:438–444.
4. Josephson ME, Harken AH, Horowitz LN. Endocardial excision—a new surgical technique for the treatment of recurrent ventricular tachycardia. *Circulation* 1979;60:1430–1439.
5. Moral J, Kehoe RF, Loeb J, et al. Extended endocardial resection for the treatment of ventricular tachycardia and ventricular fibrillation. *Ann Thorac Surg* 1982;34:538–552.
6. Ostermeyer J, Breithardt G, Borggrefe M, et al. Surgical treatment of ventricular tachycardias. Complete versus partial encircling endocardial ventriculotomy. *J Thorac Cardiovasc Surg* 1984;87:517–525.
7. Selle JG, Svenson RH, Sealy WC, et al. Successful clinical laser ablation of ventricular tachycardia: a promising new therapeutic method. *Ann Thorac Surg* 1986;42:380–384.

8. Ferguson TB Jr, Cox, JL. Surgery for supraventricular arrhythmias. In: Baue AE, Geha AS, Hammond GL, et al, eds. *Glenn's Thoracic and Cardiovascular Surgery,* 6th ed. Stamford, Conn: Appleton & Lange; 1996:2141–2180.
9. Ott DA, Garson A, Cooley DA, et al. Definitive operation for refractory cardiac tachyarrhythmias in children. *J Thorac Cardiovasc Surg* 1985;90:681–689.
10. Crawford FA Jr, Gillette PC. Pediatric electrophysiologic surgery. In: Kron IL, ed. *Innovations in Congenital Heart Surgery.* Philadelphia: Hanley & Belfus, Inc; 1989:297–310.
11. Mahomed Y, King RD, Zipes DP, et al. Surgical division of Wolff-Parkinson-White pathways utilizing the closed-heart technique: a 2-year experience in 47 patients. *Ann Thorac Surg* 1988;45:495–504.
12. Weber H, Schmitz L. Catheter technique for closed-chest ablation of an accessory atrioventricular pathway (letter). *N Engl J Med* 1983;308:653–654.
13. Scheinman MM, Evans-Bell T. Catheter ablation of the atrioventricular junction: a report of the percutaneous mapping and ablation registry. *Circulation* 1984;70:1024–1029.
14. Jackman WM, Wang X, Friday KJ, et al. Catheter ablation of accessory atrioventricular pathways (Wolff-Parkinson-White syndrome) by radiofrequency current. *N Engl J Med* 1991;324:1605–1611.
15. Cox JL. The surgical treatment of atrial fibrillation. IV. Surgical technique. *J Thorac Cardiovasc Surg* 1991;101:584–592.
16. Cox JL, Jaquiss RD, Schuessler RB, et al. Modification of the maze procedure for atrial flutter and atrial fibrillation. II. Surgical technique of the Maze III procedure. *J Thorac Cardiovasc Surg* 1995;110:485–495.
17. Tsui SS, Grace AA, Ludman PF, et al. Maze 3 for atrial fibrillation: two cuts too few? *Pacing Clin Electrophysiol* 1994;17:2163–2166.
18. Mavroudis C, Backer CL, Deal BJ, et al. Fontan conversion to cavopulmonary connection and cryoablation of arrhythmia circuit. *J Thorac Cardiovasc Surg* 1998;115:1–9.
19. Deal BJ, Mavroudis C, Backer CL, et al. A comparative study of surgical conversion for recurrent atrial tachycardia in Fontan patients: the favorable impact of arrhythmia circuit cryoablation. *Circulation.* In press.
20. Cox JL, Ferguson TB Jr. Surgery for the Wolff-Parkinson-White syndrome: the endocardial approach. *Semin Thorac Cardiovasc Surg* 1989;1:34–46.
21. Harada A, D'Agostino HJ Jr, Schuessler RB, et al. Potential distribution mapping. New method for precise localization of intramural septal origin of ventricular tachycardia. *Circulation* 1988;78:137–147.
22. Lowe JE. Surgical treatment of the Wolff-Parkinson-White syndrome and other supraventricular tachyarrhythmias. *J Cardiac Surg* 1986;1:117–134.
23. Guiraudon GM, Klein GJ, Sharma AD, et al. Closed-heart technique for Wolff-Parkinson-White syndrome. Further experience and potential limitations. *Ann Thorac Surg* 1986;42:651–657.
24. Mahomed Y, King RD, Zipes DP, et al. Surgical division of Wolff-Parkinson-White pathways utilizing the closed-heart technique: a 2-year experience in 47 patients. *Ann Thorac Surg* 1988;45:495–504.
25. Guiraudon GM, Klein GJ, Sharma AD, et al. Surgery for the Wolff-Parkinson-White syndrome: the epicardial approach. *Semin Thorac Cardiovasc Surg* 1989;1:21–33.
26. Bromberg BI, Mavroudis C, Cox, JL. Surgical management of pediatric arrhythmias. In: Emmanouilides GC, Riemenschneider TA, Allen HD, et al, eds. *Moss and Adams' Heart Disease in Infants, Children, and Adolescents Including the Fetus and Young Adult.* Baltimore: Williams & Wilkins; 1994:468–480.

27. Pritchett ELC, Anderson RW, Benditt DG, et al. Reentry within the atrioventricular node: surgical cure with preservation of atrioventricular conduction. *Circulation* 1979;60:440–446.

28. Holman WL, Ikeshita M, Lease JG, et al. Elective prolongation of atrioventricular conduction by multiple discrete cryolesions: a new technique for the treatment of paroxysmal supraventricular tachycardia. *J Thorac Cardiovasc Surg* 1982;84:554–559.

29. Holman WL, Ikeshita M, Lease JG, et al. Cryosurgical modification of retrograde atrioventricular conduction: implications for the surgical treatment of atrioventricular nodal reentry tachycardia. *J Thorac Cardiovasc Surg* 1986;91:826–834.

30. Ross DL, Johnson DC, Denniss AR, et al. Curative surgery for atrioventricular junction ("AV nodal") reentrant tachycardia. *J Am Coll Cardiol* 1985;6:1383–1392.

31. Gielchinsky I. Personal communication to Crawford FA Jr, Gillette PC. Pediatric electrophysiologic surgery. In: Kron IL, Mavroudis C, eds. *Innovations in Congenital Heart Surgery.* Philadelphia: Hanley & Belfus, Inc; 1989:297–310.

32. Case CL, Crawford FA, Gillette PC, et al. Successful surgery for atrioventricular reentrant tachycardia in a small child. *Am Heart J* 1988;116:187–189.

33. Cox JL. Surgery for cardiac arrhythmias. In: Braunwald E, ed. *Heart Disease Update 13 to Heart Disease: A Textbook of Cardiovascular Medicine,* 3rd ed. Philadelphia: WB Saunders Co; 1991:295–322.

34. Kugler JD, Baisch SD, Cheatham JP, et al. Improvement of left ventricular dysfunction after control of persistent tachycardia. *J Pediatr* 1984;105:543–548.

35. Gillette PC, Smith RT, Garson A Jr, et al. Chronic supraventricular tachycardia: a curable cause of congestive cardiomyopathy. *JAMA* 1985;253:391–392.

36. Bromberg BI, Dick M II, Snider AR, et al. Tachycardia related cardiomyopathy in children: response to control of the arrhythmia. *J Interven Cardiol* 1989;2:211–218.

37. Walsh EP, Saul JP, Hulse JE, et al. Transcatheter ablation of ectopic atrial tachycardia in young patients using radiofrequency current. *Circulation* 1992;86:1138–1146.

38. Dorostkar PC, Dick M II, Serwer GA, et al. Radiofrequency ablation for the treatment of persistent junctional reciprocating tachycardia. *Circulation* 1992;86(suppl I):581. Abstract.

39. Gillette PC, Wampler DG, Garson A, et al. Treatment of atrial automatic tachycardia by ablation procedures. *J Am Coll Cardiol* 1985;6:405–409.

40. Balaji S, Johnson TB, Sade RM, et al. Management of atrial flutter after the Fontan operation. *J Am Coll Cardiol* 1994;23:1209–1215.

41. Ferrans VJ, McAllister HA, Haese WH. Infantile cardiomyopathy with histiocytoid change in cardiac muscle cells. *Circulation* 1976;53:708–719.

42. Zeigler VL, Gillette PC, Crawford FA Jr, et al. New approaches to treatment of incessant ventricular tachycardia in the very young. *J Am Coll Cardiol* 1990;16:681–685.

43. Fish FA, Gillette PC, Benson DW Jr. Proarrhythmia, cardiac arrest and death in young patients receiving encainide and flecainide. *J Am Coll Cardiol* 1991;18:356–365.

44. Garson A Jr, Smith RT Jr, Moak JP, et al. Incessant ventricular tachycardia in infants: myocardial hamartomas and surgical cure. *J Am Coll Cardiol* 1987;10:619–626.

45. Garson A Jr, Gillette C, Titus JL, et al. Surgical treatment of ventricular tachycardia in infants. *N Engl J Med* 1984;310:1443–1445.

46. Campbell RM, Hammon JW Jr, Echt DS, et al. Surgical treatment of pediatric cardiac arrhythmia. *J Pediatr* 1987;110:501–508.

47. Harken AH, Horowitz LN, Josephson ME. Surgical correction of recurrent sustained ventricular tachycardia following complete repair of tetralogy of Fallot. *J Thorac Cardiovasc Surg* 1980;80:779–781.
48. Horowitz LN, Vetter VL, Harken AH, et al. Electrophysiologic characteristics of sustained ventricular tachycardia occurring after repair of tetralogy of Fallot. *Am J Cardiol* 1980;46:446–452.
49. Deal BJ, Scagliotti D, Miller SM, et al. Electrophysiologic drug testing in symptomatic ventricular arrhythmias after repair of tetralogy of Fallot. *Am J Cardiol* 1987;59:1380–1385.
50. Downar E, Harris L, Kimber S, et al. Ventricular tachycardia after surgical repair of tetralogy of Fallot: results of intraoperative mapping studies. *J Am Coll Cardiol* 1992;20:648–655.
51. Cox JL, Bardy GH, Damiano RJ Jr, et al. Right ventricular isolation procedures for non-ischemic ventricular tachycardia. *J Thorac Cardiovasc Surg* 1985;90:212–224.
52. Kron J, Oliver RP, Norsted S, et al. The automatic implantable cardioverter defibrillator (AICD) in young patients. *Circulation* 1990;82(suppl II):389. Abstract.
53. Boineau JP, Schuessler RB, Mooney CR, et al. Natural and evoked atrial flutter due to circus movement in dogs. Role of abnormal atrial pathways, slow conduction, nonuniform refractory period distribution and premature beats. *Am J Cardiol* 1980;45:1167–1181.
54. Cox JL, Schuessler RB, Boineau JP. The surgical treatment of atrial fibrillation. I. Summary of the current concepts of the mechanisms of atrial flutter and atrial fibrillation. *J Thorac Cardiovasc Surg* 1991;101:402–405.
55. Cox JL, Canavan TE, Schuessler RB, et al. The surgical treatment of atrial fibrillation. II. Intraoperative electrophysiologic mapping and description of the electrophysiologic basis of atrial flutter and atrial fibrillation. *J Thorac Cardiovasc Surg* 1991;101:406–426.
56. Cox JL, Schuessler RB, D'Agostino JH, et al. The surgical treatment of atrial fibrillation. III. Development of a definitive surgical procedure. *J Thorac Cardiovasc Surg* 1991;101:569–583.
57. Ferguson TB Jr, Schuessler RB, Hand DE, et al. Lessons learned from computerized mapping of the atrium: surgical for atrial fibrillation and atrial flutter. *J Electrocardiol* 1993;26:210–219.
58. Cox JL, Boineau JP, Schuessler RB, et al. A review of surgery for atrial fibrillation. *J Cardiac Electrophysiol* 1991;2:541–561.
59. Cox JL, Boineaur JP, Schuessler RB, et al. Five year experience with the Maze procedure for atrial fibrillation. *Ann Thorac Surg* 1993;56:814–824.
60. Cox JL. Combined treatment of mitral stenosis and atrial fibrillation with valvuloplasty and a left atrial Maze procedure (reply). *J Thorac Cardiovasc Surg* 1994;107:622–624.
61. Cox JL. Surgical treatment of atrial fibrillation (reply). *J Thorac Cardiovasc Surg* 1992;104:1492–1494.
62. Cox JL. Evolving applications of the Maze procedure for atrial fibrillation. *Ann Thorac Surg* 1993;55:578–580.
63. Kawaguchi AT, Kosakai Y, Isobe F, et al. Risk and benefit of combined Maze procedure for atrial fibrillation associated with valvular heart disease. *J Am Coll Cardiol* 1994;23:459.
64. Shyu K, Cheng J, Chen J, et al. Recovery of atrial function after atrial compartment operation for chronic atrial fibrillation in mitral valve disease. *J Am Coll Cardiol* 1994;24:392–398.

65. Kono T, Sabbah HN, Rosman H, et al. Left atrial contribution to ventricular filling during the course of evolving heart failure. *Circulation* 1992;86:1317–1322.
66. McCarthy PM, Cosgrove DM, Castle LW, et al. Combined treatment of mitral regurgitation and atrial fibrillation with valvuloplasty and the Maze procedure. *Am J Cardiol* 1992;71:483–486.
67. DeFauw JJ, Guiraudon GM, van Hemel NM, et al. Surgical therapy of paroxysmal atrial fibrillation with the "corridor" operation. *Ann Thorac Surg* 1992;53:564–570.
68. Brodman RF, Frame R, Fisher JD, et al. Combined treatment of mitral stenosis and atrial fibrillation with valvuloplasty and a left atrial Maze procedure (letter). *J Thorac Cardiovasc Surg* 1994;107:622.
69. Hioki M, Ikeshita M, Iedokoro Y, et al. Successful combined operation for mitral stenosis and atrial fibrillation. *Ann Thorac Surg* 1993;55:776–778.
70. Sueda T, Shikata H, Orihashi K, et al. Modified left atrial isolation for chronic atrial fibrillation associated with mitral valve disease. *Ann Thorac Surg.* In press.
71. Itoh T, Okamoto H, Ogawa Y, et al. Left atrial function after the Cox's Maze operation concomitant with mitral valve operation. *Ann Thorac Surg* 1995;60:354–359.
72. Graffigna A, Pagani F, Minzioni G, et al. Left atrial isolation associated with mitral valve operation. *Ann Thorac Surg* 1992;54:1093–1098.
73. Blitz A, McLoughlin D, Gross J, et al. Combined Maze procedure and septal myectomy in a septuagenarian. *Ann Thorac Surg* 1992;54:364–365.
74. Bonchek LI, Burlingame MW, Worley SJ, et al. Cox/Maze procedure for atrial septal defect with atrial fibrillation: management strategies. *Ann Thorac Surg* 1993;55:607–610.
75. Mavroudis C, Zales VR, Backer CL, et al. Fenestrated Fontan with delayed catheter closure. Effects of volume loading and baffle fenestration on cardiac index and oxygen delivery. *Circulation* 1992;86(suppl II):85–92.
76. Puga FJ, Chiavarelli M, Hagler DJ. Modifications of the Fontan operation applicable to patients with left atrioventricular valve atresia or single atrioventricular valve. *Circulation* 1987;76(suppl III):53–60.
77. Bridges ND, Lock JE, Castaneda AR. Baffle fenestration with subsequent transcatheter closure. Modification of the Fontan operation for patients at increased risk. *Circulation* 1990;82:1681–1689.
78. Marcelletti C, Corno A, Giannico S, et al. Inferior vena cava-pulmonary artery extracardiac conduit. A new form of right heart bypass. *J Thorac Cardiovasc Surg* 1990;100:228–232.
79. Peters NS, Sommerville J. Arrhythmias after the Fontan procedure. *Br Heart J* 1992;68:199–204.
80. Gelatt M, Hamilton RM, McCrindle BW, et al. Risk factors for atrial tachyarrhythmias after the Fontan operation. *J Am Coll Cardiol* 1994;24:1735–1741.
81. Case CL, Gillette PC, Zeigler V, et al. Problems with permanent atrial pacing in the Fontan patient. *Pacing Clin Electrophysiol* 1989;12:92–96.
82. Triedman JK, Saul JP, Weindling SN, et al. Radiofrequency ablation of intra-atrial reentrant tachycardia after surgical palliation of congenital heart disease. *Circulation* 1995;91:707–714.
83. Kalman JM, Van Hare GF, Olgin JE, et al. Ablation of "incisional" reentrant atrial tachycardia complicating surgery for congenital heart disease. Use of entrainment to define a critical isthmus of conduction. *Circulation* 1996;93:502–512.
84. Lesh MD, Van Hare GF, Epstein LM, et al. Radiofrequency catheter ablation of atrial arrhythmias. Results and mechanisms. *Circulation* 1994;89:1074–1089.

85. Johnsrude CL, Deal BJ, Backer CL, et al. Short term follow-up of transmural atrial pacing leads in patients with postoperative congenital heart disease. *Pacing Clin Electrophysiol* 1997;20:1131.

86. Hoyer MH, Beerman LB, Ettedgui JA, et al. Transatrial lead placement for endocardial pacing in children. *Ann Thorac Surg* 1994;58:97–101.

87. Kao JM, Alejos JC, Grant PW, et al. Conversion of atriopulmonary to cavopulmonary anastomosis in management of late arrhythmias and atrial thrombosis. *Ann Thorac Surg* 1994;58:1510–1514.

88. McElhinney DB, Reddy VM, Moore P, et al. Revision of previous Fontan connections to extracardiac or intraatrial conduit cavopulmonary anastomosis. *Ann Thorac Surg* 1996;62:1276–1282.

89. Kreutzer J, Keane JF, Lock JE, et al. Conversion of modified Fontan procedure to lateral atrial tunnel cavopulmonary anastomosis. *J Thorac Cardiovasc Surg* 1996;111:1169–1176.

90. Vitullo DA, DeLeon SY, Berry TE, et al. Clinical improvement after revision in Fontan patients. *Ann Thorac Surg* 1996;61:1797–1804.

91. Cox JL. Intraoperative computerized mapping techniques. In: Brugada P, Wellens HJJ, eds. *Cardiac Arrhythmias: Where to Go From Here?* Mount Kisco NY: Futura; 1987.

92. Cox JL. The surgical management of cardiac arrhythmias. In: Sabiston DC Jr, Spencer FC, eds. *Surgery of the Chest.* 5th ed. Philadelphia, Pa: WB Saunders Co, 1990:1872.

93. Cox JL, Holman WL, Cain ME. Cryosurgical treatment of AV reentrant tachycardia. *Circulation* 1987;76:1331.

94. Lowe JE, Hendry PJ, Packer DL, et al. Surgical management of chronic ectopic atrial tachycardia. *Semin Thorac Cardiovasc Surg* 1989;1:64.

95. Williams JM, Ungerleider RM, Loffler GK, et al. Left atrial isolation: new technique for the treatment of supraventricular arrhythmias. *J Thorac Cardiovasc Surg* 1980;80:374–375.

96. Harada A, D'Agostino HJ Jr, Schuessler RB, et al. Right atrial isolation: a new surgical treatment for SVT. I. Surgical technique and electrophysiologic effects. *J Thorac Cardiovasc Surg* 1988;95:644–645.

97. Ferguson TB Jr, Cox JL. Successful surgical treatment for atrial fibrillation. *Prim Cardiol* 1992;18:15–25.

98. Ferguson TB Jr. The future of arrhythmia surgery. *J Cardiovasc Electrophysiol* 1994;5:621–634.

Device Therapy for Arrhythmias

Christopher L. Case, MD
Mary C. Sokoloski, MD
and Paul C. Gillette, MD

Background

This chapter deals with implantable devices that are used to control pediatric arrhythmias. Use of internal or implanted devices for arrhythmia control involves a unique set of complex technical, therapeutic, legal, and ethical issues.

Issues of device reliability and patient safety are of utmost importance for devices that are implanted in patients. Since these implanted machines deliver therapy that is not monitored on-line by medical personnel, therapeutic errors and side effects can occur outside the immediate governance of the prescribing doctor. Since these devices are implanted in human tissues, reliability over time is sometimes difficult to ascertain. The human body is an "extremely hostile environment,"[1] where the interaction between device and human physiology can be unpredictable. This interaction, over time, can produce disease processes that are unanticipated and irreversible. Merely because of its presence, the device can be wrongly implicated as a possible etiology for a particular medical malady. The medical-legal controversy over silicone breast implants affords an overview of the complex implications of implantation medicine.[2]

The use of implantable devices for arrhythmia control involves an invasive procedure, which introduces risk even before therapy is instituted.

From Deal B, Wolff G, Gelband H, (eds.). *Current Concepts in Diagnosis and Management of Arrhythmias in Infants and Children.* Armonk, NY: Futura Publishing Co., Inc.; © 1998.

Reversing the therapy is sometimes only possible by another invasive procedure that may incur an even greater risk.

Not least of the unique aspects of device arrhythmia therapy are psychological issues that may be more devastating than the physical scar produced by the implantation surgery. In children where issues of body image can change with psychological development, the choice of device therapy for a pediatric arrhythmia may have far-reaching and complex effects.

Similar to drug therapy, but in contrast to ablation procedures, device therapy never "cures" the arrhythmia. Ablation therapy is unique in its application to arrhythmias in that the "perfect" result implies no ongoing treatment. Device therapy, like medicines, only "control" arrhythmias. In most cases, device therapy (with the exception of antibradycardia pacing used to inhibit tachycardia episodes) requires the occurrence of the arrhythmia to deliver its therapy. In contrast, drug therapy inhibits the arrhythmia. Thus, due to their different treatment strategies, drug therapy and device therapy can be complements for many arrhythmia conditions. In general, however, because ablation and device therapy are both invasive, it is reasonable to use ablation therapy over device therapy if the two are comparable in efficacy and secondary effects.

There are other unique aspects of device therapy for arrhythmias as it applies to the pediatric patient. Few (if any) of these devices are designed and developed with children in mind. These machines are designed to treat adult disease processes and are skillfully adapted by pediatric practitioners for use in children. Due to the various levels of expertise of pediatric practitioners when dealing with devices, care must be taken in the selection of a device that it is appropriate for the needs of the child and the expertise of the physician. Although there are some absolute indications for the use of implantable device therapy in children (ie, pacemaker therapy for surgically required heart block), there are some conditions where device therapy is attractive, yet not the only therapeutic option available (ie, antitachycardia pacing for postoperative atrial muscle reentry tachycardia). The pediatric patient with an antiarrhythmia device must have 24-hour access to care with experienced personnel.

With these thoughts as a backdrop, this chapter deals with three areas of arrhythmia device therapy in children: (1) pacemaker therapy for bradycardia, (2) antitachycardia pacing, and (3) implantable defibrillators. Each area has unique aspects in pediatrics that warrant separate discussions.

Antibradycardia Pacing

Pacemaker implantation to treat bradycardia is by far the most frequent device therapy performed for pediatric arrhythmia control. In fact, there is no recognized chronic pharmacologic therapy for cardiac bradycardia with the exception of medical therapy for cardioinhibitory syncope. Pacemaker therapy is the treatment of choice for chronic cardiac brady-cardia needing intervention. Starting in the early 1970s and continuing into the 1990s, cardiac pacing became "user-friendly" in the pediatric age, so that the child in the late 1990s with a cardiac pacing system can be expected to live an active, productive life, unencumbered by the implanted arrhythmia device.[3–9]

Indications

Indications for chronic pacing therapy for pediatric cardiac bradycar-dia are outlined in the American Heart Association/American College of Cardiology (AHA/ACC) guidelines.[10] The guidelines generally deal with indications for pacemaker insertion in the adult patient, but do address some pediatric concerns. In this publication, indications for pacemaker implantation were grouped according to the following classifications: class I, where there is general agreement that a pacemaker should be implanted; class II, where pacemakers are frequently used but there is divergence of opinion regarding the necessity for implantation; and class III, where there is general agreement that pacemakers are unnecessary.[10]

Common sense dictates that cardiac pacing is indicated in pediatric patients who have bradycardia that is life threatening, potentially life threat-ening, or causes symptoms. Bradycardia in children is caused by diseases of the sinus node (SN) (rare) and/or atrioventricular (AV) function (most common). The bradycardia may be congenital [ie, complete AV block, long QT syndrome (LQTS)] or acquired (postoperative AV block, drug-induced sinus bradycardia). In most pediatric centers, the majority of pacemakers are inserted due to bradycardia secondary to conduction disturbances as a result of surgical intervention for congenital heart disease. A retrospective review of 6000 patients who underwent open repair of congenital heart defects at a high-volume pediatric surgical center showed a 2.2% incidence of conduction abnormalities necessitating postoperative permanent car-diac pacing.[11] In this study, indications for pacing were early AV block in 55%, late-onset AV block in 31%, and sick sinus syndrome in 14%. Correc-tion of a ventricular septal defect alone or in combination with other anom-alies was present in 67% of the patients; atrial surgery accounted for 21% of the children requiring pacing. It is generally agreed that surgically ac-quired AV block (beyond second-degree type I) that persists 14 days post-operatively requires permanent cardiac pacing.

Indications for permanent cardiac pacing from surgically acquired sinus bradycardia are more controversial. In general, pacing is indicated for children with sinus bradycardia and symptoms (fatigue, exercise in-tolerance) or signs of ventricular dysfunction as assessed by history, phys-ical examination, chest radiograph, or echocardiogram. Symptoms of fatigue and/or exercise intolerance may be difficult to verify in a child as they are frequently confounded by other circumstances. Signs of poor cardiac function in the postoperative patient with congenital heart disease can be caused by residual hemodynamic lesions. Although there is not universal agreement, we consider pacing for sinus bradycardia in the asymptomatic postoperative child who has nighttime heart rates less than 30 beats per minute (bpm), daytime heart rates less than 40 bpm, and/or 3-second pauses. In the presence of coexistent tachycardia necessitating drug therapy, our indications are more liberal (see antitachycardia pacing). Many patients with postoperative congenital heart disease have atrial and/or ventricular tachyarrhythmias secondary to their repair. Tachycardia treatment with antiarrhythmic agents sometimes results in acquired bradycardia due to drug effects on a compromised SN, AV node (AVN), or His-Purkinje system. In this situation, some advocate pacing when medications beyond digoxin are required for tachycardia control, yet this indication is not seen as absolute by all and, thus, is a class II indication according to current AHA/ACC guidelines.[10] Underlying bradycardia may provide the milieu for the development of atrial tachycardia; occasionally, providing a regular atrial rate may prevent episodes of atrial tachycardia.[12] Finally, evidence suggests that regularization of cardiac rhythm may augment cardiac output and prevent declining ventricular performance.[13]

Cardiac pacing indications for children with structurally normal hearts usually involve the syndrome of congenitally complete AV block. Recent data indicate that virtually all patients with this disease entity will ultimately require permanent cardiac pacing to avoid an increased incidence of sudden cardiac death.[14] In the absence of symptoms, criteria were developed to help guide the timing of pacemaker insertion. Wide QRS escape rate and/or block below the His bundle are absolute criteria for pacemaker insertion. A daily average ventricular rate in a child of <50 bpm or an awake rate of <45 bpm are relative indications, as is the presence of a long QT interval or ventricular ectopy. Ventricular dysfunction and/or exercise intolerance with congenital complete AV block would be signs and symptoms that would warrant pacemaker insertion at any age. Once again, however, decreased exercise performance may be a multifaceted problem in children. Many children with complete AV block may have enlarged cardiac silhouettes on chest radiographs and increased left ventricular volume on echocardiogram due to an increased stroke volume.

Other genetic conditions that may necessitate cardiac pacing include the LQTS and Kearns-Sayre syndrome. Children with Kearns-Sayre syndrome have external ophthalmoplegia and bifascicular block, which can progress to complete block and sudden cardiac death. Thus, the diagnosis of this syndrome in a child is a definite indication for permanent cardiac pacing.[15]

Some children with LQTS have sinus bradycardia as a component of their conduction abnormality. This bradycardia can predispose the patient to ventricular instability. Cardiac pacing was recognized as a component of therapy for long QT patients, especially for those with symptoms despite β-blocker therapy or bradycardia-dependent torsades de pointes. A recent study of patients with LQTS secondary to a sodium channel abnormality showed that these patients have an increased shortening of their QT intervals in response to an increased heart rate, suggesting that there is a subset of long QT patients where pacing may be a most important therapy.[16]

There are some very controversial uses of pacing in certain pediatric disease processes. One deserving mention is the use of pacing in certain forms of neurocardiogenic syncope. Some believe there is no place for pacing in this condition,[17-19] while others reported some beneficial effects in children with severe cardioinhibitory forms of neurocardiogenic syncope.[20-22]

Types of Pacemakers

The types and models of pacemakers that are available to the practitioner for use in the pediatric patient are vast. The choice as to the most appropriate pulse generator, lead system, pacing mode, and route of pacing is multifactorial. The pacing mode is best described by the North American Society of Pacing and Electrophysiology (NASPE)/British Pacing Guidelines pacemaker code (Table 1). Single-chamber, fixed-rate pacemakers are rarely recommended, due to the availability of rate-responsive and dual-chamber pacing. The most common sensor for rate responsiveness detects activity; others sense blood temperature or minute ventilation. The rate-responsive pacemaker provides an increased cardiac output with exercise; the pacemaker rate is programmed to increase the heart rate linearly up to a programmed maximum of 150–180 bpm. The factors used to determine which mode of pacing is best for the patient include the type of arrhythmia, the cardiac hemodynamic status, the percent of time the patient will need pacing, long-term pacing and cardiac expectations, and battery longevity. In general, poor cardiac status, greater pacing time requirement, and more abnormal cardiac structure dictate the need for "physiological" pacing modalities that provide AV synchrony. For the postoperative patient with AV block, physiological needs may necessitate using dual chamber pacing modes (DDD or DDD-R) depending on SN competence; alternatively, single-chamber ventricular pacing with rate responsiveness may be adequate.

In the patient with SN disease secondary to postoperative congenital heart disease, and normal AVN function, atrial pacing may be sufficient (AAI or AAI-R). Patients with congenital complete AV block usually are best served with dual chamber pacing to guarantee more physiological car-

Table 1

Revised NASPE/BPG Pacemaker Code

		Position Category		
I Chamber(s) Paced	II Chamber(s) Sensed	III Response to sensing	IV Programmability; rate modulation	V Antitachyarrhythmia function
O = none	O = none	O = none	O = none	O = none
A = atrium	A = atrium	T = triggered	P = simple programmable	P = pacing (antitachyarrhythmia)
V = ventricle	V = ventricle	I = inhibited	M = multi-programmable	S = shock
D = dual (A + V)	D = dual (A + V)	D = dual (T + I)	C = communicating	D = dual (P + S)
Manufacturers' designation only	S = single (A or V)	S = single (A or V)	R = rate modulation	

diac conduction and hemodynamics. In infants and small children, many centers prefer epicardial rate-responsive ventricular (VVIR) or dual-chamber (DDD-R) pacemakers until the child reaches adolescence.

The leads of the pacing system can be placed via the transvenous or epicardial approach. The advantages of the transvenous placement of the lead system include avoidance of a thoracotomy, greater lead longevity, and better sensing and pacing function.[23] However, the evolution of steroid-eluting epicardial leads greatly diminished the difference between epicardial and transvenous lead systems.[24,25] Some argue that epicardial systems should be used in small children to preserve the transvenous route for later pacing requirements, with concern that early transvenous pacing may lead to venous thrombosis. The recent availability of steroid-eluting epicardial leads allows dual-chamber pacing in infants and children with improved threshold and lead longevity. We used the epicardial approach in infancy alone and favor the transvenous pacing route for all children over 8 kg. Due to the risk of systemic embolization, the presence of intracardiac shunts is a significant limitation for transvenous pacing. A good contrast echocardiogram prior to pacemaker placement should always be performed to document the integrity of the atrial and ventricular septa.

Overall, a pacing system should be chosen that gives the patient the most physiological response and the greatest battery longevity without compromising future pacemaker procedures. Within reason, the mode and system should also be chosen in accordance with the expertise of the follow-up physician and facility.

Pacemaker Basics: Equipment

The working "pacemaker unit" consists of a pulse generator and its attached pacemaker lead. The pulse generator contains integrated circuits or "chips," which are actual microprocessors with random access memory (RAM). These microprocessors contain pacing and sensing algorithms as well as the stored program settings. Also, within the pulse generator is a source of electrical current, a timer to measure intervals, and an output circuit that will accumulate energy from the battery and hold it for release to the heart via the electrode system. The sensing component of the pulse generator contains amplifiers and filters that clarify the local myocardial depolarization. Filtering tends to rid the intrinsic electrogram of signals resulting from myopotentials, external sources of electrical magnetic interference, and T waves. A major portion of the pulse generator is the power source. Since its introduction in the early 1970s, the lithium alloy power cell is the industry standard. This power source has a number of characteristics that make it attractive as an implantable pulse generator. It has a high-energy density, and, due to the nature of its chemical reaction, internal energy losses are low, maximizing its shelf-life. Most importantly, this power source can be hermetically sealed, adding to the stability of the pulse generator. The decline of the lithium cell's voltage before the end of life of the pulse generator is gradual, generally occurring over a 6-month period. This allows increased flexibility in patient/management schemes when pacemaker replacement is needed.

Lead systems for cardiac pacing are composed of one or more electrodes, a fixation device, conducting wires, an insulating system, and connector. Each of these components is important in the proper functioning of a lead system. There are two different lead designs (bipolar and unipolar), and each design dictates how and where the lead is placed on the heart. Each of these leads has a cathode electrode, which is usually located at its tip. In the case of the bipolar lead, the anode electrode is located more proximally along the electrode shaft, usually in the form of a ring parallel to the long axis of the shaft. These electrodes are usually made of platinum. In the case of a unipolar lead, the catheter electrode is once again at the tip of the lead and is the only electrode incorporated into the lead proper. The pulse generator functions as the anode electrode in this pacing system. Unipolar leads are generally used if the lead is placed on the epicardial surface of the heart. Bipolar leads are usually used with transvenous pacing systems. There are a number of differences between the pacing and sensing properties of a unipolar versus bipolar leads. In general, the stimulus artifact on the electrocardiogram (ECG) is larger with a unipolar lead system. The possibility of extra cardiac pacing rarely occurs with bipolar systems but occasionally occurs with unipolar systems. The selectivity of sensing is much higher with a bipolar system than with a unipolar system. The electrogram size obtained from a bipolar system is generally larger than that from a unipolar system.

Bipolar leads can be fixed to the endocardium of the heart with active devices, ie, screws that fix the lead tip into the myocardium. There are also passive lead fixation systems that use tines to entrap the lead in the trabeculations of the right ventricle (RV). Epicardial leads can be sewn on the heart or affixed to the heart via barbs that extend from the electrode lead interface. The common conductor material used in all leads is a coil of nickel cobalt alloy. Lead connectors usually come in 5-mm or 6-mm measurements. In general, the 5-mm insulated shoulder can be adapted to attach to a larger style header (part of the pulse generator into which the leads insert) by using an adapter sleeve to enlarge the connector. Incorporating the larger connector to the smaller header is more problematic. Insulating material for leads is generally made of polyurethane or silicone rubber. Development of polyurethane leads made it easier to place two electrodes in a single vein because of the decrease in lead diameter afforded by this material.

At the time of implantation of the pacemaker, a piece of equipment commonly referred to as a pacing system analyzer (PSA) is used to test the properties of the implanted lead system. This piece of equipment measures acute thresholds, sensing thresholds, and lead resistances so the integrity of the implanted lead system can be verified prior to conclusion of the procedure. In follow-up of a pacemaker, a pacemaker programmer (usually specific for the brand type of pacemaker inserted) is needed to test the parameters of a pacemaker. These programmers usually consist of a wand, which is attached via a cord to the programmer. The wand is placed over the pacemaker and communicates with the pulse generator via electromagnetic waves. The programmer is a small computer that can send information and retrieve data from the pulse generator, thus programming values for pacemaker function.

Pacemaker Basics: Programming

Pacemaker programming procedures are performed at regular intervals to monitor pacemaker function and to change programmed pacemaker settings. Depending on the pacemaker, there is a variety of information that the pacemaker measures and stores. This information can be obtained at a pacemaker check. The number of sensed (intrinsic) depolarizations of the atrium and ventricle as well as the number of paced events can be assessed. Information concerning the integrity of the lead system (resistance) can also be measured. The pacemaker program settings including the mode, rate, the sensitivity, the pulse width, and refractory periods may be changed. Intracardiac electrograms may also be recorded.

At a typical pacemaker check, the pacing mode of the pacemaker is verified. Depending on the pacemaker, and the number of leads used, the mode of the pacemaker can be changed. The pacing rate can also be verified and changed. The core of most pacemaker checks involves checking the pacemaker's stimulation and sensing thresholds. The *stimulation threshold* is the minimal output required to stimulate the myocardium consistently. This is checked by varying the pulse width (milliseconds), voltage (millivolts), or current (mA) depending on the capacity of the individual device. The pacemaker is programmed to increase the rate until consistent capture is evident; the output is then decreased until capture is no longer present. The threshold is the minimum output that stimulates the myocardium as recorded on the ECG. The usual way to check the stimulation threshold of a pacemaker is to maintain a constant voltage and decrease the pulse width until capture is lost. Then the pulse width is increased until capture is obtained consistently. This point of consistent capture is the stimulation threshold. The sensitivity threshold is also checked at a typical pacemaker evaluation. *Sensitivity* is defined as the minimal amount of intrinsic cardiac depolarization (measured in millivolts) that will be consistently recognized by the pacemaker's sensing amplifiers. This testing is done during the patient's intrinsic underlying rhythm. The millivolts are gradually increased until the pacemaker inappropriately tries to stimulate the myocardium. Both the stimulation threshold and sensitivity threshold are attained in the atrium and ventricle if two leads are used in the pacing system.

Pacemaker Complications

Complications of pacemaker implantation are uncommon, yet can be serious. The most feared complication is the role of infection due to the nature of implanting a "foreign object" (pulse generator and lead) in the body. Serious pacemaker infection usually necessitates explanting the pacemaker system, administering systemic antibiotics, and reimplanting a new system after the infection is controlled. Superficial pacemaker pocket infection can usually be handled without explantation of the pacing system. Other complications during pacemaker implantation include the possibility of excessive bleeding from the formation of the pacemaker pocket or problems obtaining transvenous access for lead placement. Occasionally, a lead placed in the transvenous route may migrate, causing pacemaker malfunction. Periodic x-rays during pacemaker follow-up can track subtle lead migration. Lead malfunction may occur in a transvenous system due to entrapment of the transvenous lead between the clavicle and first rib, causing a fracture of the lead. Epicardial leads may malfunction due to excessive scarring around the lead electrode causing sensing and/or pacing (exit block) problems. In general, with vigorous pacemaker follow-up, problems with the lead migration and malfunction can be anticipated and remedied so as not to jeopardize the stability of the patient's rhythm.

Antitachycardia Pacing

In the late 1970s, progress in refinement of bradycardia pacing systems spurred development of implantable devices that allowed pacing for bradycardia and treatment of tachycardia. The impetus for designing an implantable antitachycardia pacemaker was based on the electrophysiological (EP) fact that reentrant arrhythmias can be terminated by delivering a critically timed extrastimulus that enters the reentrant circuit and interrupts tachycardia by changing the conduction time or refractory period of the circuit. From clinical experience with temporary intravenous catheter and transesophageal pacing, the principles of pace termination of arrhythmias were explored. Pace termination of a reentrant arrhythmia was found to be dependent on several definable factors. The smaller the reentry circuit, the farther away the reentry circuit is from the pacing impulse, and, the more rapid the tachycardia rate, the more difficult it is to terminate the tachycardia.

Effective antitachycardia therapy for reentrant arrhythmias is based on two principles. First, the pathological tachycardia has to be effectively recognized. This tachycardia recognition has to be both sensitive and specific. Proper arrhythmia recognition is based on the use of a bipolar sensing system that recognizes low-amplitude atrial signals but is not influenced by far-field erroneous signals. Once these signals are recognized, the frequency and pattern must be identified as physiological (sinus tachycardia) or pathological [ie, atrial flutter (AF), AV reentry tachycardia]. This "recognition" is accomplished by the use of algorithms, which, singularly or in combination, examine the rate of the tachycardia, its onset characteristics, and the rate stability of the signals. Using these principles, pathologic tachycardia can be distinguished from physiological states of sinus tachycardia.

Once the tachycardia state is recognized, effective antitachycardia pacing requires delivering therapy, usually a prescribed pacing sequence consisting of 1–128 extrastimuli. The pacing protocol can be refined by varying the number, rate, and decrementing intervals of the extrastimuli. Between an individual therapy, the pacemaker again uses its recognition algorithm to decide if a therapy was successful. The prescribed pacing therapy can be repeated or changed after recognition of a failed termination. Thus, successful antitachycardia pacemaker function is dependent on a dual function of the antitachycardia device: (1) sensitive and specific tachycardia recognition and (2) efficacious tachycardia termination with critically timed extrastimuli.

Clinical Uses of Antitachycardia Pacing

Theoretically, any reentrant rhythm, regardless of its site of origin (atrial, junctional, or ventricular) can be treated with an implantable automatic antitachycardia pacemaker. In reality, implantable antitachycardia pacemakers were used mostly to treat specific supraventricular rhythms. The use of antitachycardia pacing for reentrant ventricular tachycardias (VT) evolved to become established as one component of the therapy delivered by most third-generation implantable cardioverter-defibrillators (ICDs; see below).

Approximately 85% of supraventricular tachycardias (SVT) in pediatric patients involve reentry, using either accessory AV connections or dual AVN pathways. Implantable atrial antitachycardia pacemakers were used to treat patients with these two entities. However, in the 1990s, catheter ablation became the nonpharmacologic treatment of choice for these arrhythmias, and antitachycardia pacing was not indicated; in certain situations it may be contraindicated.

The most experience with the use of antitachycardia pacing in the pediatric age group involves the treatment of atrial reentry tachycardia, which is acquired after surgery for congenital heart disease involving extensive suture lines in atrial tissues. Patients who had an atrial septal defect (ASD) closure, a Senning or Mustard repair of transposition of the great vessels, or a Fontan procedure often are plagued by this tachycardia. Atrial reentry tachycardia is a primary atrial tachycardia that is reentrant in nature. The etiology is thought to be a by-product of multiple circuits in the atrium caused by atrial suturing and scarring and/or atrial enlargement. In a single patient, there can be multiple circuits and, thus, multiple tachycardia morphologies. In one study, mostly comprised of postoperative pediatric patients, uncontrolled atrial reentry tachycardia was a risk factor for cardiac death.[26]

Pharmacologic treatment of atrial reentry tachycardia was problematic. Not only is nonefficacy of class I and class III drugs common, but proarrhythmia may be responsible for worsening the atrial arrhythmias or provoking ventricular arrhythmias. Since this arrhythmia is common in patients with abnormal structural and functional heart disease, antiarrhythmic therapy may exacerbate preexisting sinus bradycardia (necessitating bradycardia pacing) and also compromise myocardial function. Many patients need combination drug therapy for tachycardia control.

Strategies were adopted that use antitachycardia pacing to treat postoperative atrial reentry tachycardia. Experience was first gained with its use in the Mustard or Senning patient. The majority of these patients with atrial reentry can be treated with the use of antitachycardia pacing and digoxin therapy.[27] Similarly, most patients with atrial reentry tachycardia following ASD closure can be controlled by antitachycardia pacing and no medications.[28]

Patients with the Fontan operation and atrial reentry tachycardia are difficult to manage, even with the use of antitachycardia pacing. In our experience, antitachycardia pacing is rarely the sole effective treatment for these patients, and most will require additional strong antiarrhythmic therapy (class I or III medications) to help control the rhythm.[29] Newer modifications of the Fontan procedure incorporating less native atrial tissue in the high-pressure Fontan anastomosis may decrease the incidence of this rhythm disturbance. Conversely, if atrial pacing is necessary in these patients, Fontan modifications (lateral tunnel) may render the patient less suitable for atrial pacing via the transvenous route due to a paucity of tissue for lead implantation.

Devices

There is only one automatic atrial antitachycardia pacemaker available for use in the United States, the Intertach II model 262–12 (Intermedics, Angleton, Tex), the third in a series of antitachycardia pacemakers that started in the late 1970s. The current Intertach II is suitably sized, even for an infant. The pacemaker is used in the bipolar configuration because of the need to recognize very rapid and small atrial depolarizations.

The pacemaker can perform standard bradycardia pacing with a very wide range of outputs (voltage and pulse width). Sensitivity can be set as low as 0.5 mV, with a variably programmable atrial refractory period to allow for sensing of signals that are small and at short cycle lengths (CLs). Tachycardia can be solely monitored, or monitored and treated with a programmable therapy.

With the Intertach II, pathological tachycardias can be recognized using one of nine algorithms. The criteria of atrial rate, onset, and stability of atrial rate are used alone or in combination to determine if the tachycardia is pathological. The algorithms that combine rate and onset of rate are best suited in the pediatric patient to distinguish pathological reentrant atrial tachycardias from physiological sinus tachycardias. Reentrant atrial tachycardias will not only have a fast rate but also have a sudden onset (δ-rate change) that can be programmed to facilitate accurate recognition.

Tachycardia termination is accomplished by the use of pacing algorithms. Programmable features of the algorithms include (1) number of pulses; (2) delay between the last tachycardia beat and the first paced beat; (3) pacing CL; (4) number of attempts; (5) autodecrementing; (6) scanning; and (7) minimum CL. It is possible to set a primary and secondary tachycardia termination algorithm. The primary and secondary mode can be totally different, except they must have a common minimum pacing CL.

Some patients with complex heart disease (post-Fontan) have multiple tachycardia circuits that need to be addressed with aggressive tachycardia pacing algorithms. The more aggressive the protocol (ie, the faster the CL and the greater the number of pulses), the more likely it is to induce atrial fibrillation. In general, the atrial fibrillation will break quickly, and an atrial paced rhythm will ensue. Patients with less serious heart disease (ASDs) generally have fewer atrial arrhythmia circuits, and an 8- to 16-beat burst at 70% of the tachycardia CL will invariably terminate the arrhythmia.

The Intertach II also will store tachycardia information, such as the number of times the device sensed the high rate and/or sudden onset criteria, the number of successful termination events, and the CL of the most recent tachycardia event.

Evaluation of the Patient for Antitachycardia Pacing

In the 1990s, preoperative evaluation of the pediatric patient for whom antitachycardia pacing is an option usually involves a postoperative patient with congenital heart disease and atrial reentry tachycardia.

A good history, physical, and noninvasive evaluation are necessary prior to implantation. This evaluation includes an echocardiogram for identifying structural abnormalities (baffle obstruction for the Fontan/

Mustard patient) that may underlie the arrhythmia. Sometimes ameliorating structural abnormalities can greatly lessen tachycardia occurrences.[26] Evaluation should include assessment of intracardiac shunts.

Noninvasive arrhythmia workup includes an ECG and a Holter monitor for verifying the mechanism of the tachycardia. Although atrial reentry tachycardia is the most common SVT in some patients after surgery for congenital heart disease, these same children can have SVT mediated by abnormal automaticity (atrial ectopic tachycardia) or reentry through an accessory connection or AVN reentry tachycardia. These specific tachycardias, as discussed before, are treated by ablation procedures. Examination of the Holter recording can also reveal coexistent sinus bradycardia and junctional rhythm that precedes and may precipitate atrial reentry tachycardia. In these cases, sometimes atrial antibradycardia pacing may provide some protection against episodes of atrial reentry tachycardia, and the antitachycardia pacing modality can be utilized as a backup to control the tachyarrhythmia.

Exercise testing may be important to assess the chronotropic response of the SN during exertion. This rate may be similar to the rate of the atrial reentry tachycardia. In this case, detection algorithms must employ rate onset and/or rate stability criteria to help distinguish the pathological from the physiological.

Noninvasive EP evaluation should also include some assessment of AVN function via ECG, Holter, or stress testing. It is important to make sure that coexisting bradycardia is not on the basis of AVN disease.

Electrophysiology Evaluation and Implantation Technique

Prior to implantation, careful review of operative notes should be performed to ascertain the exact systemic venous anatomy and type of baffle anastomosis that were fashioned. This is especially important in the patient with a Fontan procedure. Certain variations of the Fontan procedure could preclude atrial pacing (an external conduit Fontan) or somewhat limit access to the atrial tissues for pacing (lateral tunnel Fontan). Systemic venous anatomy in the patient with single ventricle physiology can be complex, with left superior vena cava (SVC), absent right SVC, and variations of these vena cava as they empty into the heart (right atrium, left atrium, pulmonary artery, coronary sinus). If the systemic venous anatomy, the type of Fontan anastomosis, or the presence of intracardiac shunts are not clear from the echocardiogram or operative notes, angiography is indicated. If the hemodynamic status is unclear from the noninvasive workup, it should be investigated by catheterization prior to pacemaker implantation.

An invasive EP study is necessary prior to antitachycardia pacemaker implantation. This study should confirm the mechanism of the tachycardia, the number of tachycardia morphologies, the hemodynamic consequences of the tachycardias, and their correlations with the clinical tachycardia(s). Every tachycardia should be assessed in terms of termination with pacing. This assessment should include recording various pacing algorithms as well as different catheter positions needed to facilitate overdrive pacing. These catheter positions can guide the subsequent placement of the permanent pacing lead.

In general, if only one reentrant tachycardia can be induced and it can be adequately mapped, catheter ablation may be a better alternative than antitachycardia pacing for arrhythmia control. The more multiple and complex the tachycardia circuits, the more antitachycardia pacing becomes the therapy of choice over catheter ablation.

If antitachycardia pacing is chosen and the transvenous route is feasible, the pacemaker can be implanted in the catheterization laboratory after the EP study (Figure 1). During this procedure, especially in the Fontan patient, lead insertion may be more problematic than in other pediatric transvenous pacemaker procedures. Blood loss can be more than usual due to placing the lead in a high-pressure Fontan circuit. Obtaining reliable acute pacing and sensing thresholds may be complicated by scarred atrial tissue, a paucity of atrial tissue (lateral tunnel Fontan) or difficult lead access to the heart (abnormal venous anatomy). We exclusively use screw-in leads for transvenous antitachycardia pacing. For sensing thresholds, electrogram testing is done to obtain a large atrial depolarization (greater than 2 mV) and a small far-field "R" wave (less than 0.5 mV). These parameters are not always possible in Fontan patients. A pacing threshold is determined by decreasing the voltage at 0.5-millisecond pulse width. A threshold of 1 V is very good, but often one must be satisfied with a 2- or 2.5-V threshold.

In patients with the Mustard or Senning procedure, the lead is usually placed on the roof of the systemic venous atrium. This avoids placing the lead on the left lateral atrial wall and the consequent possibility of phrenic nerve stimulation. Transvenous lead placement for the Fontan patient depends on the particular atriopulmonary anastomosis. In these patients, care also must be taken to avoid possible right phrenic nerve stimulation.

If antitachycardia pacing is necessary and the transvenous route is not possible or contraindicated, epicardial antitachycardia pacing is feasible. We usually place two unipolar leads and connect them to an adaptor so bipolar pacing and sensing is possible. Access is obtained via a left thoracotomy, and leads are placed on the "less diseased" left atrium. Like any pacing technique performed via epicardial leads, pacing and sensing functions of epicardial antitachycardia pacing systems are more problematic than those obtained for transvenous systems; a course of oral steroids postoperatively may improve chronic pacing and sensing thresholds.

A

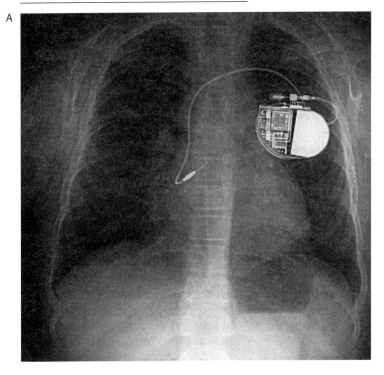

B

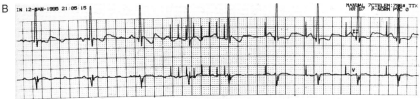

Figure 1. A: Chest radiograph of a 5-year-old child s/p Fontan operation with re-fractory atrial reentry tachycardia. An antitachycardia pacemaker was placed to help control his arrhythmia. **B**: ECG of an antitachycardia pacemaker overdriving AF. Note that after conversion of the AF there is atrial bradycardia pacing.

After placement of the antitachycardia pacemaker and prior to dis-charge, a noninvasive atrial stimulation study can be performed through the pacemaker. During this noninvasive EP study, tachycardias can be in-duced, and detection and therapy algorithms can be fine tuned. Prior to discharge, consideration is given to instituting chronic anticoagulation therapy (aspirin and/or coumadin) for Fontan patients who have trans-venous leads through their low-flow Fontan circuit.

Follow-up of these patients with antitachycardia pacemakers depends on the severity of their arrhythmia, the efficacy of the pacemaker in controlling the tachycardia, concomitant pharmacologic therapy, and the severity of the structural heart disease. Due to these factors, in the chronic phase of treatment, the follow-up can vary from monthly to yearly. Most well-controlled children are evaluated twice a year.

Implantable Cardioverter-Defibrillators

The success of ICDs in saving lives of adult patients with malignant ventricular arrhythmias was one impetus for extending the use of this therapy into the pediatric age group. The collective pediatric ICD experience is limited, yet there are some emerging trends suggesting that pediatric ICD therapy will continue to expand. Similar to the initial application of pacemaker therapy to children, technical modifications in the physical dimensions of ICDs and their lead systems continue to make this therapy more "user friendly" for the small, young patient.

Sudden Cardiac Death in the Young

The main purpose of ICDs is to prevent sudden cardiac death from ventricular arrhythmias. In adult patients with coronary artery disease, sudden cardiac death due to ventricular arrhythmias is a public health problem of momentous proportions. However, in the pediatric population, sudden cardiac death is rare, with an estimated frequency of 1–13 events per 100,000 patient years.[30–32] There are some fundamental differences between adults and children in the documented arrhythmogenic mechanism of cardiac arrest. In most pediatric patients without heart disease, asystole rather than ventricular fibrillation (VF) (77% vs. 11%) is the most commonly documented terminal arrhythmia.[33] However, in the presence of preexisting heart disease, children are more likely to have ventricular arrhythmias as a cause of sudden death.[34] The implications of this fact vis-à-vis ICD therapy is that the arrhythmia mechanism of a cardiac arrest episode in a child (especially if preexisting heart disease is absent) cannot be assumed. For these reasons, most ICDs in the pediatric population were implanted in individuals with preexisting structural or electrical cardiac anomalies.

History of Implantable Cardioverter-Defibrillators Therapy

The first defibrillator implanted in a human was reported in 1980.[35] In 1985, these devices were approved by the FDA for the treatment of malignant ventricular arrhythmias that are not due to reversible causes. The first-generation ICDs were nonprogrammable devices that could only deliver high-energy shocks after sensing ventricular arrhythmias. Second-generation devices are minimally programmable and allow for ventricular pacing (VVI mode); some have limited telemetry functions. The impetus for second-generation devices was based on the fact that 15% of ICD patients had coexistent conduction abnormalities that required pacing for bradycardia.[36] Currently, third-generation ICDs are being implanted with the capacity for antitachycardia pacing, low-energy cardioversion, defibrillation, and bradycardia pacing. In addition, third-generation devices have the capacity for "tiered therapy" to progressively advance from antitachycardia pacing to low-energy cardioversion and, finally, maximum energy defibrillation. Thus, therapy for certain arrhythmias can be sequenced from "least" to "most" aggressive. In contrast to first-generation devices (committed), newer ICDs are termed "noncommitted" because, prior to delivering their therapy, they reconfirm the presence of the arrhythmia, preventing the delivery of painful therapies for self-terminating arrhythmias. In addition, third-generation ICDs are highly programmable devices with extensive memory and telemetry functions that greatly aid in the diagnosis and treatment of device malfunction as well as arrhythmia substrates that are in the process of changing. Data logging and electrogram storage capacity greatly facilitated device troubleshooting.

Finally, third-generation devices have the capacity to induce arrhythmias by various pacing maneuvers. The ability to induce tachycardia facilitates the assessment of the efficacy of the ICD's programmed therapy algorithms.

Hardware

An ICD system consists of the device itself and a lead system. The device, in its external appearance, resembles a large pacemaker. Early ICDs weighed over 200 g, and current models weigh half as much. The lead system and its complexity is mostly dependent on the route of implantation. Initial ICDs were all implanted via a thoracotomy approach, with defibrillator leads consisting of patches (at least two) that were sewn on the epicardial surface of the heart. With time, other positions for the patch electrodes in the thorax were used, ie, subcutaneously or on the pericardium. Critical to the sensing function of the ICD is a bipolar sensing lead system. Most ICDs implanted via a thoracotomy require two screw-in ventricular leads that are attached to the ICD to function in the bipolar sensing mode. A combination of the screw-in ventricular leads and/or the patch electrodes can be used for ventricular pacing functions. In some epicardial systems, as many as five leads are required to accomplish all programmed functions. The original ICD device was so large that it required implantation in the abdomen.

In 1993, nonthoracotomy ICD systems, small enough for subpectoral implantation, were approved for implantation. Transvenous lead systems were developed in which all ICD functions (sensing, pacing, cardioversion, and

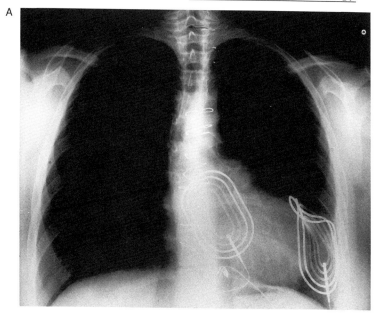

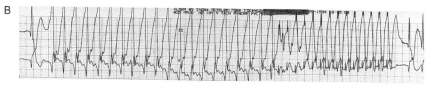

Figure 2. A: Chest radiograph of a 10-year-old child s/p repair of double outlet RV with an epicardial defibrillator system. The patches are sewn onto the epicardium of the heart via a thoracotomy. The defibrillator device (not pictured) is implanted in the abdomen. **B**: Telemetry strip documenting successful overdrive termination of monomorphic VT by an implanted third-generation cardioverter/defibrillator with antitachycardia pacing capacity.

defibrillation) can be performed with a single lead in the RV apex. The ICD sensing and pacing functions are performed by electrodes and the coil at the distal end of the lead; cardioversion/defibrillator function is performed by using the coil on the same lead and the ICD device itself. The simplicity of this ICD configuration is in stark contrast to earlier epicardial systems (Figure 2).

How Do Implantable Cardioverter-Defibrillators Work?

The main purpose of ICDs is to constantly monitor cardiac electrical activity and recognize and then terminate ventricular arrhythmias. Tachy-

C

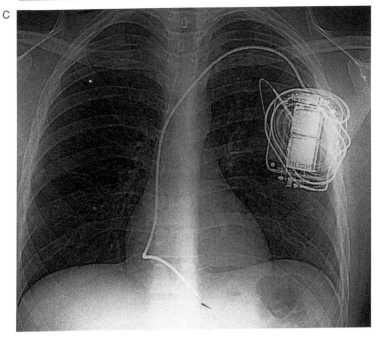

D

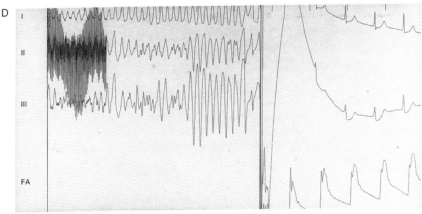

Figure 2. C: Chest radiograph of a 16-year-old male with a single-lead transvenous defibrillator system placed to help control arrhythmias secondary to the LQTS. **D**: Prior to discharge, successful defibrillator capacity of the device is verified in the catheterization laboratory.

cardia recognition features of ICDs are much like those used in antitachycardia pacing (see previous sections). Most ICDs use parameters of tachycardia rate, onset, and rate stability to distinguish VT from other tachycardias. Current ICDs cannot consistently distinguish SVT from VT.

Some sensing algorithms, using rate stability and probability density function (CPI devices), can help distinguish various types of SVT from VT. However, delivery of therapy for SVT episodes is a common reason for inappropriate device function.[37] The therapy programmed for a specific ventricular arrhythmia that meets detection criteria can include antitachycardia pacing, low-energy cardioversion, or defibrillation; individual programming obviously depends on the nature of the ventricular arrhythmia. Approximately 70% to 80% of VTs in adults can be successfully treated with antitachycardia pacing and/or low-energy cardioversion, depending on the rate of the VT.[38] Defibrillation energy discharge can be reserved for very fast VT or VF in the case of nonefficacy of the primary therapy or for arrhythmia acceleration by a less aggressive therapy. Programming progressively more aggressive therapies is termed "tiered therapy."

Implantation Technique

The general sequence for ICD implantation is very much dependent on patient age, diagnoses, and preferred route of implantation. Prior to implantation, all patients require an invasive EP study that should yield the following information: (1) arrhythmia diagnosis, (2) its suitability for various therapies, and (3) underlying cause (reversible or nonreversible). If an ICD is determined to be the indicated therapy during that EP study, and a transvenous system is preferred, the procedure can be immediately performed. If an epicardial ICD system is mandated, this is accomplished in the operating room.

Implantation of the device is accomplished with this general sequence. First, the lead system is implanted. Then, adequate pacing and sensing functions of the lead system are verified. Subsequently, the "defibrillation threshold" (DFT) is checked. This is generally accomplished by fibrillating the heart and verifying the level of energy needed to defibrillate. In general, an acceptable DFT is at least less than half the maximal energy value that the chosen ICD can deliver. Once the DFT is deemed acceptable, the device is attached to the lead system and, once again, the efficacy of defibrillation is verified.

After patient recovery and prior to discharge, the ICD function is again tested, usually in the catheterization laboratory. Using the ICDs built-in diagnostic and arrhythmia-induction capacities, the patient's arrhythmias are induced, and the accuracy of the ICDs sensing function and the efficacy of programmed therapies can be verified. Obviously, depending on the patient's state of sedation and autonomic tone, the induced arrhythmia's characteristics and ICD function may or may not exactly mimic the patient's future clinical use of the device. Nonetheless, decisions regarding arrhythmia recognition and therapy algorithms and/or the need for concomitant pharmacologic therapy are made at this session.

Follow-up, once the patient is discharged, depends on many factors, including patient age, diagnosis, the presence of concomitant drug therapy, requirements of the ICD device, patient recognition of arrhythmia therapy (shock), and psychological factors. For all pediatric patients, follow-up is at least monthly following implantation until the child and parents are comfortable with the new therapy. Any time the patient recognizes that therapy was delivered, we recommend a follow-up visit. In the chronic stage, routine follow-up is usually at 3-month or 6-month intervals.

Depending on the diagnosis and age of the child, restrictions on activity are similar to those advised for a pediatric pacemaker patient. In the presence of good hemodynamics and a well-controlled arrhythmia, the patient is told to avoid all activities that could result in a direct physical blow to the ICD device.

Pediatric Implantable Cardioverter-Defibrillators Experience

Published data concerning ICD therapy in children are sparse, although one of the first patients who had an ICD placed was a 16-year-old male with arrhythmia symptoms suggestive of RV dysplasia.[35] Children comprise less than 2% of the total ICD population, and most children with ICDs usually have structural or electrical heart disease. According to a recent survey of pediatric ICD data,[39] indications for ICDs in children included 80% who are sudden cardiac arrest survivors, 10% who had VT where a suitable alternative therapy could not be found, and 10% with a clinical history of heart disease and syncope with a family history of sudden death. Sixty percent of the young patients had a diagnosis of cardiomyopathy (two thirds hypertrophic, one third dilated), 25% had electrical system disease (LQTS and/or primary VF), and 15% had repaired congenital heart disease (aortic stenosis, tetralogy of Fallot, or post-Mustard or post-Senning repair of transposition of the great arteries). Most of these patients had thoracotomy systems; recently, however, a report of the successful use of nonthoracotomy systems in a group of young patients was published.[40]

Postimplantation, ICD utilization of children mirrors that of the adult population, with 38% of patients receiving appropriate therapy at 1 year, 50% at 2 years, and 60% at 3 years. The post-ICD sudden cardiac death rate in these pediatric patients was 2% at 30 days, 3% at 1 year, 5% at 2 years, and 10% at 5 years. Similar to adult data, total cardiac death rate in this population was higher at all times (3%, 5%, 7%, and 15%), reflecting nonarrhythmogenic death mechanisms secondary to a poor cardiac status. In this pediatric population, post-ICD mortality correlated with impaired ventricular function and prior history of ICD discharge. Operative and perioperative complications occurred in 20% of this young ICD population. Included in these complications were intraoperative death (1% with intractable VF), high DFTs (5%), wound infections with or without device erosion (9%), and pneumothorax or effusions (5%). At follow-up, 20% of the population received "inappropriate ICD therapy." Reasons for these inappropriate therapies included supraventricular rhythm sensing (sinus tachycardia, AF, AV reciprocating SVT), nonsustained VT, and technical problems, such as lead malfunction and programming errors.

When considering ICD therapy in children, a few technical considerations are pertinent. In general, transvenous, subpectoral implants should be reserved for those over 40 kg (~10 years of age). When in doubt about size, use of an epicardial system with an abdominal ICD is preferable in view of the potential longevity of a young child's ICD requirements, saving the subpectoral transvenous ICD approach for the older child. If a transvenous route is chosen, careful review of venous anatomy and the presence of residual atrial or ventricular intracardiac shunts should be undertaken, especially in the presence of postoperative congenital heart disease. SVC anatomy in patients with congenital heart disease can be complex, and the presence of residual cardiac shunts limits transvenous lead placement due to the possibility of systemic embolism. DFTs, especially in children with congenital heart disease and cardiomyopathy, may be unpredictable. One should be prepared to use additional lead configurations in unusual positions to compensate for cardiac chamber malpositions and coronary anomalies.

Inappropriate discharges in children are a predictable problem due to overlap between the typical rates of sinus tachycardia and VT. A careful assessment of the sinus mechanism of each patient via Holter and stress test can help select specific tachycardia recognition algorithms to avoid inappropriate therapy delivery. We found that a combination of nonsustained VT seen in some long QT patients and the sinus tachycardia that surrounds these nonsustained VT events often can meet criteria for ICD discharge, and can take an obvious psychologic toll on a young child. Often, VT in children is very fast, over 200 bpm. For these reasons, we found the use of antitachycardia pacing in our young population to be limited and prefer the use of low-energy cardioversion as a less aggressive initial therapy.

Finally, in patients with postoperative congenital heart disease and episodes of cardiac arrest, it is important to keep in mind the multiplicity of possible arrhythmogenic mechanisms. AF with a rapid ventricular response is possible after virtually any repair of congenital heart disease, as is the abrupt onset of complete heart block, which may be transient. Assumption of a ventricular origin of the arrhythmia, even in patients who had a tetralogy repair, may lead to a misguided use of current-day ICDs. Similarly, it is important to keep in mind that ventricular arrhythmias are known to be an important mechanism of cardiac arrest in those postoperative congenital heart disease patients primarily prone to atrial arrhythmias (Senning/Mustard, Fontan patient).

Future Implantable Cardioverter-Defibrillators Developments

Similar to the history of pediatric pacemaker therapy, future use of ICDs in the young population will increase. Driven by technical advances (miniaturization) and expanding applications of ICD therapy (atrial defibrillators), implantable devices in children with a variety of cardiac disease states will cease to be a rarity.

References

1. The PCD® Tachyarrhythmia Control Device. Model 7217B Technical Manual. Medtronic, 1992;87.
2. Sanchez-Guerrero J, Colditz GA, Karlson EW, et al. Silicone breast implants and the risk of connective-tissue diseases and symptoms. *N Engl J Med* 1995;332:1666–1670.
3. Serwer GA, Mericle JM. Evaluation of pacemaker pulse generator and patient longevity in patients aged 1 day to 20 years. *Am J Cardiol* 1987;59:824–827.
4. Kugler JD, Danford DA. Pacemakers in children: an update. *Am Heart J* 1989;117:665–679.
5. Kerstjens-Frederikse MWS, Bink-Boelkens MTE, de Jongste MJL, et al. Permanent cardiac pacing in children: morbidity and efficacy of follow-up. *Int J Cardiol* 1991;33:207–214.
6. Friedman RA. Pacemakers in children: medical and surgical aspects. *Tex Heart Inst J* 1992;19:178–184.
7. Bernstein AD, Parsonnet V. Survey of cardiac pacing and defibrillation in the United States in 1993. *Am J Cardiol* 1996;78:187–196.
8. Rao V, Williams WG, Hamilton RH, et al. Trends in pediatric cardiac pacing. *Can J Cardiol* 1995;11:993–999.
9. Kusumoto FM, Goldschlager N. Cardiac pacing. *N Engl J Med* 1996;334:89–98.
10. Guidelines for implantation of cardiac pacemakers and antiarrhythmia devices. A report of the American College of Cardiology/American Heart Association Task Force on Assessment of Diagnostic and Therapeutic Cardiovascular Procedures (Committee on Pacemaker Implantation). *J Am Coll Cardiol* 1991;18:1–13.
11. Goldman BS, Williams WG, Hill T, et al. Permanent cardiac pacing after open heart surgery: congenital heart disease. *Pacing Clin Electrophysiol* 1985;8:732–739.
12. Gillette PC, Wampler DG, Shannon C, et al. Use of atrial pacing in a young population. *Pacing Clin Electrophysiol* 1985;8:94–100.
13. Vince JV, Tyers GFO, Kerr CR. Transvenous atrial pacing in the management of sick sinus syndrome following surgical treatment of the univentricular heart: case report and review. *Pacing Clin Electrophysiol* 1986;9:441–448.
14. Michaëlsson M, Jonzon A, Riesenfeld T. Isolated congenital complete atrioventricular block in adult life. A prospective study. *Circulation* 1995;92:442–449.
15. Polak PE, Zijlstra F, Roelandt JR. Indications for pacemaker implantation in the Kearns-Sayre syndrome. *Eur Heart J* 1989;10:281–282.
16. Schwartz PJ, Priori SG, Locati EH, et al. Long QT syndrome patients with mutations of the *SCN5A* and *HERG* genes have differential responses to Na$^+$ channel blockade and to increases in heart rate. Implications for gene-specific therapy. *Circulation* 1995;92:3381–3386.

17. Perry JC, Friedman RA, Moak JP, et al. Bradycardia and syncope in children not controlled by pacing: beta-adrenergic sensitivity. *Pacing Clin Electrophysiol* 1991;14:391–394.

18. Sra JS, Jazayeri MR, Avitall B, et al. Comparison of cardiac pacing with drug therapy in the treatment of neurocardiogenic (vasovagal) syncope with bradycardia or asystole. *N Engl J Med* 1993;328:1085–1090.

19. Deal BJ, Streipes M, Scagliotti D. et al. The medical therapy of cardioinhibitory syncope in pediatric patients. Pacing Clin Electrophysiol 1997;7:1759–1761.

20. Porter CJ, McGoon MD, Espinosa RE, et al. Apparent breath-holding spells associated with life-threatening bradycardia treated by permanent pacing. *Pediatr Cardiol* 1994;15:260. Abstract.

21. Menozzi C, Brignole M, Lolli G, et al. Follow-up of asystolic episodes in patients with cardioinhibitory, neurally mediated syncope and VVI pacemaker. *Am J Cardiol* 1993;72:1152–1155.

22. Oslizlok P, Allen M, Griffin M, et al. Clinical features and management of young patients with cardioinhibitory response during orthostatic testing. *Am J Cardiol* 1992;69:1363–1365.

23. Kratz JM, Gillette PC, Crawford FA, et al. Atrioventricular pacing in congenital heart disease. *Ann Thorac Surg* 1992;54:485–489.

24. Hamilton R, Gow R, Bahoric B, et al. Steroid-eluting epicardial leads in pediatrics: improved epicardial thresholds in the first year. *Pacing Clin Electrophysiol* 1991;14:2066–2072.

25. Johns JA, Fish FA, Burger JD, et al. Steroid-eluting epicardial pacing leads in pediatric patients: encouraging early results. *J Am Coll Cardiol* 1992;20:395–401.

26. Garson A Jr, Bink-Boelkens M, Hesslein PS, et al. Atrial flutter in the young: a collaborative study of 380 cases. *J Am Coll Cardiol* 1985;6:871–878.

27. Gillette PC, Wampler DG, Shannon C, et al. Use of cardiac pacing after the Mustard operation for transposition of the great arteries. *J Am Coll Cardiol* 1986;7:138–141.

28. Case CL, Gillette PC, Zeigler VL, et al. Successful treatment of congenital atrial flutter with antitachycardia pacing. *Pacing Clin Electrophysiol* 1990;13:571–573.

29. Case CL, Gillette PC, Zeigler VL, et al. Problems with permanent atrial pacing in the Fontan patient. *Pacing Clin Electrophysiol* 1989;12:92–96.

30. Molander N. Sudden natural death in later childhood and adolescence. *Arch Dis Child* 1982;57:572–576.

31. Neuspiel DR, Kuller LH. Sudden and unexpected death in childhood and adolescence. *JAMA* 1985;254:1321–1325.

32. Driscoll DJ, Edwards JE. Sudden unexpected death in children and adolescents. *J Am Coll Cardiol* 1985;5:118B–121B.

33. Eisenberg M, Bergner L, Hallstrom A. Epidemiology of cardiac arrest and resuscitation in children. *Ann Emerg Med* 1983;12:672–674.

34. Walsh CK, Krongrad E. Terminal cardiac electrical activity in pediatric patients. *Am J Cardiol* 1983;51:557–561.

35. Mirowski M, Reid PR, Mower MM, et al. Termination of malignant ventricular arrhythmias with an implanted automatic defibrillator in human beings. *N Engl J Med* 1980;303:322–324.

36. Estes NAM III. Overview of the implantable cardioverter-defibrillator. In: Estes NAM III, Manolis AS, Wang PJ, eds. *Implantable Cardioverter-Defibrillators. A Comprehensive Textbook.* New York: Marcel Dekker, Inc; 1994;635–653.

37. Callans DJ, Hook BG, Kleiman RB, et al. Unique sensing errors in third-generation implantable cardioverter-defibrillators. *J Am Coll Cardiol* 1993;22:1135–1140.

38. Saksena S, Chandran P, Shah Y, et al. Comparative efficacy of transvenous cardioversion and pacing in patients with sustained ventricular tachycardia: a prospective, randomized, crossover study. *Circulation* 1985;72:153–160.
39. Silka MJ, Kron J, Dunnigan A, et al. Sudden cardiac death and the use of implantable cardioverter-defibrillators in pediatric patients. The Pediatric Electrophysiology Society. *Circulation* 1993;87:800–807.
40. Kron J, Silka MJ, Ohm O-J, et al. Preliminary experience with nonthoracotomy implantable cardioverter defibrillators in young patients. The Medtronic Transvene Investigators. *Pacing Clin Electrophysiol* 1994;17:26–30.

Index